CLINICAL DECISION MAKING

Case Studies in Medical-Surgical, Pharmacologic, and Psychiatric Nursing

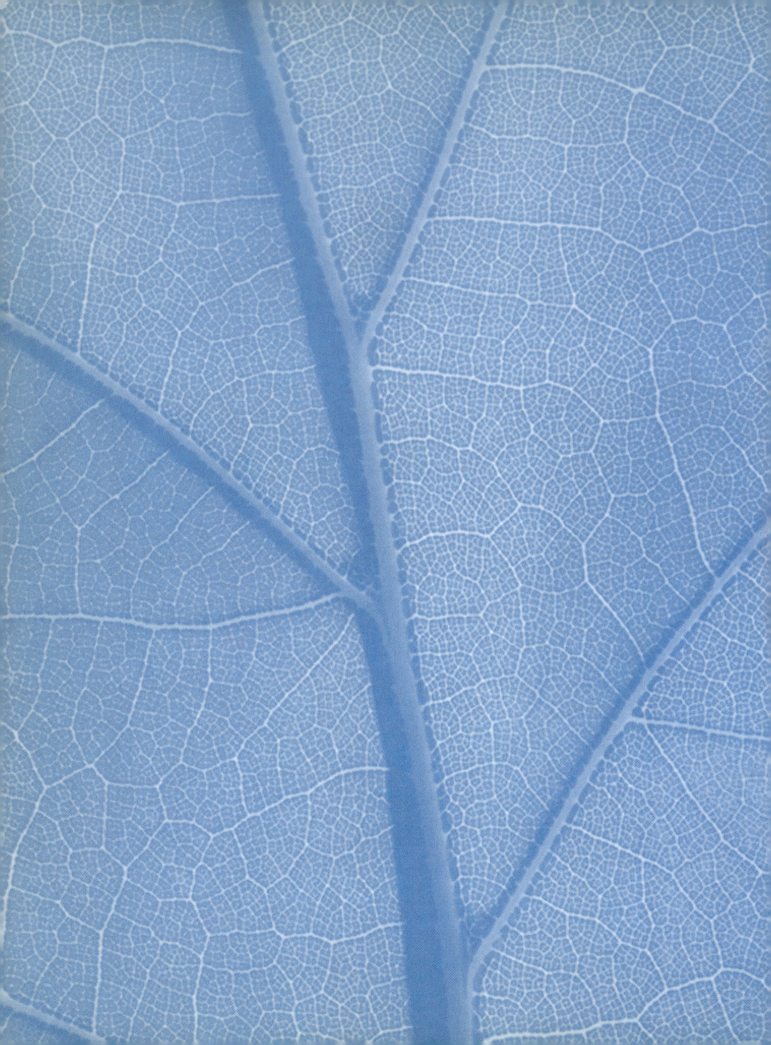

CLINICAL DECISION MAKING

Case Studies in Medical-Surgical, Pharmacologic, and Psychiatric Nursing

Gina M. Ankner
RN, MS, ANP-BC

Hyacinth Martin
BSN, MA, MSEd, MPS, RNBC

Betty K. Richardson
PhD, RN, CNS-MHP, BC, LPC, LMFT

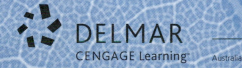

DELMAR
CENGAGE Learning™

Australia   Canada   Mexico   Singapore   Spain   United Kingdom   United States

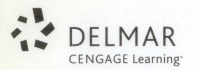

DELMAR
CENGAGE Learning™

Clinical Decision Making: Case Studies in Medical-Surgical, Pharmacologic, and Psychiatric Nursing
Gina M. Ankner, Hyacinth Martin, and Betty K. Richardson

Vice President, Career and Professional Editorial: Dave Garza

Director of Learning Solutions: Matthew Kane

Acquisitions Editor: Maureen Rosener

Managing Editor: Marah Bellegarde

Product Manager: Patricia Gaworecki

Editorial Assistant: Meaghan O'Brien

Vice President, Career and Professional Marketing: Jennifer McAvey

Marketing Director: Wendy Mapstone

Marketing Manager: Michele McTighe

Marketing Coordinator: Scott Chrysler

Production Director: Carolyn Miller

Production Manager: Andrew Crouth

Content Project Manager: Anne Sherman

Art Director: Jack Pendleton

Library of Congress Control Number: 2008930306

ISBN-13: 978-1-435-43985-6
ISBN-10: 1-4354-3985-6

Delmar Cengage Learning
5 Maxwell Drive
Clifton Park, NY 12065-2919
USA

Cengage Learning products are represented in Canada by Nelson Education, Ltd.

For your lifelong learning solutions, visit **delmar.cengage.com**

Visit our corporate website at **cengage.com**

Notice to the Reader
Publisher does not warrant or guarantee any of the products described herein or perform any independent analysis in connection with any of the product information contained herein. Publisher does not assume, and expressly disclaims, any obligation to obtain and include information other than that provided to it by the manufacturer. The reader is expressly warned to consider and adopt all safety precautions that might be indicated by the activities described herein and to avoid all potential hazards. By following the instructions contained herein, the reader willingly assumes all risks in connection with such instructions. The publisher makes no representations or warranties of any kind, including but not limited to, the warranties of fitness for particular purpose or merchantability, nor are any such representations implied with respect to the material set forth herein, and the publisher takes no responsibility with respect to such material. The publisher shall not be liable for any special, consequential, or exemplary damages resulting, in whole or part, from the readers' use of, or reliance upon, this material.

Printed in the United States of America
1 2 3 4 5 6 7 12 11 10 09 08

Contents

Part 2   The Respiratory and Immune Systems 181

Part 3   The Cardiovascular and Lymphatic Systems 215

Part 4   The Nervous System 265

Part 5   The Endocrine System 281

Section 1
Medical-Surgical Nursing

Comprehensive Table
of Variables

Case Study	Gender	Age	Setting	Ethnicity	Culture	Preexisting Conditions	Coexisting Conditions	Communication	Disability	Socioeconomic Status	Spirituality	Pharmacologic	Psychosocial	Legal	Ethical	Alternative Therapy	Prioritization	Delegation
Part One: The Digestive System																		
1	F	46	Hospital	White American			X			X		X						
2	F	46	Hospital	White American			X			X	X	X		X			X	X
3	F	33	Hospital	White American						X	X	X						X
4	M	44	Hospital	White American		X	X		X			X					X	
5	F	63	Hospital	White American		X	X			X		X						
Part Two: The Urinary System																		
1	F	56	Hospital	Hispanic		X	X			X		X					X	X
2	F	56	Hospital	Hispanic		X	X			X				X			X	
Part Three: The Respiratory System																		
1	F	38	Walk-in	White American		X				X							X	
2	M	25	Hospital	Black American			X					X					X	
3	M	75	Hospital	Jewish American	X	X	X	X	X	X	X	X		X		X	X	
4	M	67	Primary care	White American		X	X		X	X	X	X			X			
5	M	90	Hospital	Irish American														
Part Four: The Cardiovascular System and the Blood																		
1	F	20	Hospital	Asian American	X	X						X		X			X	
2	M	58	Rehabilitation unit	Asian American		X		X		X		X					X	
3	F	71	Hospital	Russian		X				X		X				X		
4	F	88	Primary care	White American	X	X	X		X	X		X		X	X		X	
5	M	42	Hospital	White American		X												
6	F	67	Hospital	Black American	X	X				X		X					X	
7	F	70	Home	Black American	X		X			X		X		X		X		
8	F	20	Hospital	Black American	X			X				X					X	
9	F	55	Hospital	White American					X					X				
Part Five: The Skeletal System																		
1	M	81	Hospital	Portuguese	X	X	X		X	X				X	X			
2	F	77	Hospital	Black American	X	X	X		X	X		X						X

#	Sex	Age	Setting	Ethnicity
3	M	73	Hospital	White American
Part Six: The Muscular System				
1	M	81	Hospital	White American
2	F	48	Primary care	White American
Part Seven: The Integumentary System				
1	F	70	Home	White American
2	M	57	Hospital	White American
3	F	72	Hospital	White American
4	M	32	Primary care	White American
5	M	55	Hospital	Black American
Part Eight: The Nervous/Neurological System				
1	F	59	Hospital	Black American
2	M	85	Long-term care	Native American
3	F	92	Hospital	White American
4	F	35	Hospital	White American
5	M	73	Home	White American
Part Nine: The Endocrine/Metabolic System				
1	M	81	Long-term care	White American
2	M	61	Hospital	Mexican American
3	F	88	Hospital	White American
Part Ten: The Reproductive System				
1	F	45	Hospital	Black American

Section 2
Pharmacologic Nursing

Comprehensive Table of Variables

Comprehensive Table of Variables: Pharmacologic Nursing

Case Study	Gender	Age	Setting	Ethnicity/Culture	Preexisting Conditions	Coexisting Conditions	Lifestyle	Communication	Disability	Socioeconomic	Spiritual/Religious	Pharmacologic	Psychosocial	Legal	Ethical	Alternative Therapy	Prioritization	Delegation
Part One: The Digestive and Urinary Systems																		
1	M	64	Hospital	White American	×	×	×				×	×	×			×	×	×
2	M	34	Clinic	Japanese/Asian			×	×			×	×	×			×	×	×
3	M	52	"Outpatient, urology clinic"	Mexican American	×	×	×	×			×		×	×	×	×	×	×
4	F	35	Hospital	White American	×	×	×	×			×	×	×		×	×	×	×
5	F	60	Hospital	Black American		×	×				×	×	×		×		×	×
6	M	38	Hospital	Black American/West Indian			×				×	×	×			×	×	×
7	M	40	Hospital	Jewish American			×		×	×	×	×	×		×		×	×
8	M	64	Hospital	White American			×				×	×	×				×	
Part Two: The Respiratory and Immune Systems																		
1	M	76	Skilled nursing facility	White American		×	×		×	×	×		×				×	×
2	F	32	"Clinic, tertiary care center of medical center"	Black/South African	×		×	×	×	×	×	×	×	×	×	×	×	×
3	M	50	Hospital	White American	×	×	×		×	×	×	×	×	×	×	×	×	×
4	M	55	Hospital	Black American	×	×	×			×	×	×	×	×	×	×	×	×
5	F	60	Hospital	African/Nigerian		×	×				×	×	×			×	×	×
6	M	62	Hospital	Italian/American		×	×	×			×		×				×	×
7	M	42	Hospital	Black American	×	×	×				×	×	×	×	×	×	×	×
8	M	40	Hospital	Hispanic American		×	×		×		×	×	×				×	×
Part Three: The Cardiovascular and Lymphatic Systems																		
1	M	65	ER	Black American	×	×	×			×	×	×	×		×	×	×	×
2	F	68	Outpatient	White American	×	×	×			×	×	×	×	×	×	×	×	×
3	M	78	Hospital	Black American	×	×	×				×	×	×				×	×
4	F	56	Hospital	Black American			×	×			×	×	×		×	×	×	×
5	F	60	Hospital	Hispanic American	×	×	×				×	×	×		×		×	
6	M	66	Hospital	White American			×				×	×	×			×	×	×

#	Sex	Age	Setting	Ethnicity
7	M	56	Hospital	Hispanic American
8	M	54	Outpatient	White American
9	F	64	Hospital	Black American
10	M	60	Hospital clinic	White Portuguese
11	M	72		White American
12	M	72	Adult home/hospital	Black American/West Indian

Part Four: The Nervous System

#	Sex	Age	Setting	Ethnicity
1	M	30	Clinic	Hispanic American
2	F	38	Hospital	White American
3	F	24	ER	Black American/West Indian
4	F	42	Hospital	mixed race

Part Five: The Endocrine System

#	Sex	Age	Setting	Ethnicity
1	F	30	Office	Black American/West Indian
2	F	42	Hospital	Native American/Argentina
3	M	20	Hospital	Hispanic American
4	F	50	Hospital	White American
5	F	56	Office	Black American/West Indian

Part Six: The Musculoskeletal and Reproductive Systems

#	Sex	Age	Setting	Ethnicity
1	F	25	Clinic	Native American
2	M	32	Hospital	Black American/West Indian
3	M	64	Hospital	White American
4	F	58	Clinic	Black American
5	F	40	Hospital	Black American
6	M	30	Hospital	Black American

Section 3
Psychiatric Nursing

Comprehensive Table
of Variables

Case Study	Gender	Age	Setting	Ethnicity	Culture	Preexisting Conditions	Coexisting Conditions	Communication	Disability	Socioeconomic Status	Spirituality	Pharmacologic	Psychosocial	Legal	Ethical	Alternative Therapy	Prioritization	Delegation
Part One: The Client Experiencing Schizophrenia and Other Psychotic Disorders																		
1	F	34	Psychiatric hospital	Hungarian American	X		X					X	X	X	X			X
2	M	48	Clinic	American Indian/White American	X	X	X			X		X	X	X	X	X		
Part Two: The Client Experiencing Anxiety																		
1	M	26	Outpatient	White American	X		X			X		X	X	X				
2	F	50	Center	Mexican American	X		X				X	X	X		X	X		
3	F	19	Psychiatric hospital	White American	X							X	X					
4	F	25	Hospital	Central American	X		X						X	X	X			
Part Three: The Client Experiencing Depression or Mania																		
1	M	14	Psychiatric hospital	Black American	X		X			X	X	X	X	X	X		X	X
2	F	35	Inpatient psych. hosp.	Central American				X		X		X	X	X	X			X
3	F	13	Psychiatric hospital	White American	X		X			X	X				X	X	X	X
4	F	41	Hospital	German	X							X	X	X	X			
Part Four: The Client Who Abuses Chemical Substances																		
1	M	42	Hospital	White American	X		X			X	X		X	X	X		X	X
2	F	51	Home	White American	X	X	X			X	X	X	X	X	X	X		
3	M	19	Office	White American	X					X				X	X	X		
4	F	13	School nurse	White American	X	X			X	X			X		X			X
Part Five: The Client with a Personality Disorder																		
1	F	27	Office	White American	X		X			X	X		X		X		X	
2	M	39	Center	White American	X					X		X	X	X	X	X	X	
3	M	55	Home	White American	X	X				X				X	X	X	X	
4	M	62	Clinic	White American			X			X	X		X	X	X			
5	F	22	Center	White American	X		X			X	X				X		X	X
6	M	36	ER	White American			X								X			
7	M	32	Clinic	Black/White American	X		X					X	X		X	X	X	X

Part Six: The Client Experiencing a Somatoform, Factitious, or Dissociative Disorder

#	Sex	Age	Setting	Ethnicity
1	F	15	ER	White/Chilean American
2	F	51	Home	African American
3	F	34	Psychiatric unit	White American
4	F	31	Office	White American

Part Seven: The Client with Disorders of Self-Regulation

#	Sex	Age	Setting	Ethnicity
1	F	26	Psychiatric hospital	White American
2	F	21	Hospital	East Asian/White American
3	M	25	Local jail	White American

Part Eight: Special Populations: The Child, Adolescent, or Elderly Client

#	Sex	Age	Setting	Ethnicity
1	M	13	Center	White American
2	M	14	Hospital	White American
3	F	8	School nurse	White American
4	F	7	School nurse	Asian American
5	M	5	Children's unit	Asian American
6	F	7	School nurse	White American
7	F	89	Home	Black American
8	M	15	School	White/Black American
9	M	7	Center	White American

Part Nine: Survivors of Violence or Abuse

#	Sex	Age	Setting	Ethnicity
1	F	10	Home	White American
2	M	77	Gerontologist's office	White American
3	M	11	School infirmary	White/Hispanic American

Reviewers

Patricia N. Allen, MSN, APRN-BC
Clinical Assistant Professor
Indiana University School of Nursing
Bloomington, Indiana

Ann K. Beckett, PhD, RN
Assistant Professor
Oregon Health and Science University School of Nursing
Portland, Oregon

Jane E. Bostick, PhD, APRN, BC
Assistant Professor of Clinical Nursing
University of Missouri–Columbia
Sinclair School of Nursing
Columbia, Missouri

Bonita E. Broyles, RN, BSN, PhD
Associate Degree Nursing Faculty
Piedmont Community College
Roxboro, North Carolina

Joyce Campbell, MSN, APRN, BC, CCRN
Associate Professor
Chattanooga State Technical Community College
Chattanooga, Tennessee

Marianne Curia, MSN, RN
Assistant Professor
University of St. Francis
Joliet, Illinois

Karen K. Gerbasich, RN, MSN
Faculty Assistant Professor
Ivy Tech Community College
South Bend, Indiana

Kimberly M. Gregg, MS APRN, BC
Adult Mental Health Clinical Nurse Specialist
Altru Health Systems
Instructor
University of North Dakota
Grand Forks, North Dakota

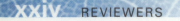

Mary Beth Kiefner, RN, MS
Nursing Program Director
Nursing Faculty, Illinois Central College
East Peoria, Illinois

Joan Piper Mader, RN, MSN
Associate Professor or Nursing
College of the Mainland
Texas City, Texas

Bethany Phoenix, RN, PhD, CNS
Associate Clinical Professor
Coordinator, Graduate Program in Psychiatric/Mental Health Nursing
University of California, San Francisco
San Francisco, California

Charlotte R. Price, EdD, RN
Professor and Chair
Augusta State University Department of Nursing
Augusta, Georgia

Amanda M. Reynolds, MSN
Associate Professor
Grambling State University
Grambling, Louisiana

Mari A. Smith, DSN, RN, CCRN
Professor
School of Nursing, Middle Tennessee State University
Murfreesboro, Tennessee

Linda Stafford, PhD, RN, CS
Division Head, Psychiatric Mental Health Nursing
The University of Texas Health Science Center at Houston
School of Nursing
Houston, Texas

Darla R. Ura, MA, RN, APRN, BC
Clinical Associate Professor
Department of Adult and Elder Health Nursing
School of Nursing, Emory University
Atlanta, Georgia

Preface

Delmar Cengage Learning's Case Studies Series was created to encourage nurses to bridge the gap between content knowledge and clinical application. The products within the series represent the most innovative and comprehensive approach to nursing case studies ever developed. Each title has been authored by experienced nurse educators and clinicians who understand the complexity of nursing practice as well as the challenges of teaching and learning. All of the cases are based on real-life clinical scenarios and demand thought and "action" from the nurse. Each case brings the user into the clinical setting, and invites him or her to utilize the nursing process while considering all of the variables that influence the client's condition and the care to be provided. Each case also represents a unique set of variables, to offer a breadth of learning experiences and to capture the reality of nursing practice. To gauge the progression of a user's knowledge and critical thinking ability, the cases have been categorized by difficulty level. Every section begins with basic cases and proceeds to more advanced scenarios, thereby presenting opportunities for learning and practice for both students and professionals.

All of the cases have undergone expert review to ensure that as many variables as possible are represented in a truly realistic manner and that each case reflects consistency with realities of modern nursing practice.

How to Use This Book

Every case begins with a table of variables that are encountered in practice, and that must be understood by the nurse in order to provide appropriate care to the client. Categories of variables include age; gender; setting; ethnicity; pre-existing conditions; coexisting conditions; cultural, communication considerations, disability, socioeconomic, spiritual, pharmacological, psychosocial, legal, ethical, prioritization, and delegation considerations; and alternative therapy. If a case involves a variable that is considered to have a significant impact on care, the specific variable is included in the table. This allows the user an "at a glance" view of the issues that will need to be considered to provide care to the client in the scenario. The table of variables is followed by a presentation of the case, including the history of the client, current condition, clinical setting, and professionals involved. A series of questions follows each case that ask the user to consider how she would handle the issues presented within the scenario. Suggested answers and rationales are provided for remediation and discussion.

Organization

The cases are grouped into parts based on topics. Within each part, cases are organized by difficulty level from easy, to moderate, to difficult. This classification is somewhat subjective, but they are based upon a developed standard. In general, difficulty level has been determined by the number of variables that impact the case and the complexity of the client's condition. Colored tabs are used to allow the user to distinguish the difficulty levels more easily. A comprehensive table of variables is also provided for reference, to allow the user to quickly select cases containing a particular variable of care.

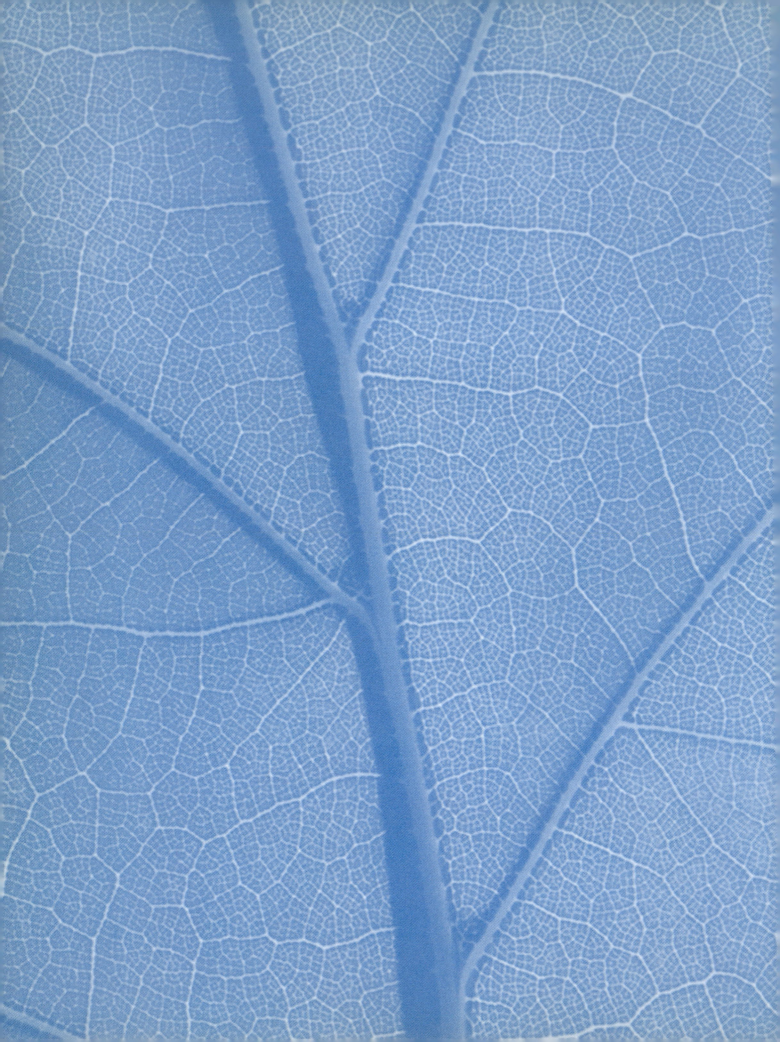

SECTION 1

CLINICAL DECISION MAKING

Case Studies in Medical-Surgical Nursing

Gina M. Ankner

RN, MS, ANP-BC

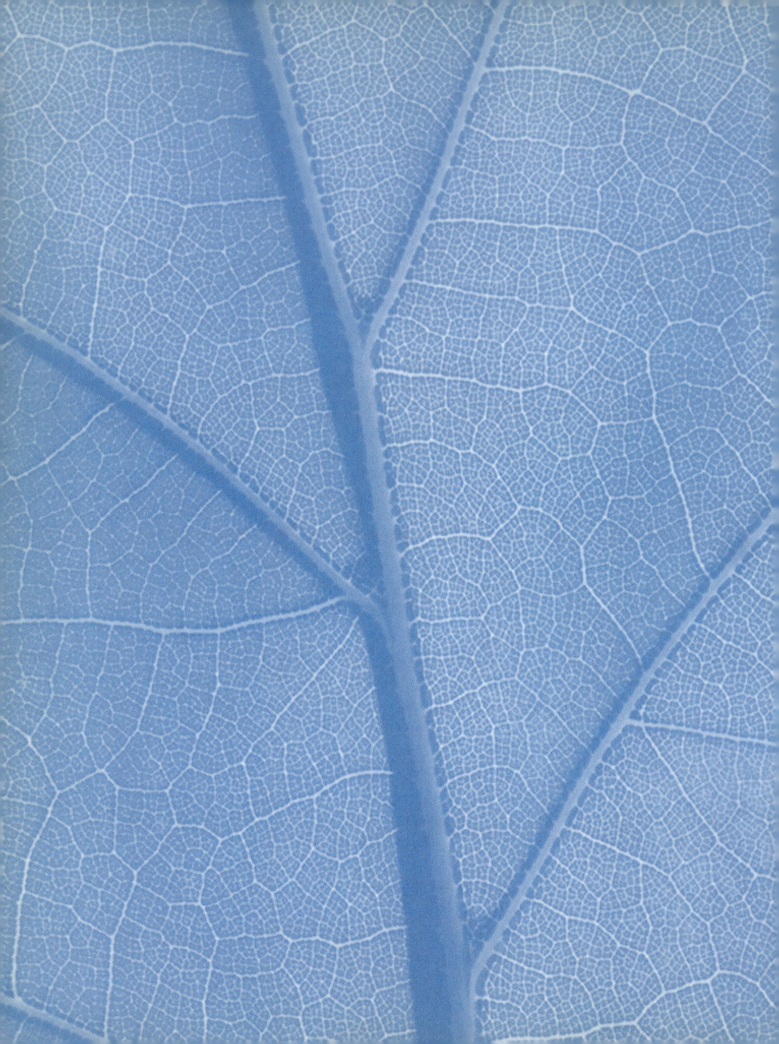

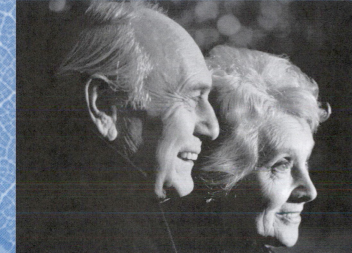

## PART ONE

The Digestive System

GENDER

Female

AGE

46

SETTING

- Hospital

ETHNICITY

- White American

CULTURAL CONSIDERATIONS

PREEXISTING CONDITION

COEXISTING CONDITION

- Urinary tract infection (UTI)

COMMUNICATION

DISABILITY

SOCIOECONOMIC

- Married. No children.

SPIRITUAL/RELIGIOUS

PHARMACOLOGIC

- Cefoxitin sodium (Mefoxin); metronidazole (Flagyl); morphine sulfate; diphenoxylate hydrochloride with atropine sulfate (Lomotil); propantheline bromide (Pro-Banthine); acetaminophen (Tylenol)

LEGAL

ETHICAL

ALTERNATIVE THERAPY

PRIORITIZATION

DELEGATION

MODERATE

THE DIGESTIVE SYSTEM

Level of difficulty: Moderate

Overview: This case requires the nurse to recognize the clinical presentation of diverticular disease. The nurse is asked to compare the presenting symptoms of other differential diagnoses to those of diverticulitis. Diagnostic testing and the treatment of diverticulitis are discussed.

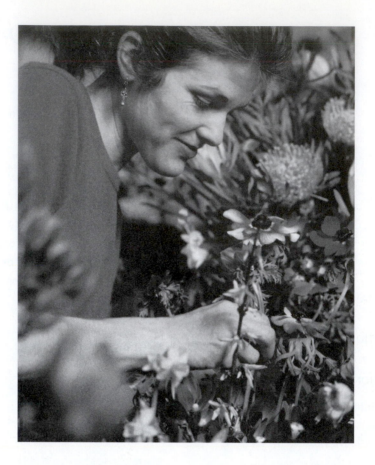

Client Profile

Mrs. Dolan is a 46-year-old female who presented to the emergency department with complaints of episodic abdominal pain, a low-grade fever, and diarrhea for almost two weeks. Mrs. Dolan was on vacation in another country when she developed pain in the left lower quadrant of her abdomen. Mrs. Dolan delayed seeking health care because of fear of the country's unfamiliar medical system and the assumption that bad water or food she had while on vacation must have given her a stomach "bug." Mrs. Dolan also reports a recent onset of painful urination.

Case Study

Upon examination in the emergency room, Mrs. Dolan is found to be dehydrated with a fever of 102.5°F (39.2°C). Vital signs are blood pressure (BP) 106/58, pulse 88, and respiratory rate of 22. Her potassium (K^+) level is 2.8 mEq/L, erythrocyte sedimentation rate (ESR) is 37 mm/hr, and white blood cell (WBC) count is 16,000 cells/mm^3. A urinalysis showed a positive urinary tract infection (UTI) and an abdominal/pelvic computed tomography (CT) scan revealed diverticulitis with a question of an ileus.

Mrs. Dolan is admitted and started on intravenous (IV) fluid of D51/2 normal saline (NS) with 20 meq of potassium chloride (KCl) at 50 cc per hour. Two IV antibiotics (cefoxitin sodium and metronidazole) are prescribed. Her admitting orders include nothing by mouth (NPO), bed rest, IV morphine sulfate for pain management, stools to be checked for occult blood, strict intake and output

(I & O), and repeat blood work in the morning to monitor her K^+. Her height and weight on admission are 5 feet 7 inches and 170 lbs (77.3 kg). She is prescribed diphenoxylate hydrochloride with atropine sulfate, propantheline bromide, and acetaminophen as "as needed" pro re nata (prn) medications.

Questions

1. How does diverticulitis differ from diverticulosis?

2. Summarize the pathophysiology of acute and chronic diverticulitis.

3. Describe the predisposing risk factors for diverticulitis. Identify any contributing factors for the development of diverticulitis in Mrs. Dolan's case.

4. The emergency department health care provider also considered that Mrs. Dolan's symptoms could be indicative of a diagnosis of gastroenteritis. Briefly describe the clinical features of gastroenteritis and diverticulitis. How are the clinical presentations of these diagnoses similar?

5. What is the usual source of the bacteria that leads to the development of gastroenteritis?

6. Explain how Mrs. Dolan's symptoms may be related to her urinary tract infection.

7. The emergency department health care provider considered several differential diagnoses for Mrs. Dolan and a diagnosis of diverticulitis was determined. What diagnostic test confirmed Mrs. Dolan's diagnosis of acute diverticulitis?

8. Mrs. Dolan's abdominal/pelvic CT scan revealed diverticulitis with a question of an ileus. What is an ileus?

9. Briefly explain why a barium enema, sigmoidoscopy, and colonoscopy are not considered appropriate diagnostic tests for a client with suspected acute diverticulitis.

10. Discuss the medical management for a client with acute diverticulitis.

11. The admitting health care provider explains to Mr. and Mrs. Dolan that some clients require surgery if conservative treatment does not resolve the acute episode of diverticulitis. What are the indications for surgical intervention?

12. Discuss the rationale for including prn orders for diphenoxylate hydrochloride with atropine sulfate, propantheline bromide, and acetaminophen in Mrs. Dolan's treatment plan.

13. When collaborating with Mrs. Dolan to develop a plan of care, what outcome goals will be nursing care priorities?

14. Mrs. Dolan requests morphine sulfate. What should be the initial nursing action?

EASY

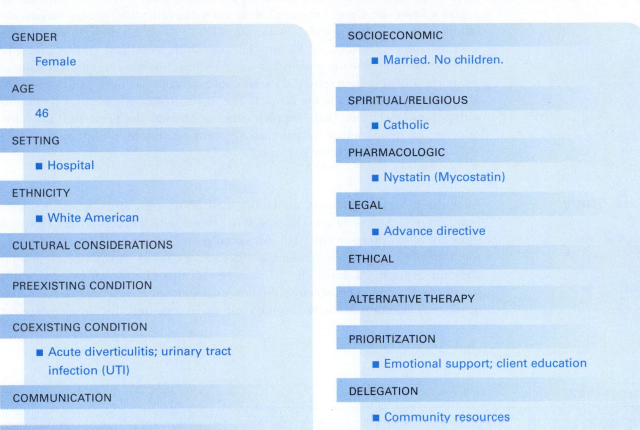

GENDER

Female

AGE

46

SETTING

■ Hospital

ETHNICITY

■ White American

CULTURAL CONSIDERATIONS

PREEXISTING CONDITION

COEXISTING CONDITION

■ Acute diverticulitis; urinary tract infection (UTI)

COMMUNICATION

DISABILITY

SOCIOECONOMIC

■ Married. No children.

SPIRITUAL/RELIGIOUS

■ Catholic

PHARMACOLOGIC

■ Nystatin (Mycostatin)

LEGAL

■ Advance directive

ETHICAL

ALTERNATIVE THERAPY

PRIORITIZATION

■ Emotional support; client education

DELEGATION

■ Community resources

THE DIGESTIVE SYSTEM

Level of difficulty: Easy

Overview: This case requires the nurse to prepare Mr. and Mrs. Dolan for Mrs. Dolan's emergent surgical procedure. Following surgery, the nurse must provide discharge teaching to educate Mrs. Dolan on the care of her temporary colostomy. Priority nursing considerations for the client living with a colostomy are reviewed.

Client Profile

Mrs. Dolan is a 46-year-old female who presented to the emergency department three days ago with complaints of abdominal pain, fever, and diarrhea for almost two weeks. Upon examination in the emergency room, Mrs. Dolan was found to be dehydrated with a potassium (K⁺) level of 2.8 mEq/L, erythrocyte sedimentation rate (ESR) of 37 mm/hr, and white blood cell (WBC) count of 16,000 cells/mm³. She was positive for a urinary tract infection and an abdominal/pelvic computed tomography (CT) scan confirmed the diagnosis of diverticulitis. Mrs. Dolan was admitted to the hospital. She was started on intravenous (IV) fluids with potassium chloride (KCl) supplementation. She was also prescribed IV antibiotics and morphine sulfate for pain management. She has been nothing by mouth (NPO) since admission three days ago.

Case Study

After three days of IV fluids, antibiotics, and bowel rest, Mrs. Dolan's K⁺ level is 3.7 mEq/L, ESR is 30 mm/hr, and WBC count is 15,000 cells/mm³. Her vital signs are blood pressure (BP) 114/68, radial pulse/heart rate (HR) 102, respiratory rate (RR) 18, and temperature of 103°F (39.4°C). Mrs. Dolan has a follow-up abdominal/pelvic CT scan. The CT scan reveals that Mrs. Dolan's diverticultitis has not responded to conservative medical management and an abscess has developed. Surgical intervention is necessary and she is scheduled for surgery the next morning.

Questions

1. Briefly discuss the potential complications associated with acute diverticulitis.

2. Which assessment findings are of concern in Mrs. Dolan's case?

3. Describe Mrs. Dolan's preoperative care needs.

4. What are the potential complications associated with abdominal surgery that Mrs. Dolan should be informed of prior to giving consent for the surgical procedure?

5. Describe the purpose of the following advance directive alternatives: *living will, health care proxy, durable power of attorney.*

6. During the immediate postoperative phase of Mrs. Dolan's care, what should the nurse assess?

7. What is a *stoma* and how are the following three types of stomas surgically created: *end stoma, double-barrel stoma,* and *loop stoma?*

8. Generate two to three key points to address when providing Mrs. Dolan with colostomy care education regarding each of the following: *stoma assessment, skin protection, pouch care, diet, medications, sexuality issues,* and *community resources.*

9. Prioritize three nursing diagnoses appropriate for the client living with a colostomy.

10. It has been three weeks since discharge, and Mrs. Dolan and her husband are eating at a restaurant. Mrs. Dolan is trying to decide between the following three meal choices: (a) corned beef and cabbage, (b) spaghetti with tomato sauce, and (c) salmon with baked potato. Which meal should Mrs. Dolan chose in order to follow the nurse's instructions regarding appropriate diet guidelines?

Ms. Winnie

GENDER

Female

AGE

33

SETTING

- Hospital

ETHNICITY

- White American

CULTURAL CONSIDERATIONS

PREEXISTING CONDITION

COEXISTING CONDITION

- Flulike symptoms for one week.

COMMUNICATION

DISABILITY

SOCIOECONOMIC

- Recently promoted to project manager.

SPIRITUAL/RELIGIOUS

- Jehovah's Witness

PHARMACOLOGIC

- Norgestimate/ethinyl estradiol (Ortho Tri-Cyclen); ibuprofen (Advil); pantoprazole (Protonix); prochlorperazine (Compazine); omeprazole (Prilosec)

LEGAL

ETHICAL

ALTERNATIVE THERAPY

PRIORITIZATION

DELEGATION

- Delegating within the scope of assistant nursing personnel responsibilities.

MODERATE

THE DIGESTIVE SYSTEM

Level of difficulty: Moderate

Overview: This case requires recognition of the signs and symptoms of a gastrointestinal (GI) bleed and characteristics of upper versus lower GI tract bleeding. The nurse provides client education in preparation for a diagnostic procedure and explains the significance of the results. The procedure for administering a blood transfusion is reviewed. Discharge instructions are given.

Client Profile

Ms. Winnie is a 33-year-old woman who presented to the emergency department. She states, "I have been so sick. It must be the flu. Everyone at work has it. I am achy and tired. I keep vomiting and have not been able to keep anything down for the past three days. After a while, it is just these violent dry heaves since there is nothing more in my stomach to throw up. Tonight I vomited twice within three hours and it was red like blood. I got scared and came in."

Case Study

Ms. Winnie's vital signs are BP 110/60, HR 88, RR 20, Temp. 100.5°F(38°C). Her skin is clammy and pale. Lab results are WBC 11,800 cells/mm^3, RBC 3.31 million/μL, Hgb 11 g/dL, Hct 34%, platelets 150,000 mm^3, K 3.8 mEq/L, Na 140 mEq/L. An electrocardiogram (ECG, EKG) shows normal sinus rhythm. A kidneys, ureters, and bladder (KUB) abdominal X-ray is done, and she will have an esophagogastro-duodenoscopy (EGD) at 7:00 A.M. the next day. She is admitted with the diagnosis of probable upper GI bleed. Ms. Winnie expresses concern to the nurse, "Do you think I'll be in the hospital long? I have been managing an important project for the past few months at the company I work for, and although my boss has been pretty understanding about me being out sick for the past few days, there is an important deadline coming up next week. Being in the hospital long may jeopardize my job." She is started on intravenous (IV) fluids of normal saline (NS) at 100 cc per hour. Pantoprazole continuous IV drip and prochlorperazine as needed for nausea and vomiting are prescribed. Ms. Winnie is to have strict monitoring of her intake and output and her vital signs assessed every two hours. She will be on bed rest. Her stools are to be tested for occult blood. She will have a complete blood count (CBC) assessed every six hours.

Results of the KUB are reported as a nonspecific gas pattern with moderate amount of stool throughout the colon with no acute abnormality noted. The EGD reveals a normal duodenum with no vascular anomalies, ulceration, or inflammation. There is a normal appearing gastric mucosa with no erosive changes, ulcer, or mass. A small Mallory-Weiss tear is noted.

Questions

1. The nurse asks Ms. Winnie if she takes any medications at home. Ms. Winnie states, "I take Ortho Tri-Cyclen once a day and I was taking Advil three to four times a day for the aches and pains of being sick." Should the nurse suggest to the health care provider that these two medications be included in Ms. Winnie's admission orders?

2. Identify four nursing diagnoses that are appropriate for Ms. Winnie upon admission.

3. Which lab results are abnormal and what is the significance of the abnormal results in Ms. Winnie's case?

4. Distinguish between the characteristics of upper and lower GI bleeding.

5. It is 1:00 A.M. and Ms. Winnie is settled into her room on the nursing unit. She asks the nurse,

"Do you have some saltine crackers and ginger ale to try and help settle my stomach?" Should the nurse give Ms. Winnie something to eat?

6. The nurse recognizes the above situation as a teaching opportunity. How might the nurse explain why an EGD has been prescribed for Ms. Winnie and what she can expect during the procedure?

7. What are the nursing responsibilities after Ms. Winnie has the EGD and returns to her room?

8. Discuss the Mallory-Weiss tear found during Ms. Winnie's EGD. What is a Mallory-Weiss tear? What are the common symptoms of a Mallory-Weiss tear and what causes it?

9. Which factors determine if blood products will be administered to a patient with GI tract bleeding secondary to a Mallory-Weiss tear?

Questions (continued)

10. If a transfusion is needed and Ms. Winnie's blood type is A positive, what are compatible blood types? Explain why a person can only receive compatible blood types.

11. Although unlikely with a Mallory-Weiss tear, the nurse realizes that if Ms. Winnie's bleeding does not resolve she may need a blood transfusion. The nurse has not administered blood in a while and reviews the agency policy and procedure. Place the following 10 steps of administering a blood transfusion in the proper order:

- Monitor vital signs per agency policy.
- Obtain blood products from the blood bank. Keep in mind that a packed red blood cell (PRBC) transfusion is to be completed within four hours of removal from refrigeration.
- Remain with the client during the first fifteen to thirty minutes of the transfusion (infusion of the first 50 ml of blood product) to assess for adverse reactions.
- Administer the blood product using appropriate filter tubing. Filters remove aggregates and possible contaminants. If blood is to be diluted, use only normal saline.
- Verify the medical prescription for type of blood product, dose, and transfusion time.
- Discontinue the transfusion when complete, and dispose of the bag and tubing properly.
- Document type of blood product infused, time of infusion, and any adverse reactions.
- Obtain venous access with a larger-bore needle (19-gauge).
- Assess baseline vital signs, urine output, skin color, and history of transfusion reactions.
- With another registered nurse, verify the client by name and identification number, check blood product compatibility, and note expiration time. Do not use the client's room number as a form of client identification.

12. Later in the shift, the nurse is looking through Ms. Winnie's chart and comments to herself, "I think I may have reviewed the policy and procedure book for nothing." Why does the nurse believe she may not need to know how to administer blood to Ms. Winnie after all?

13. Which aspects of Ms. Winnie's plan of care could the registered nurse assign to assistive nursing personnel such as a certified nursing assistant (CNA)?

14. Should Ms. Winnie be concerned about her job? What do you anticipate will be her length of stay in the hospital?

15. If it is determined that Ms. Winnie has a bacterial infection and she is discharged with a prescription for an antibiotic, what teaching is appropriate regarding the use of an antibiotic with an oral contraceptive?

Mr. Cummings

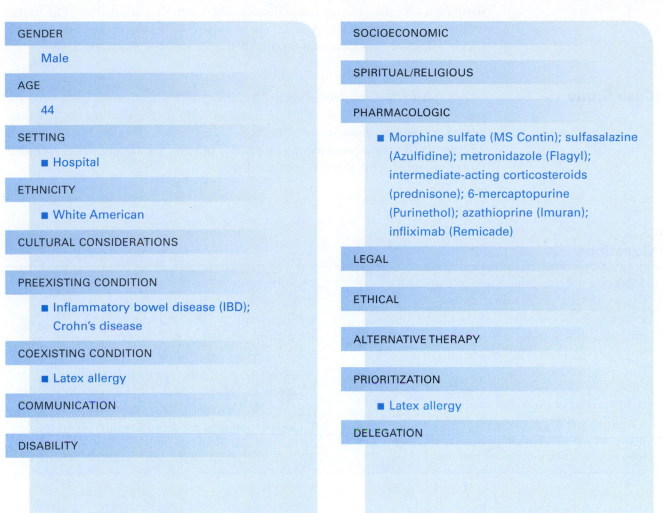

GENDER

Male

AGE

44

SETTING

- Hospital

ETHNICITY

- White American

CULTURAL CONSIDERATIONS

PREEXISTING CONDITION

- Inflammatory bowel disease (IBD); Crohn's disease

COEXISTING CONDITION

- Latex allergy

COMMUNICATION

DISABILITY

SOCIOECONOMIC

SPIRITUAL/RELIGIOUS

PHARMACOLOGIC

- Morphine sulfate (MS Contin); sulfasalazine (Azulfidine); metronidazole (Flagyl); intermediate-acting corticosteroids (prednisone); 6-mercaptopurine (Purinethol); azathioprine (Imuran); infliximab (Remicade)

LEGAL

ETHICAL

ALTERNATIVE THERAPY

PRIORITIZATION

- Latex allergy

DELEGATION

THE DIGESTIVE SYSTEM

Level of difficulty: Moderate

Overview: This case requires the nurse to differentiate between the characteristics of Crohn's disease and ulcerative colitis. Treatment options for Crohn's disease are reviewed. The nurse must provide safe care for a client with a latex allergy.

Client Profile

Mr. Cummings is a 44-year-old male admitted with lower right quadrant abdominal pain, nausea, and vomiting for four days. His past medical history is significant for inflammatory bowel disease (IBD) with Crohn's disease. The health care provider suspects Mr. Cummings is experiencing an exacerbation of his Crohn's disease. Mr. Cummings is scheduled for a series of diagnostic tests.

Case Study

Prior to Mr. Cummings's admission to the nursing unit, his room is prepared according to a latex-free protocol. Mr. Cummings is NPO in preparation for a barium enema, a colonoscopy, and to rest his bowel. The nurse caring for Mr. Cummings has identified pain management as a priority of care. Mr. Cummings is receiving morphine sulfate (MS Contin) with good effect.

Questions

1. What is inflammatory bowel disease (IBD)? Discuss the incidence and prevalence of IBD.

2. Discuss how the physiology of Crohn's disease differs from that of ulcerative colitis.

3. Briefly discuss the manifestations that are common to both Crohn's disease and ulcerative colitis and then discuss the manifestations that are characteristic of each disease.

4. Discuss the treatment options the health care provider will consider to help treat a Crohn's disease exacerbation. Consider common

medications prescribed, activity, diet, and surgical interventions.

5. Briefly explain the manifestations characteristic of the three types of latex reactions.

6. What precautions should the nurse take when caring for a client with an allergy to latex?

7. Explain why the hospital dietician should be aware of Mr. Cummings's allergy to latex.

8. List five potential nursing diagnoses the nurse should include in Mr. Cummings's plan of care.

Mrs. Bennett

GENDER

Female

AGE

63

SETTING

- Hospital

ETHNICITY

- White American

CULTURAL CONSIDERATIONS

PREEXISTING CONDITION

- Malabsorption syndrome (celiac disease); chronic wounds; pancreatitis with a pancreatic resection; depression

COEXISTING CONDITION

- Stage III coccyx pressure ulcer

COMMUNICATION

DISABILITY

- Has been on disability for the past five years.

SOCIOECONOMIC

- Cared for in a nursing home for the past five years.

SPIRITUAL/RELIGIOUS

PHARMACOLOGIC

- Allergy to erythromycin, tetracycline, tape, pneumococcal polysaccharide (pneumonia) vaccine

LEGAL

ETHICAL

ALTERNATIVE THERAPY

PRIORITIZATION

DELEGATION

- Collaboration with dietician and assistive nursing personnel.

THE DIGESTIVE SYSTEM

Level of difficulty: Difficult

Overview: This case requires the nurse to consider the holistic effects of malabsorption syndrome on the client's health and quality of life. Symptoms of nutrient deficiencies are reviewed. The impact of poor nutrition on wound healing is discussed. The nurse must be attentive to the safety risks specific to this client. Priority nursing diagnoses are identified.

DIFFICULT

Client Profile

Mrs. Bennett is a 63-year-old woman with a history of malabsorption syndrome secondary to celiac disease. She is 5 foot 6 inches tall and weighs 79 pounds. She arrives in the emergency department from a nursing home with an elevated temperature and a decreased blood pressure and heart rate from her baseline. Her oxygen saturation is 89% on room air. She has a stage III pressure ulcer on her coccyx.

Case Study

Laboratory tests in the emergency department reveal Mrs. Bennett's white blood cell (WBC) count is 12,000 cells/mm^3, red blood cell (RBC) count is 3.16 million/mm^3, hemoglobin (Hgb) 8.9 g/dL, hematocrit (Hct) 25.7%, mean cell (or corpuscular) volume (MCV) 70.8 μm^3, mean cell (or corpuscular) hemoglobin (MCH) 20 pg, ferritin 7 mg/L, iron (Fe) 30 μg/L, total iron binding capacity (TIBC) 496 μg/dL, and transferrin 195 mg/dL. Her potassium (K$^+$) is 1.7 mEq/L, sodium (Na^{2+}) 128 mEq/L, chloride (Cl$^-$) 79 mmol/L, calcium (Ca^{2+}) 7.8 mg/dL, and protein 4.0 g/dL. Mrs. Bennett is admitted to the telemetry unit. She is placed on 4 liters of oxygen by nasal cannula. Her oxygen saturation improves to 96%. A regular diet is prescribed, with strict intake and output documentation and calorie counts. Since she will be primarily on bed rest, compression boots, graduated compression stockings (TEDs), and heel protectors are prescribed. Her dressing change documentation for the wound on her coccyx indicates that during each shift, the wound is to be irrigated with 250 cc of normal saline (NS), Mesalt rope moistened with NS is to be packed in the wound and in the areas of undermining, and then the entire wound is to be covered with Mesalt gauze dressings.

Questions

1. A colleague is not familiar with malabsorption syndrome. How would you explain what this condition is?

2. Intrigued, the colleague asks, "How would you know if you had malabsorption? What are the symptoms?" How would you answer?

3. If Mrs. Bennett were to have a deficiency of each of the following nutrients, what symptoms might she experience?

1. calcium
2. magnesium
3. iron
4. folic acid
5. protein
6. niacin (nicotinic acid)
7. vitamin A (Retinol)
8. vitamin B$_1$ (thiamine)
9. vitamin B$_2$ (riboflavin)
10. vitamin B$_{12}$
11. vitamin C (ascorbic acid)
12. vitamin D
13. vitamin K

4. What would the nurse expect to find during assessment of Mrs. Bennett's HEENT (head, eyes, ears, nose, and throat), skin, abdomen, and extremities?

5. The nurse assesses Mrs. Bennett for Trousseau's and Chvostek's sign. What is the nurse looking for and if positive, what do these signs indicate?

6. The nurse is concerned that a regular diet is prescribed for Mrs. Bennett. The nurse calls Mrs. Bennett's health care provider to discuss the concern and suggest an alternate diet. What foods are allowed on a regular diet and which type of diet will the nurse suggest instead?

7. The nurse calls the dietician to discuss the scheduling of Mrs. Bennett's meals. What type of scheduling will the nurse suggest?

8. Why has Mrs. Bennett been admitted to a telemetry unit?

9. Intravenous (IV) potassium chloride is prescribed. Should the initial dose be administered as an IV push ("bolus dose") to help begin to

Questions (continued)

correct Mrs. Bennett's critically low potassium (K^+) level of 1.7 mEq/L? Explain your answer.

10. Before hanging Mrs. Bennett's potassium, the nurse asks the assistive nursing personnel what Mrs. Bennett's urine output has been during the shift. Why is the nurse concerned about the client's urine output?

11. A type & cross match of two units of packed red blood cells (PRBC) has been added to Mrs. Bennett's medical treatment plan. Explain what it means to "type & cross match" and the rationale for including a PRBC transfusion in Mrs. Bennett's plan.

12. Mrs. Bennett says to the nurse "The other day I overheard my doctor tell someone I had nontropical sprue. As much as I wish I was on a tropical vacation somewhere and not in the hospital, there is nothing warm and relaxing about what I have. What was he talking about?" Explain which disease the health care provider was discussing.

13. Briefly explain the significance of Mrs. Bennett's history of pancreatitis with a pancreatic resection to her present condition.

14. Which factors for proper wound healing are inadequate in Mrs. Bennett's case?

15. Mrs. Bennett has a prescription to obtain a wound culture during the next dressing change. Should the nurse obtain the wound sample before or after irrigating the wound with normal saline? Explain your answer.

16. Provide a rationale for including compression boots, graduated compression stockings (TEDs), and heel protectors in Mrs. Bennett's plan of care.

17. What must the nurse keep in mind when gathering supplies to do Mrs. Bennett's dressing change?

18. Identify five nursing diagnoses appropriate for Mrs. Bennett's plan of care. List the diagnoses in order of priority.

19. Which of Mrs. Bennett's allergies is of greatest concern and why?

20. Discuss the impact that a chronic illness has on a person's quality of life.

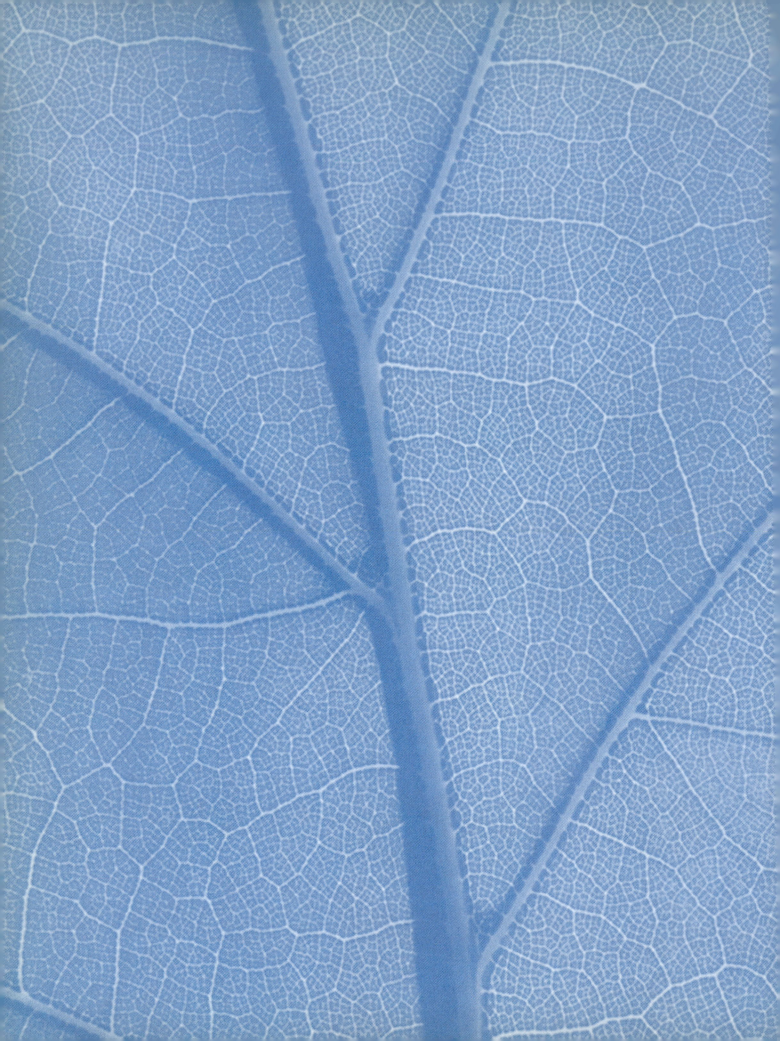

PART TWO

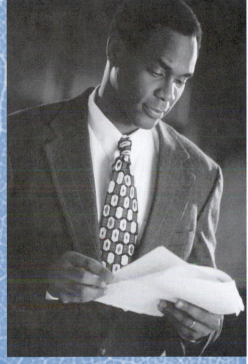

The Urinary System

Ms. Jimenez (Part 1)

GENDER

Female

AGE

56

SETTING

- Hospital

ETHNICITY

- Hispanic

CULTURAL CONSIDERATIONS

PREEXISTING CONDITION

- Motor vehicle accident (MVA) eight weeks ago with no injury; depression

COEXISTING CONDITION

- Suicide attempt; metabolic acidosis

COMMUNICATION

DISABILITY

SOCIOECONOMIC

- Financial difficulties secondary to divorce five years ago. Nonsmoker.

SPIRITUAL/RELIGIOUS

PHARMACOLOGIC

- 4-methylpyrazole (Fomepizole; Antizol); pyridoxine hydrochloride (Vitamin B_6); thiamine (Vitamin B_1); succinylcholine chloride (Anectine); levalbuterol (Xopenex); lorazepam (Ativan); propofol (Diprivan, Disoprofol); etomidate

LEGAL

ETHICAL

ALTERNATIVE THERAPY

PRIORITIZATION

- Medical stabilization

DELEGATION

THE URINARY SYSTEM

Level of difficulty: Difficult

Overview: This case addresses the medical consequences of a failed suicide attempt. The nurse's understanding of the effects of ingesting ethylene glycol (antifreeze) is essential for prioritizing care, interpreting lab and arterial blood gas results, and identifying the purpose of prescribed medications.

DIFFICULT

Client Profile

Ms. Jimenez is a 56-year-old woman who has been having financial difficulties since her divorce five years ago. She was recently involved in a motor vehicle accident (MVA) where she drove over a curb and hit a telephone pole. She did not sustain any significant injuries in the MVA. Today, Ms. Jimenez's daughter Maria returned home at 9:00 P.M. to find Ms. Jimenez sitting on the floor with a decreased level of consciousness. Maria was able to shake her mother awake. With slurred speech, Ms. Jimenez told her daughter that she drank three large glasses of antifreeze (ethylene glycol) at around 7:00 P.M. Maria called 911 and emergency medical services transported Ms. Jimenez to the local emergency department.

Case Study

Upon arrival to the emergency department, Ms. Jimenez is afebrile with a rectal temperature of 97°F (36.1°C). Her other vital signs are blood pressure 135/85, pulse 68, and respiratory rate 24. Her initial arterial blood gases (ABGs) on a 15 liters per minute non-rebreather revealed a pH of 7.19, partial pressure of carbon dioxide ($PaCO_2$) of 13 mmHg, partial pressure of oxygen (PaO_2) of 359 mmHg, bicarbonate (HCO_3^-) of 5 mEq/L, and oxygen (O_2) saturation of 100%. Ms. Jimenez is sedated in the emergency department using etomidate. She is intubated and put on a mechanical ventilator. A Foley catheter is inserted. She receives succinylcholine chloride, lorazepam, and propofol. Her oxygen saturation is 92% on an FIO_2 (fraction of inspired oxygen) of 70%. The health care provider's physical examination reveals no abnormal findings. The neurological exam is deferred because Ms. Jimenez is intubated and sedated. An electrocardiogram (ECG, EKG) shows that Ms. Jimenez is in a normal sinus rhythm. A chest X-ray (CXR) shows no infiltrate and proper endotracheal tube placement.

A urinalysis shows a specific gravity of 1.010, a small amount of occult blood, 3 to 5 white blood cells per high-power field (HPF), a few bacteria per HPF, and a moderate amount of uric acid crystals and urine calcium oxalate crystals. A urine culture & colony count was negative (no growth). Her blood alcohol level is less than 10 mg/dL. Her ethylene glycol level is 36 mg/dL. Her complete blood count (CBC) is within normal limits except for a mean cell volume (MCV) of 79.2 μm^3. Troponin level is 0 ng/mL, creatine kinase (CK) is 182 U/L, and creatine kinase cardiac isoenzyme (CK-MB) is within normal limits (WNL). Serum osmolality is 392 mOsm/Kg. Her electrolytes are WNL except for a serum bicarbonate of 7 mEq/L. She has an anion gap of 29 mEq/L, blood urea nitrogen (BUN) of 25 mg/dL, and creatinine of 1.4 mg/dL. Her liver function tests are WNL.

Ms. Jimenez is admitted to the intensive care unit (ICU) and prescribed intravenous (IV) fluids of normal saline with 2 ampules of bicarbonate at 125 cc per hour. The medications prescribed for her include 4-methylpyrazole IV every 12 hours, intramuscular (IM) pyridoxine 5 mg, thiamine 100 mg IM, and levalbuterol treatments. Lab work prescribed includes CBC, electrolytes, ethylene glycol levels, basic metabolic panel (BMP), creatinine level, acetone level, and urinalysis.

In the ICU at the bedside, a Quinton dialysis catheter is surgically inserted in the right internal jugular vein for emergency dialysis and placement of the Quinton catheter is confirmed by CXR.

Questions

1. What is ethylene glycol? What products contain ethylene glycol?

2. Discuss the potential effects of ingesting ethylene glycol (antifreeze).

3. What is a "half-life"? Explain the half-life of ethylene glycol and how ethylene glycol is cleared from the body.

4. Ms. Jimemez's ethylene glycol level is 36 mg/dL. Is there a safe amount of ethylene glycol that can be consumed by an adult? What is the lethal dose of ethylene glycol?

5. Discuss the rationale for why Ms. Jimenez is receiving 4-methylpyrazole. What is a drawback of this medication?

6. If 4-methylpyrazole is not available, what is the next most effective treatment for ethylene glycol poisoning? Discuss how this treatment is administered and what should be monitored during administration.

7. If Maria had come home earlier and Ms. Jimenez was found within an hour of drinking the antifreeze, what four interventions could have been considered to decrease the progression of the toxic effects of the ethylene glycol?

8. Briefly describe the indication for each of the following medications Ms. Jimenez received during her initial medical treatment: pyridoxine hydrochloride, thiamine, succinylcholine chloride, levalbuterol, lorazepam, propofol, and etomidate.

9. Why were intravenous (IV) fluids of normal saline with 2 ampules of bicarbonate at 125 cc per hour prescribed as part of the medical management of Ms. Jimenez?

10. Complete an analysis of Ms. Jimenez's initial arterial blood gas (ABG) results while on 15 liters of oxygen via non-rebreather. Are her ABGs consistent with those expected for a person with an ethylene glycol overdose?

11. Why was Ms. Jimenez intubated and placed on a mechanical ventilator?

12. Ms. Jimenez is on a mechanical ventilator set on assist-control of 14, respiratory rate of 28, volume 650, oxygen 40%, and a positive end-expiratory pressure (PEEP) of 5. What does each ventilator setting indicate?

13. The respiratory rate on a mechanical ventilator is usually set between 10 and 14 breaths per minute. Why is the rate for Ms. Jimenez set at 28 breaths per minute?

14. Which of Ms. Jimenez's laboratory results below are most significant in the determination of a diagnosis of ethylene glycol poisoning?

- Urinalysis: specific gravity of 1.010, small amount of occult blood, 3 to 5 white blood cells per HPF, a few bacteria per HPF, a moderate amount of uric acid crystals, and urine calcium oxalate crystals.
- Urine culture & colony count was negative (no growth).
- Serum osmolality is 392 mOsm/Kg.
- Bicarbonate of 7 mEq/L.
- Anion gap of 29 mEq/L.
- BUN of 25 mg/dL.
- Creatinine of 1.4 mg/dL.

15. Explain how a Wood lamp could be used to help confirm the ingestion of ethylene glycol.

16. Briefly explain what Ms. Jimenez's troponin, CPK, and CK-MB indicate.

17. Why did Ms. Jimenez's prescribed laboratory tests include an assessment of her liver function?

18. What is a Quinton catheter and why was one inserted?

19. Prioritize three nursing diagnoses that are appropriate to include in Ms. Jimenez's plan of care.

Ms. Jimenez (Part 2)

GENDER

Female

AGE

56

SETTING

- Hospital

ETHNICITY

- Hispanic

CULTURAL CONSIDERATIONS

PREEXISTING CONDITION

- Motor vehicle accident (MVA) eight weeks ago with no injury; depression

COEXISTING CONDITION

- Suicide attempt with ethylene glycol (antifreeze) poisoning

COMMUNICATION

DISABILITY

SOCIOECONOMIC

- Financial difficulties secondary to divorce five years ago. Nonsmoker.

SPIRITUAL/RELIGIOUS

PHARMACOLOGIC

LEGAL

- Safety sitter

ETHICAL

ALTERNATIVE THERAPY

PRIORITIZATION

- Client safety

DELEGATION

- Psychiatric consult; Social services

MODERATE

THE URINARY SYSTEM

Level of difficulty: Moderate

Overview: The client ingested ethylene glycol two days ago and has been medically stabilized. The long-term effects of ethylene glycol poisoning are discussed. The nurse is asked to explain the stages of acute renal failure and the function of hemodialysis. Collaborative resources to assist the client following discharge are identified.

Client Profile

Ms. Jimenez is a 56-year-old woman who has been having financial difficulties since her divorce five years ago. She was recently involved in a motor vehicle accident (MVA) where she drove over a curb and hit a telephone pole. She did not sustain any significant injuries in the MVA. Two days ago, Ms. Jimenez's daughter Maria returned home at 9:00 P.M. to find Ms. Jimenez sitting on the floor with a decreased level of consciousness. Maria was able to shake her mother awake. With slurred speech, Ms. Jimenez told her daughter that she drank three large glasses of antifreeze (ethylene glycol) at around 7:00 P.M. Maria called 911 and emergency medical services transported Ms. Jimenez to the local emergency department.

Case Study

It is forty-eight hours after her arrival in the emergency department. Ms. Jimenez has undergone twelve hours of emergency dialysis, has been extubated, and is medically stable for transfer to a medical-surgical nursing unit. A safety sitter remains in Ms. Jimenez's room at all times. Ms. Jimenez is alert and oriented but has a flat affect. She is not remorseful for her actions and states, "I had hoped I would be successful this time." A psychiatrist sees Ms. Jimenez for a consultation. The psychiatric assessment reveals that she has been planning the poisoning for a few weeks. She states, "I was hoping I would die quickly and it would look like an accident." Ms. Jimenez states that she has made attempts in the past to overdose on medications. She did not seek care at the hospital when these suicide attempts were not successful. She has been depressed since divorcing her husband five years ago. Since her divorce, she has not paid taxes and there have been mounting financial bills with the Internal Revenue Service. As a result, her wages are being garnished (money is withheld from her paycheck and sent to a creditor). She reports, "On the outside I appear bright and upbeat but on the inside I am so lonely and sad and just don't want to go on anymore." She wonders how she will pay for her medical care now. "I had not planned on the poison not working and needing dialysis. I bet dialysis is expensive."

Questions

1. Explain acute renal failure (ARF).

2. Discuss the characteristics and causes of the three types of ARF.

3. Considering the conditions that cause ARF, which type of ARF is Ms. Jimenez experiencing?

4. What characteristics and laboratory data define the four phases of acute renal failure, and what is the approximate duration of each phase?

5. It has been four days since admission. According to the definitions provided in the response to question 4, which phase of acute renal failure is Ms. Jimenez experiencing?

6. While the nurse is assessing the Quinton catheter insertion site, Ms. Jimenez asks what dialysis is and how long she will need to do it. Her initial dialysis treatment was twelve hours long, and she is wondering if she will always have to be "hooked up" to the machine that long each time. How should the nurse respond?

7. On admission, Ms. Jimenez's creatinine was 1.4 mg/dL and her blood urea nitrogen (BUN) was 25 mg/dL. Ms. Jimenez has repeat creatinine and BUN labs drawn two days after admission. The results are a creatinine of 4.7 mg/dL and a BUN of 24 mg/dL. A day later, her creatinine is 8.5 mg/dL with a BUN of 57 mg/dL. Are these results getting better or worse since admission? Discuss why.

8. The following potassium values are reported: on admission, 3.6 mEq/L; forty-eight hours after admission, 4.0 mEq/L; and seventy-two hours after admission, 4.2 mEq/L. What potential cardiovascular change is of greatest concern to the nurse?

Questions (continued)

9. Identify five priority nursing diagnoses that are appropriate to include in Ms. Jimenez's plan of care.

10. Why has a safety sitter been included as part of Ms. Jimenez's plan of care?

11. What are two collaborative services to consider when planning Ms. Jimenez's discharge?

12. Discuss how Ms. Jimenez's recent MVA may relate to her current admission.

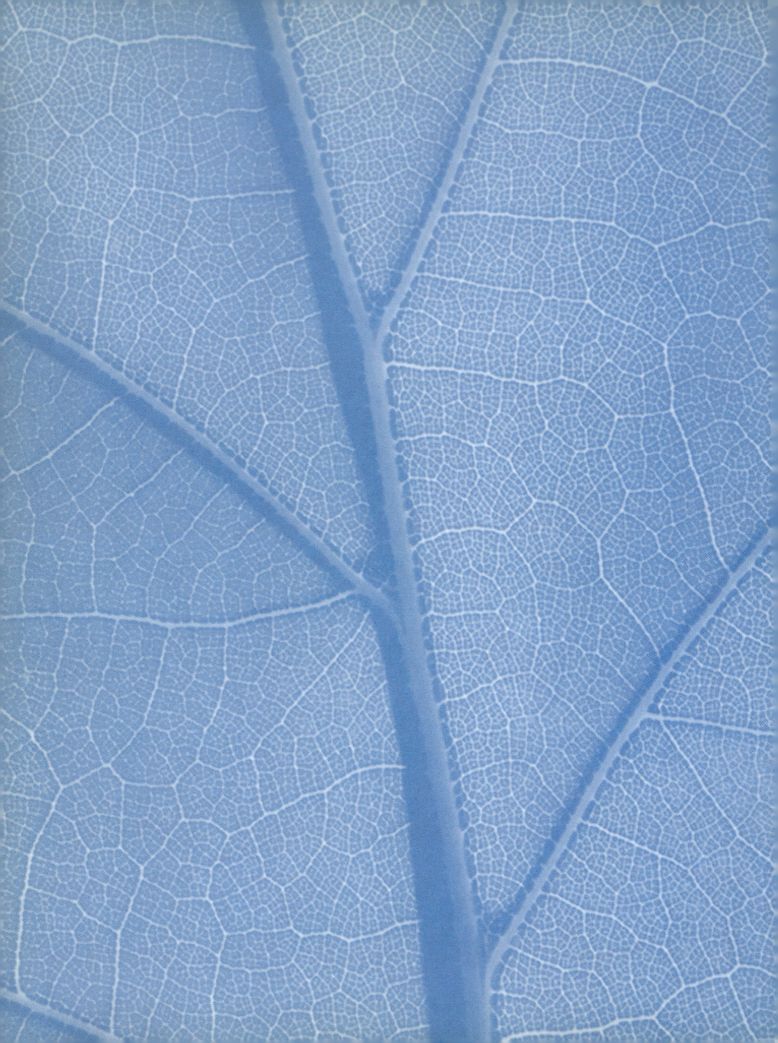

PART THREE

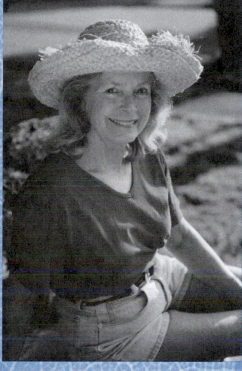

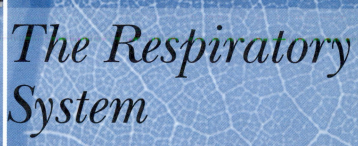

The Respiratory System

Mrs. Hogan

GENDER

Female

AGE

38

SETTING

■ Walk-in health care center

ETHNICITY

■ White American

CULTURAL CONSIDERATIONS

PREEXISTING CONDITION

■ Mild persistent asthma

COEXISTING CONDITION

COMMUNICATION

DISABILITY

SOCIOECONOMIC

■ Husband employed in asbestos removal.

SPIRITUAL/RELIGIOUS

PHARMACOLOGIC

■ Albuterol (Proventil, Ventolin); beclomethasone dipropionate (Beconase)

LEGAL

ETHICAL

ALTERNATIVE THERAPY

PRIORITIZATION

■ Ensuring a patent airway; monitoring for status asthmaticus.

DELEGATION

THE RESPIRATORY SYSTEM

Level of difficulty: Easy

Overview: This case requires that the nurse recognize appropriate interventions for an asthma attack and understand the actions of respiratory medications. The nurse must assess the triggers specific to this patient and provide teaching to reduce the patient's risk of another exacerbation. Priority nursing diagnoses and outcome goals are identified.

Client Profile

Mrs. Hogan is a 38-year-old woman brought to a walk-in health care center by her neighbor. Mrs. Hogan is in obvious respiratory distress. She is having difficulty breathing with audible high-pitched wheezing and is having difficulty speaking. Pausing after every few words to catch her breath, she tells the nurse, "I am having a really bad asthma attack. My chest feels very tight and I cannot catch my breath. I took my albuterol and Vanceril, but they are not helping." Mrs. Hogan hands her neighbor her cell phone and asks the neighbor to dial a telephone number. "That number is my husband's boss. My husband just started working for an asbestos removal company about a month ago. He is usually on the road somewhere. Can you ask his boss to get a message to him that I am here?"

Case Study

While auscultating Mrs. Hogan's lung sounds, the nurse hears expiratory wheezes and scattered rhonchi throughout. Mrs. Hogan is afebrile. Her vital signs are blood pressure 142/96, pulse 88, and respiratory rate 34. Her oxygen saturation on room air is 86%. Arterial blood gases (ABGs) are drawn. Mrs. Hogan is placed on 2 liters of humidified oxygen via nasal cannula. She is started on intravenous (IV) fluids and receives an albuterol nebulizer treatment.

Questions

1. What other signs and symptoms might the nurse note during assessment of Mrs. Hogan?

2. In what position should the nurse place Mrs. Hogan and why?

3. Identify at least five signs and symptoms that indicate that Mrs. Hogan is not responding to treatment and may be developing status asthmaticus (a life-threatening condition).

4. Mrs. Hogan states that she took her albuterol and beclomethasone prior to coming to the walk-in health care center. How do these medications work?

5. Briefly discuss the common adverse effects Mrs. Hogan may experience with the albuterol nebulizer treatment.

6. Physiologically, what is happening in Mrs. Hogan's lungs during an asthma attack?

7. In order of priority, identify three nursing diagnoses that are appropriate during Mrs. Hogan's asthma exacerbation.

8. Write three outcome goals for Mrs. Hogan's diagnosis of ineffective breathing pattern.

9. Mrs. Hogan has responded well to the albuterol nebulizer treatment. Her breathing is less labored, and she appears less anxious. The nurse asks Mrs. Hogan what she was doing when the asthma attack began. Mrs. Hogan says "Nothing special. I was doing the laundry." What other questions might the nurse ask (and why) to assess the cause of Mrs. Hogan's asthma exacerbation?

10. What are some other questions the nurse might ask to get a better sense of Mrs. Hogan's asthma?

11. The nurse asks Mrs. Hogan to describe step-by-step how she uses her inhalers. Mrs. Hogan describes the following steps: "First I shake the inhaler well. Then I breathe out normally and place the mouthpiece in my mouth. I take a few breaths and then while breathing in slowly and deeply with my lips tight around the mouthpiece, I give myself a puff. I hold my breath for a count of five and breathe out slowly as if I am blowing out a candle. I wait a minute or two and then I repeat those steps all over again for my second puff." Which step(s) is/are of concern to the nurse and why?

12. Briefly discuss three nursing interventions to help decrease Mrs. Hogan's risk of another asthma exacerbation.

GENDER

Male

AGE

25

SETTING

- Hospital

ETHNICITY

- Black American

CULTURAL CONSIDERATIONS

PREEXISTING CONDITION

COEXISTING CONDITION

COMMUNICATION

DISABILITY

SOCIOECONOMIC

SPIRITUAL/RELIGIOUS

PHARMACOLOGIC

- Heparin; lidocaine (Xylocaine)

LEGAL

ETHICAL

ALTERNATIVE THERAPY

PRIORITIZATION

- Critical arterial blood gases

DELEGATION

THE RESPIRATORY SYSTEM

Level of difficulty: Easy

Overview: This case provides the nurse with an opportunity to convey an understanding of the arterial blood gas testing method and practice the skill of acid-base analysis/arterial blood gas results interpretation.

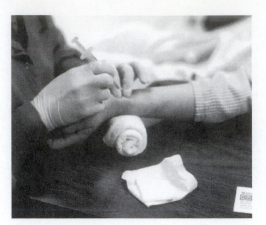

Insert the needle with the bevel up at a 45° angle

Client Profile   **William** is a newly graduated registered nurse. He will begin working on a respiratory nursing unit next week. During orientation to his role, he will learn how to collect an arterial blood gas (ABG) sample. He is given five sets of ABG results to practice acid-base analysis/arterial blood gas results interpretation. William must determine acid-base balance, determine if there is compensation, and decide whether each client is hypoxic.

Case Study   The five sets of arterial blood gas results are:

1. pH 6.95 $PaCO_2$ 48 mmHg HCO_3^- 23 mEq/L SaO_2 95% PaO_2 79 mmHg
2. pH 7.48 $PaCO_2$ 44 mmHg HCO_3^- 30 mEq/L SaO_2 88% PaO_2 70 mmHg
3. pH 7.48 $PaCO_2$ 31 mmHg HCO_3^- 19 mEq/L SaO_2 93% PaO_2 82 mmHg
4. pH 7.35 $PaCO_2$ 42 mmHg HCO_3^- 26 mEq/L SaO_2 95% PaO_2 83 mmHg
5. pH 7.53 $PaCO_2$ 31 mmHg HCO_3^- 35 mEq/L SaO_2 90% PaO_2 57 mmHg

Questions

1. Describe the purpose of the arterial blood gas (ABG) test.

2. Describe the client preparation that is necessary prior to drawing an ABG sample. Is written client consent (a consent form) required prior to drawing the blood sample?

3. List the equipment the nurse must gather prior to collecting the ABG sample.

4. List the steps for obtaining an ABG sample from a radial artery. Include how to perform a modified Allen's test to assess ulnar circulation.

5. What are the potential complications of the ABG collection procedure?

6. Discuss the nursing responsibilities after the ABG sample is obtained.

7. Explain how an ABG sample should be transported to the laboratory for processing.

8. How long does it take to obtain ABG results?

9. Briefly discuss at least five factors that can cause false ABG results.

10. What are the normal ranges for each of the ABG components in an adult: pH, partial pressure of carbon dioxide ($PaCO_2$), bicarbonate (HCO_3^-), oxygen saturation (SaO_2), and partial pressure of oxygen (PaO_2)?

11. What are the critical/panic values for each of the ABG components in an adult: pH, $PaCO_2$, HCO_3^-, SaO_2, and PaO_2?

12. How are the oxygen saturation (SaO_2) and partial pressure of oxygen (PaO_2) ABG components

Questions (continued)

used to assess the client's respiratory status? What are four factors to consider when interpreting the PaO_2?

13. Sometimes the partial pressure of carbon dioxide, oxygen saturation, and partial pressure

of oxygen results are documented/reported as "$PaCO_2$, SaO_2, and PaO_2." Other times the results are documented as "PCO_2, O_2 sat and PO_2" (without the "a"). What is the difference?

14. Help William analyze each set of ABG results. Determine whether each value is high, low, or within normal limits; interpret the acid-base balance; determine if there is compensation; and indicate whether the client is hypoxic.

1. pH 6.95	$PaCO_2$ 48 mmHg	HCO_3^- 23 mEq/L	SaO_2 95%	PaO_2 79 mmHg
2. pH 7.48	$PaCO_2$ 44 mmHg	HCO_3^- 30 mEq/L	SaO_2 88%	PaO_2 70 mmHg
3. pH 7.48	$PaCO_2$ 31 mmHg	HCO_3^- 19 mEq/L	SaO_2 93%	PaO_2 82 mmHg
4. pH 7.35	$PaCO_2$ 42 mmHg	HCO_3^- 26 mEq/L	SaO_2 96%	PaO_2 83 mmHg
5. pH 7.53	$PaCO_2$ 31 mmHg	HCO_3^- 35 mEq/L	SaO_2 90%	PaO_2 57 mmHg

15. Identify three appropriate nursing diagnoses for a client having an ABG sample obtained.

GENDER

Male

AGE

75

SETTING

- Hospital

ETHNICITY

- Jewish American

CULTURAL CONSIDERATIONS

- Perception and expression of pain.

PREEXISTING CONDITION

- Chronic obstructive pulmonary disease (COPD) (emphysema), hypertension (HTN) well controlled by enalapril (Vasotec).

COEXISTING CONDITION

- Lower back pain

COMMUNICATION

DISABILITY

- Needs assistance of one person while ambulating due to unsteady gait and dyspnea on exertion.

SOCIOECONOMIC

SPIRITUAL/RELIGIOUS

- Judaism

PHARMACOLOGIC

- Acetaminophen (Tylenol); albuterol (AccuNeb, Proventil, Ventolin); enalapril (Vasotec); oxycodone/acetaminophen (Percocet)

LEGAL

ETHICAL

ALTERNATIVE THERAPY

- Nonpharmacologic interventions for respiratory distress and pain management.

PRIORITIZATION

- Difficulty breathing; pain management

DELEGATION

MODERATE

THE RESPIRATORY SYSTEM

Level of difficulty: Moderate

Overview: This case requires that the nurse recognize the signs and symptoms of activity intolerance and respiratory distress and how symptoms differ in the client who has COPD. The nurse considers both pharmacologic and nonpharmacologic interventions to manage respiratory distress and pain. Cultural/spiritual perceptions of pain and pain management are discussed. The nurse must provide discharge teaching regarding safe use of oxygen in the home.

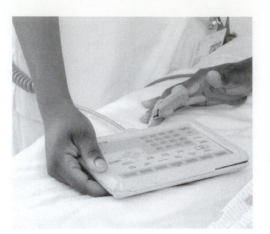

Client with Pulse Oximeter

Client Profile

Mr. Cohen is a 75-year-old male admitted with an exacerbation of chronic obstructive pulmonary disease (emphysema). He has been keeping the head of the bed up for most of the day and night to facilitate his breathing which has resulted in lower back pain. Acetaminophen (Tylenol) was not effective in reducing his pain, so the health care provider has prescribed oxycodone/acetaminophen (Percocet) one to two tablets PO every four to six hours as needed for pain. Mr. Cohen is on 2 liters of oxygen by nasal cannula. He can receive respiratory treatments of albuterol (AccuNeb, Proventil, Ventolin) every six hours as needed. Mr. Cohen needs someone to walk beside him when he ambulates because he has an unsteady gait and often needs to stop to catch his breath.

Case Study

The nurse enters the room and finds Mr. Cohen hunched over his bedside table watching television. He says this position helps his breathing. His lung sounds are clear but diminished bilaterally. Capillary refill is four seconds and slight clubbing of his fingers is noted. His oxygen saturation is being assessed every two hours to monitor for hypoxia. Each assessment reveals oxygen saturation at rest of 90% to 94% on 2 liters of oxygen by nasal cannula.

After breakfast, Mr. Cohen complains of lower back pain that caused him increased discomfort while ambulating to the bathroom. He describes the pain as a dull ache and rates the pain a "6" on a 0–10 pain scale. He requests two Percocet tablets. The nurse assesses Mr. Cohen's vital signs (blood pressure 150/78, pulse 90, respiratory rate 26) and gives the Percocet as prescribed. Forty-five minutes later, Mr. Cohen states the Percocet has helped relieve his back pain to a "2" on a 0–10 pain scale and he would like to take a walk in the hall. The nurse checks his oxygen saturation before they leave his room, and it is 92%. Using a portable oxygen tank, the nurse walks with Mr. Cohen from his room to the nurse's station (approximately 60 feet). Mr. Cohen stops to rest at the nurse's station because he is short of breath. His oxygen saturation at the nurse's station is 86%. After a few deep breaths and rest, his oxygen saturation rises to 91%. Mr. Cohen walks back to his room where he sits in his recliner to wait for lunch. His oxygen saturation is initially 87% when he returns and then 91% after a few minutes of rest. Expiratory wheezes are heard bilaterally when the nurse assesses his lung sounds. While Mr. Cohen waits for lunch to arrive, the nurse calls respiratory therapy to give Mr. Cohen his albuterol treatment. The respiratory treatment and rest relieves his acute shortness of breath. His oxygen saturation is now 93%, and his lung sounds are clear but diminished bilaterally.

Questions

1. Briefly define chronic obstructive pulmonary disease (COPD). What pathophysiology is occurring in the lungs of a client with emphysema?

2. What are five signs and symptoms of respiratory distress the nurse may observe in a client with COPD?

3. Describe the physical appearance characteristics of a client with emphysema.

4. Are Mr. Cohen's oxygen saturation readings normal? Explain your answer.

5. Explain the effects that acute pain can have on an individual's respiratory pattern and cardiovascular system.

6. List five nonpharmacologic interventions that the nurse could implement to help decrease Mr. Cohen's difficulty breathing.

7. How would the nurse measure the effectiveness of the interventions suggested in question number 6?

8. Explain why the nurse did not increase Mr. Cohen's oxygen to help ease his shortness of breath.

9. Discuss the cultural/spiritual considerations the nurse should keep in mind while creating a plan of care for Mr. Cohen's pain management.

10. What are three nonpharmacologic nursing interventions to help manage Mr. Cohen's pain?

11. How would the nurse measure the effectiveness of the interventions suggested in question number 10?

12. Should the nurse be concerned about the adverse effects of respiratory depression and hypotension when giving oxycodone/acetaminophen (Percocet) to Mr. Cohen? Why or why not?

13. What are three nursing diagnoses that address physical and/or physiological safety concerns for Mr. Cohen?

14. Mr. Cohen will be returning home with oxygen. List at least five safety considerations the nurse should include in discharge teaching regarding the use of oxygen in the home.

Mr. Kaberry

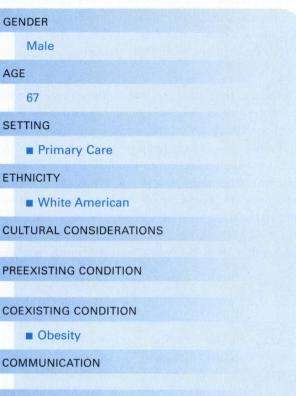

GENDER

Male

AGE

67

SETTING

■ Primary Care

ETHNICITY

■ White American

CULTURAL CONSIDERATIONS

PREEXISTING CONDITION

COEXISTING CONDITION

■ Obesity

COMMUNICATION

DISABILITY

SOCIOECONOMIC

■ Smokes a half pack of cigarettes per day for past forty years. Wife accompanied client to office visit.

SPIRITUAL/RELIGIOUS

PHARMACOLOGIC

LEGAL

ETHICAL

ALTERNATIVE THERAPY

PRIORITIZATION

DELEGATION

MODERATE

THE RESPIRATORY SYSTEM

Level of difficulty: Moderate

Overview: This case reviews the normal sleep cycle of an adult. The nurse must identify the symptoms of sleep apnea syndrome. Potential long-term complications of obstructive sleep apnea syndrome are discussed and treatment options are considered.

Client Profile

Mr. Kaberry is a 67-year-old man. He is 5 feet, 10 inches tall. Over the past five years, Mr. Kaberry has gained 50 pounds and currently weighs 260 pounds (118.2 kg). He smokes a half pack of cigarettes each day and has been a smoker for the past forty years. In the past three months, he has noticed that, despite sleeping for at least seven hours a night, he is very tired during the day. He is afraid he is ill and has made an appointment with his primary health care provider.

Case Study

While conducting an initial assessment, the nurse asks Mr. Kaberry what brought him to the provider's office. Mr. Kaberry states, "I have been so tired during the day. I realize I have put on weight over the last few years, but I am so exhausted. I work in a bank and sometimes I wish I could just put my head on my desk at and catch a quick nap. That is not like me. I usually feel rested in the morning and I never take naps during the day. There must be something wrong with me." Mrs. Kaberry adds, "If anyone should be tired it is me. He keeps me up most of the night with his snoring. I hope you can find out what is wrong with him because living with him has been unbearable lately." The nurse asks Mrs. Kaberry to explain what she means by "unbearable." Mrs. Kaberry explains that Mr. Kaberry has been short with her, "Very irritable, I guess you could say."

Questions

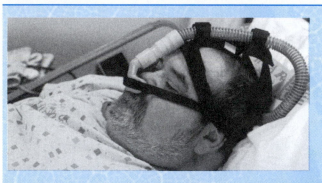

1. Describe the five stages of sleep and the normal sleep cycle of an adult.

2. How is sleep apnea syndrome defined and what are the three types of sleep apnea?

3. How does Mr. Kaberry fit the profile of the "typical" client who has sleep apnea?

4. The nurse continues the assessment of Mr. Kaberry's symptoms. List at least five other manifestations of sleep apnea the nurse should ask if he has experienced.

5. Briefly discuss Mr. Kaberry's predisposing risk factors for sleep apnea syndrome. How common is sleep apnea in the United States?

6. Discuss the anatomy and physiology that causes obstructive sleep apnea syndrome.

7. Explain how sleep apnea syndrome is diagnosed.

8. What are the potential complications associated with sleep apnea syndrome?

9. Discuss the interventions to consider when planning the medical management of Mr. Kaberry's obstructive sleep apnea. Include a discussion of continuous positive airway pressure therapy.

10. How will the nurse respond when Mrs. Kaberry asks, "Do we really need that machine? Isn't there a medication he could take to help this problem?"

11. Mr. and Mrs. Kaberry are learning how to use the continuous positive airway pressure (CPAP) machine. What are two potential side effects experienced by people using CPAP therapy and what are two interventions that can help decrease the side effects?

12. When teaching Mr. and Mrs. Kaberry how to use the CPAP machine, what relationship and body image concerns should be acknowledged?

13. Surgery may be an option for Mr. Kaberry if the symptoms of his obstructive sleep apnea do not improve with nonsurgical interventions. What surgical procedures are used to treat obstructive sleep apnea?

14. Help the nurse generate three appropriate nursing diagnoses for Mr. Kaberry.

15. Until Mr. Kaberry's sleep apnea responds to treatment and his fatigue resolves, what safety precaution(s) should the nurse suggest?

Mr. Bailey

GENDER

Male

AGE

90

SETTING

- Hospital

ETHNICITY

- Irish American

CULTURAL CONSIDERATIONS

PREEXISTING CONDITION

- Chronic obstructive pulmonary disease (COPD) (emphysema), heart failure (HF, CHF)

COEXISTING CONDITION

- Pulmonary edema, which has been worsening steadily

COMMUNICATION

- Alert and oriented x 3 with clear speech

DISABILITY

- Oxygen-dependent

SOCIOECONOMIC

- Lived independently at home prior to admission; supportive family

SPIRITUAL/RELIGIOUS

- The Last Rites; Catholic religion's beliefs regarding euthanasia and physician-assisted suicide

PHARMACOLOGIC

LEGAL

- Patient Self-Determination Act; advance directives; euthanasia; physician-assisted suicide

ETHICAL

- Euthanasia; physician-assisted suicide

ALTERNATIVE THERAPY

PRIORITIZATION

- Care of the dying client and support of the family.

DELEGATION

THE RESPIRATORY SYSTEM

Level of difficulty: Difficult

Overview: This case challenges the nurse with the client's desire to discontinue life-sustaining treatment. The nurse provides holistic end-of-life care for the client and grief support for the family. The nurse is asked to consider the ethical and legal issues surrounding euthanasia and physician-assisted suicide.

DIFFICULT

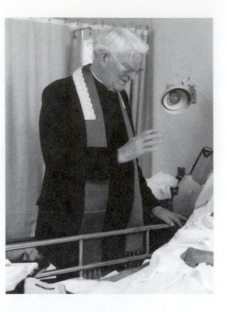

Client Profile

Mr. Bailey is a 90-year-old man admitted to the hospital with an exacerbation of chronic obstructive pulmonary disease (emphysema). He has shortness of breath and worsening pulmonary edema. Mr. Bailey is oxygen-dependent. He is alert and oriented and prior to admission he lived at home alone. His code status on admission is DNR (do not resuscitate). He has a supportive family of two daughters, two sons-in-law, a younger sister, and many grandchildren.

Case Study

The nurse caring for Mr. Bailey greets him in the morning to introduce himself and to take a set of vital signs. Mr. Bailey gets very short of breath when speaking but is able to carry on a conversation. He asks the nurse when his health care provider will be in because he has a question. The nurse tells Mr. Bailey that he anticipates the health care provider will be in shortly. The nurse asks if there is anything he can do to help Mr. Bailey before the health care provider arrives. Mr. Bailey tells the nurse that he would like to ask his doctor to remove his oxygen. The nurse asks Mr. Bailey if he understands that he needs to keep his oxygen on to breathe. Mr. Bailey says he knows this but is just so tired of being sick. Mr. Bailey explains, "I have thought about it a great deal and I am ready to die." Pausing after every few words to catch his breath, he states, "I understand that I may get better and be able to go home. But, soon enough I will be in the hospital again. I have a disease that will kill me eventually. It is not a matter of if I will die, just when. I have had a good life. I do not want to live like this any longer. I am tired of suffering. It is okay. I am ready to die." Taken back by his request and its consequence, the nurse tells Mr. Bailey that he will call his health care provider to come up and speak with Mr. Bailey as soon as possible.

Over the next few hours, most of Mr. Bailey's family arrives to visit. Together, the nurse and health care provider speak with Mr. Bailey and his family, allowing everyone to ask questions and express their thoughts. Mr. Bailey and his family fully understand that Mr. Bailey will die if the oxygen is removed. Mr. Bailey wishes to remove his oxygen. His family is obviously upset but supports his choice. The health care provider respects Mr. Bailey's wishes and turns off the oxygen and removes the nasal cannula.

Some members of Mr. Bailey's family leave his room to call other family members. His daughters, sister, and the nurse stay with Mr. Bailey. An hour and a half after the removal of his nasal cannula, Mr. Bailey dies. Many members of Mr. Bailey's family return shortly thereafter. They are sad, but thank the nurse for staying with Mr. Bailey and ask for some time alone with him to say good-bye.

Questions

1. Does this case sound unusual? If so, why?

2. What is the Patient Self-Determination Act?

3. Describe the purpose of the following advance directives: *living will, health care proxy* or *durable power of attorney,* and *advance care medical directive.*

4. Define euthanasia. Can you recall an end-of-life case brought to public attention by the media?

5. Is euthanasia the same as physician-assisted suicide? Explain your answer.

6. Would removing Mr. Bailey's oxygen be considered euthanasia or physician-assisted suicide?

7. Discuss the legal implications of euthanasia and physician-assisted suicide. Why is the state of Oregon unique?

8. Create two columns. In the first column, list at least five arguments that support euthanasia (physician-assisted suicide). In the second column, list at least five arguments against euthanasia (physician-assisted suicide).

9. What are five physical signs and symptoms the nurse may observe while caring for someone who is dying?

10. Describe at least five nursing interventions that will provide comfort for Mr. Bailey through the dying process.

11. Discuss at least five ways the nurse can support Mr. Bailey's family members in their grief.

12. What referral can the nurse offer Mr. Bailey and his family to support their spiritual well-being as they prepare for Mr. Bailey's death?

13. Discuss the religious considerations regarding the circumstances of Mr. Bailey's death.

14. What are two appropriate nursing diagnoses that address the needs of Mr. Bailey's family?

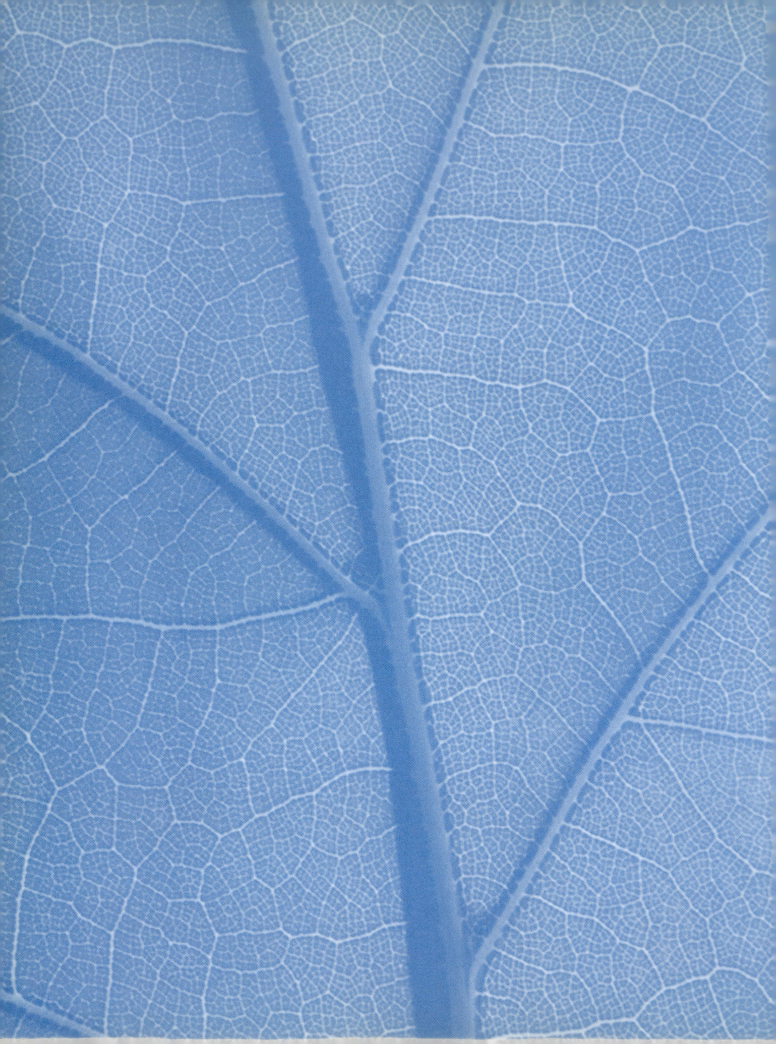

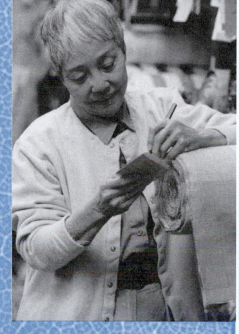

## PART FOUR

The Cardiovascular System & the Blood

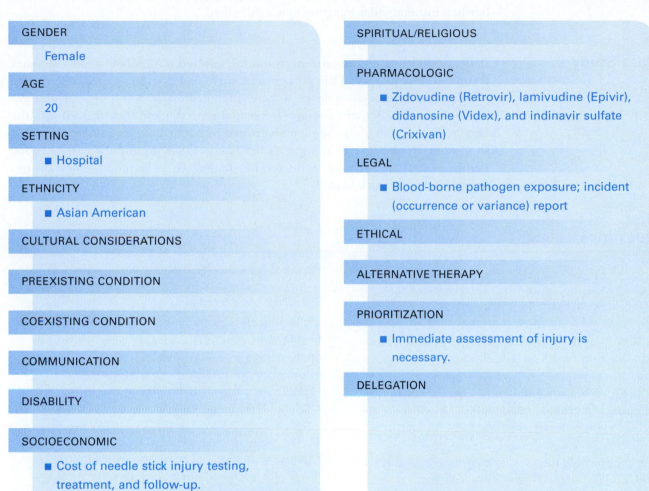

GENDER

Female

AGE

20

SETTING

■ Hospital

ETHNICITY

■ Asian American

CULTURAL CONSIDERATIONS

PREEXISTING CONDITION

COEXISTING CONDITION

COMMUNICATION

DISABILITY

SOCIOECONOMIC

■ Cost of needle stick injury testing, treatment, and follow-up.

SPIRITUAL/RELIGIOUS

PHARMACOLOGIC

■ Zidovudine (Retrovir), lamivudine (Epivir), didanosine (Videx), and indinavir sulfate (Crixivan)

LEGAL

■ Blood-borne pathogen exposure; incident (occurrence or variance) report

ETHICAL

ALTERNATIVE THERAPY

PRIORITIZATION

■ Immediate assessment of injury is necessary.

DELEGATION

THE CARDIOVASCULAR SYSTEM & THE BLOOD

Level of difficulty: Easy

Overview: This case requires that the student nurse recognize the appropriate interventions following a needle stick injury. Her risk of blood-borne pathogen exposure is considered. Testing, treatment, suggested follow-up, and the cost associated are discussed. An incident (occurrence or variance) report is completed.

Client Profile

Bethany is a 20-year-old nursing student. Although she has practiced the intramuscular injection technique in the nursing laboratory, she is nervous about giving her first intramuscular injection to a "real" client.

Case Study

Bethany has reviewed the procedure and the selected intramuscular site landmark technique. She follows all the proper steps, including donning gloves. The syringe was equipped with a safety device to cover the needle after injection, but after giving the injection, Bethany attempts to recap the needle and sticks herself with the needle through her glove. She is embarrassed to say anything in front of the client so she removes her gloves and washes her hands. Once outside the client's room, Bethany shows the nursing instructor her finger. There is blood visible on her finger where she stuck herself.

Questions

1. What should Bethany do first?

2. Discuss the appropriate interventions that the clinical agency should initiate following Bethany's needle stick injury.

3. What is the recommended drug therapy based on the level of risk of HIV exposure?

4. Which form(s) of hepatitis is Bethany most at risk for contracting? Discuss her level of risk of the form(s) of hepatitis you identified, as well as the risk of infection with HIV resulting from this needle stick.

5. Can the client's blood be tested for communicable diseases (such as hepatitis and HIV) if the client does not give consent?

6. What will be the recommendations for Bethany's follow-up antibody testing?

7. HIV test results are reported as *positive, negative,* or *indeterminate*. What does each result mean?

8. What is an incident (occurrence or variance) report, and why should Bethany and her nursing instructor complete one?

9. Discuss how Bethany could have prevented this needle stick injury.

10. Bethany's nursing instructor decides to share information with the nursing students about OSHA's "Needlestick Safety and Prevention Act." Explain OSHA's role and the safety and prevention act.

11. Discuss who is most likely responsible for the expense of Bethany's care immediately following the needle stick and any follow-up care. What risks are presented if the expense is prohibitive?

12. Identify three potential nursing diagnoses appropriate for Bethany.

Mr. Luke

GENDER

Male

AGE

58

SETTING

- Outpatient rehabilitation unit

ETHNICITY

- Asian American

CULTURAL CONSIDERATIONS

PREEXISTING CONDITION

- Left total knee replacement (TKR) five days ago.

COEXISTING CONDITION

COMMUNICATION

DISABILITY

SOCIOECONOMIC

- Smokes one pack of cigarettes per day.

SPIRITUAL/RELIGIOUS

PHARMACOLOGIC

- Enoxaparin (Lovenox); dalteparin sodium (Fragmin); warfarin sodium (Coumadin); nicotine transdermal system (Nicoderm CQ); acetylsalicylic acid (aspirin; ASA); dextran (Macrodex, Gentran)

LEGAL

ETHICAL

ALTERNATIVE THERAPY

PRIORITIZATION

- Prevention of pulmonary embolism (PE).

DELEGATION

EASY

THE CARDIOVASCULAR SYSTEM & THE BLOOD

Level of difficulty: Easy

Overview: This case requires the nurse to recognize the symptoms of a deep vein thrombosis (DVT), understand the diagnostic tests used to confirm this diagnosis, and discuss the rationale for a treatment plan. Nursing diagnoses to include in the client's plan of care are prioritized.

Client Profile

Mr. Luke is a 58-year-old man who is currently a client on an outpatient rehabilitation unit following a left TKR five days ago. This afternoon during physical therapy he complained that his left leg was very painful when walking. His left leg was noted to be swollen so he was sent to the emergency department to be examined.

Case Study

Mr. Luke's vital signs are temperature 98.1°F (36.7°C), blood pressure 110/50, pulse 65, and respiratory rate of 19. His oxygen saturation is 98% on room air. The result of a serum D-dimer is 7 µg/mL. Physical exam reveals that his left calf circumference measurement is ¾ of an inch larger than his right leg calf circumference. Mr. Luke's left calf is warmer to the touch than his right. He will have a noninvasive compression/doppler flow study (doppler ultrasound) to rule out a DVT in his left leg.

Questions

1. The health care provider in the emergency department chooses not to assess Mr. Luke for a positive Homan's sign. What is a Homan's sign and why did the health care provider defer this assessment?

2. Discuss the diagnostic cues gathered during Mr. Luke's examination in the emergency department that indicate a possible DVT.

3. Discuss Virchow's triad and the physiological development of a DVT.

4. The nurse who cared for Mr. Luke immediately following his knee surgery included appropriate interventions to help prevent venous thromboembolism when writing the postoperative plan of care. Discuss five nonpharmacological interventions the nurse included in the plan.

5. Discuss the common pharmacologic therapy options for postsurgical clients to help reduce the risk of a DVT.

6. Mr. Luke's noninvasive compression/doppler flow study (doppler ultrasound) shows a small thrombus located below the popliteal vein of his left leg. While a positive DVT is always of concern, why is the health care provider relieved that the thrombus is located there and not in the popliteal vein?

7. The preferred diagnostic test for assessing a DVT is a contrast venography. Discuss this test and its risks and benefits.

8. Mr. Luke was admitted to the hospital for observation overnight. He is being discharged back to the rehabilitation unit with the following prescribed discharge instructions:

(a) bed rest with bathroom privileges (BRP) with elevation of left leg for 72 hours;
(b) thromboembolic devices (TEDs);
(c) continue with enoxaparin 75 mg subcutaneously (SQ) every 12 hours;
(d) warfarin sodium 5 mg by mouth (PO) per day starting tomorrow;
(e) nicotine transdermal system 21 mg per day for 6 weeks, then 14 mg per day for 2 weeks, and then 7 mg per day for 2 weeks;
(f) acetylsalicylic acid 325 mg PO once daily;
(g) prothrombin time (PT) and international normalized ratio (INR) daily;
(h) occult blood (OB) test of stools;
(i) have vitamin K available; and
(j) vital signs every four hours.

Provide a rationale for each of the prescribed discharge instructions.

9. Prioritize five nursing diagnoses to include in Mr. Luke's plan of care when he returns to the rehabilitation unit.

10. What is an inferior vena cava (IVC) filter and for which clients is this filter indicated?

11. Discuss the symptoms the nurse at the rehabilitation center should watch for that could indicate that Mr. Luke has developed a PE.

12. Because of the DVT, Mr. Luke is at risk for post-phlebitic syndrome (also called post-thrombotic syndrome or PTS). Discuss the incidence, cause, symptoms, and prevention of this potential long-term complication.

Mrs. Kidway

GENDER

Female

AGE

71

SETTING

- Hospital

ETHNICITY

- Russian

CULTURAL CONSIDERATIONS

PREEXISTING CONDITION

- Heart failure (HF, CHF), pneumonia, chronic obstructive pulmonary disease (COPD), gastroesophageal reflux disease (GERD)

COEXISTING CONDITION

COMMUNICATION

- Russian speaking only; daughter speaks English.

DISABILITY

SOCIOECONOMIC

- Lives with daughter's family.

SPIRITUAL/RELIGIOUS

PHARMACOLOGIC

- Digoxin (Lanoxin); potassium chloride (KCl); atropine sulfate (Atropine); digoxin immune fab (Digibind)

LEGAL

ETHICAL

ALTERNATIVE THERAPY

- Licorice (glycyrrhiza, licorice root)

PRIORITIZATION

DELEGATION

THE CARDIOVASCULAR SYSTEM & THE BLOOD

Level of difficulty: Easy

Overview: This case requires that the nurse be knowledgeable regarding the action and pharmacokinetics of digoxin. The nurse must recognize the symptoms of digoxin toxicity and discuss appropriate treatment. The interaction between digoxin and an herbal remedy is considered. Priority nursing diagnoses for this client are identified.

Client Profile

Mrs. Kidway is a 71-year-old woman who lives at home with her daughter's family. Her daily medications prior to admission include digoxin 0.125 mg once a day.

Case Study

Mrs. Kidway arrives in the emergency room with her daughter who explains, "She was fine this morning but then this afternoon she developed terrible abdominal pain and got short of breath." Mrs. Kidway is lethargic. Her physical examination is unremarkable except for facial grimacing when palpating her abdomen. She is afebrile with a blood pressure of 105/50, pulse 60, and respiratory rate 18. Blood work on admission reveals a digoxin level of 3.8 ng/ml.

Questions

1. How does digoxin work in the body?

2. Why is Mrs. Kidway most likely taking digoxin?

3. Given Mrs. Kidway's digoxin level, explain what electrolyte imbalance is of concern.

4. During a nursing assessment of Mrs. Kidway's current medications, the nurse asks if Mrs. Kidway takes any over-the-counter medications or herbal remedies. Mrs. Kidway's daughter says, "Is licorice considered an herbal remedy? My mother started taking licorice capsules about a month ago because we heard that licorice helps decrease heartburn." Does licorice interact with digoxin? If so, explain.

5. Discuss what the terms "loading dose" and "steady state" indicate.

6. What are the onset, peak, and duration times of digoxin when it is taken orally?

7. If Mrs. Kidway was having difficulty swallowing her digoxin capsule and her health care provider changed her prescription to the elixir form of digoxin, theoretically would she still receive 0.125 mg?

8. What is a medication's "half-life"? What is the half-life of digoxin? Theoretically, if Mrs. Kidway took her digoxin at 8:00 A.M. on a Monday, when will 75% of the digoxin be cleared from her body according to the half-life? Since the half-life of digoxin is prolonged in the elderly, use the high end of the range of digoxin's half-life.

9. What is the normal therapeutic range of serum digoxin for a client taking this medication?

10. What symptoms may be noted when digoxin levels are at toxic levels?

11. At what serum digoxin range do cardiac dysrhythmias appear and what is the critical value for adults?

12. Mrs. Kidway's heart rate drops to 50 beats per minute. Her potassium is 2.1 mEq/L. She is given four vials of intravenous digoxin immune fab (reconstituted with sterile water) and admitted to the intensive care unit for monitoring. Discuss how her digoxin toxicity will be treated.

13. What are the two highest priority nursing diagnoses appropriate for Mrs. Kidway's plan of care?

Mrs. Andersson

GENDER

Female

AGE

88

SETTING

■ Primary Care

ETHNICITY

■ White American

CULTURAL CONSIDERATIONS

■ Swedish; increased risk of pernicious anemia

PREEXISTING CONDITION

■ Small bowel obstruction (SBO) with subsequent bowel resection; diverticulitis

COEXISTING CONDITION

COMMUNICATION

DISABILITY

SOCIOECONOMIC

SPIRITUAL/RELIGIOUS

PHARMACOLOGIC

■ Cyanocobalamin (oral vitamin B_{12}); cyanocobalamin crystalline (injectable vitamin B_{12}); cyanocobalamin nasal gel (Nascobal); hydrochloric acid (HCl)

LEGAL

ETHICAL

ALTERNATIVE THERAPY

PRIORITIZATION

Client safety

DELEGATION

THE CARDIOVASCULAR SYSTEM & THE BLOOD

Level of difficulty: Easy

Overview: This case requires the nurse to identify causes of vitamin B_{12} deficiency, define pernicious anemia, and discuss elements of treatment. Client education is provided regarding preventing injury when experiencing parathesias or peripheral neuropathy.

Client Profile   **Mrs. Andersson** was diagnosed with pernicious anemia at the age of 70. She has monthly appointments with her primary health care provider for treatment with vitamin B_{12} injections.

Case Study   At the age of 70, Mrs. Andersson was exhibiting weakness, fatigue, and an unexplained weight loss. A complete blood count (CBC) was done as part of her diagnostic workup. The CBC revealed red blood cell count (RBC) 3.20 million/mm^3, mean corpuscular volume (MCV) 130 μL, reticulocytes 0.4%, hematocrit (Hct) 25%, and hemoglobin (Hgb) 7.9 g/dL. Suspecting pernicious anemia, the health care provider prescribed a Shilling test. Mrs. Andersson was diagnosed with pernicious anemia and started on vitamin B_{12} injections.

Questions

1. Briefly describe the pathophysiology of pernicious anemia.

2. Identify possible causes of vitamin B_{12} deficiency.

3. Identify the possible manifestations of pernicious anemia.

4. Identify the physical assessment findings that are characteristic of pernicious anemia.

5. What are the expected results of a CBC and serum vitamin B_{12} level in a female client with pernicious anemia?

6. How does Mrs. Andersson's ethnicity relate to pernicious anemia?

7. To help make a definitive diagnosis of pernicious anemia, a Schilling test may be performed. Describe the Schilling test.

8. Mrs. Andersson understands that including foods high in vitamin B_{12} in her diet is helpful in the management of vitamin B_{12} deficiency. Identify five foods rich in vitamin B_{12}.

9. Discuss the standard dosing and desired effects of the vitamin B_{12} injections for the client with vitamin B_{12} deficiency.

10. When can Mrs. Andersson discontinue the vitamin B_{12} injections?

11. The nurse administers Mrs. Andersson's vitamin B_{12} injections using the z-tract injection method. Discuss why the nurse used this method and the steps of this injection technique.

12. Discuss other possible medications or supplements that may be indicated for the treatment of pernicious anemia.

13. During a routine visit, Mrs. Andersson tells the nurse that she has noticed a decreased sensation in her fingers. "I can pick up a cup, but I can't really feel the cup in my hand. It is a tingling sensation of sorts." What teaching should the nurse initiate to promote Mrs. Andersson's safety at home?

Mr. Thomas

GENDER

Male

AGE

42

SETTING

- Hospital

ETHNICITY

- White American

CULTURAL CONSIDERATIONS

PREEXISTING CONDITION

- Pneumonia last year; unexplained fifteen-pound weight loss over past six months

COEXISTING CONDITION

- Thrush; pneumonia; human immunodeficiency virus (HIV)

COMMUNICATION

DISABILITY

- Potential disability resulting from chronic illness.

SOCIOECONOMIC

- Married for seventeen years. Two children (ages 14 and 11 years old). Primary income provider for family.

SPIRITUAL/RELIGIOUS

PHARMACOLOGIC

LEGAL

- Infectious disease; client confidentiality; partner notification

ETHICAL

- Partner notification of exposure to HIV

ALTERNATIVE THERAPY

PRIORITIZATION

DELEGATION

MODERATE

THE CARDIOVASCULAR SYSTEM & THE BLOOD

Level of difficulty: Moderate

Overview: The nurse in this case is caring for a client who has recently learned that he is positive for the human immunodeficiency virus (HIV). Laboratory testing to monitor the progression of HIV is reviewed. The ethical and legal concerns regarding the client's decision not to disclose his HIV status to his wife or others are discussed.

Client Profile

Mr. Thomas is a 42-year-old man admitted to the hospital with complaints of shortness of breath, fever, fatigue, and oral thrush. The health care provider reviews the laboratory and diagnostic tests with Mr. Thomas and informs him that he has pneumonia and is HIV positive. Mr. Thomas believes that he contracted HIV while involved in an affair with another woman three years ago. He is afraid to tell his wife, knowing she will be angry and that she may leave him.

Case Study

The nurse assigned to care for Mr. Thomas reads in the medical record (chart) that he learned two days ago that he is HIV positive. There is a note in the record that indicates that Mr. Thomas has not told his wife the diagnosis.

To complete a functional health pattern assessment, the nurse asks Mr. Thomas if he may ask him a few questions. Mr. Thomas is willing and in the course of their conversation shares with the nurse that he believes that he contracted the HIV during an affair with another woman. He states, "How can I tell my wife about this? I am so ashamed. It is bad enough that I had an affair, but to have to tell her in this way— I just don't think I can. She is not sick at all. I will just say I have pneumonia and take the medication my health care provider gave me. I do not want my wife or anyone else to know. If she begins to show signs of not feeling well, then I will tell her. I just can't tell anyone. What will people think of me if they know I have AIDS?"

Questions

1. Briefly discuss how the HIV is transmitted and how it is not. How can Mr. Thomas prevent the transmission of HIV to his wife and others?

2. Mr. Thomas stated, "What will people think of me if they know I have AIDS?" How can the nurse explain the difference between being HIV positive and having AIDS?

3. Discuss the ethical dilemmas inherent in this case.

4. Does the health care provider have a legal obligation to tell anyone other than Mr. Thomas that he is HIV positive? If so, discuss.

5. Any loss, such as the loss of one's health, results in a grief response. Describe the stages of grief according to Kubler-Ross.

6. Discuss which stage of grief Mr. Thomas is most likely experiencing. Provide examples of Mr. Thomas's behavior that support your decision.

7. What are the laboratory tests used to confirm the diagnosis of HIV infection in an adult?

8. Discuss the function of CD4+ T cells and provide an example of how the CD4+ T-cell count guides the management of HIV.

9. Briefly explain the purpose of viral load blood tests in monitoring the progression of HIV.

10. Mr. Thomas expresses a readiness to learn more about HIV. Discuss the nurse's initial intervention when beginning client teaching and then discuss the progression of the HIV disease, including an explanation of *primary infection, categories (groups) A, B, and C,* and *four main types of opportunistic infections.*

11. Following the nurse's teaching, Mr. Thomas states, "How stupid I was to have that affair. Not only could it ruin my marriage, but it gave me a death sentence." Share with Mr. Thomas what you know about *long-term survivors, long-term nonprogressors, and highly active antiretroviral therapy (HAART).*

12. Discuss how the nurse should respond if Mr. Thomas's wife approaches him in the hall and asks, "Did the test results come back yet? Do you know what is wrong with my husband?"

13. List five possible nursing diagnoses appropriate to consider for Mr. Thomas.

Mrs. Darsana

GENDER

Female

AGE

67

SETTING

■ Hospital

ETHNICITY

■ Black American

CULTURAL CONSIDERATIONS

■ Risk of hypertension and heart disease.

PREEXISTING CONDITION

■ Hypertension (HTN)

COEXISTING CONDITION

COMMUNICATION

DISABILITY

SOCIOECONOMIC

SPIRITUAL/RELIGIOUS

PHARMACOLOGIC

■ Acetylsalicylic acid (aspirin), enoxaparin (Lovenox), GPIIb/IIIa agents, heparin sodium, morphine sulfate, nitroglycerin, tissue plasminogen activator (tPA)

LEGAL

ETHICAL

ALTERNATIVE THERAPY

PRIORITIZATION

■ Minimizing cardiac damage.

DELEGATION

MODERATE

THE CARDIOVASCULAR SYSTEM & THE BLOOD

Level of difficulty: Moderate

Overview: This case requires the nurse to recognize the signs and symptoms of an acute myocardial infarction (MI). The nurse must anticipate appropriate interventions to minimize cardiac damage and preserve myocardial function. Serum laboratory tests and electrocardiogram findings used to diagnose a myocardial infarction are discussed. Criteria to assess when considering reperfusion using a thrombolytic agent are reviewed. The nurse is asked to prioritize the client's nursing diagnoses.

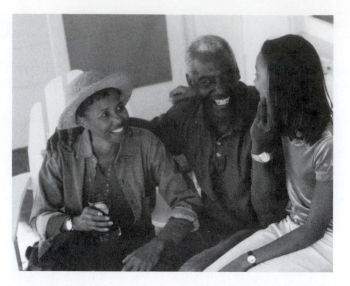

Client Profile

Mrs. Darsana was sitting at a family cookout at approximately 2:00 P.M. when she experienced what she later describes to the nurse as "nausea with some heartburn." Assuming the discomfort was because of something she ate, she dismissed the discomfort and took Tums. After about two hours, she explains, "My heartburn was not much better and it was now more of a dull pain that seemed to spread to my shoulders. I also noticed that I was a little short of breath." Mrs. Darsana told her son what she was feeling. Concerned, her son called emergency medical services.

Case Study

En route to the hospital, emergency medical personnel established an intravenous access. Mrs. Darsana was given four children's chewable aspirins and three sublingual nitroglycerin tablets without relief of her chest pain. She was placed on oxygen 2 liters via nasal cannula. Upon arrival in the emergency department, Mrs. Darsana is very restless. She states, "It feels like an elephant is sitting on my chest." Her vital signs are blood pressure 160/84, pulse 118, respiratory rate 28, and temperature 99.3°F (37.4°C). Her oxygen saturation is 98% on 2 liters of oxygen. A 12-lead electrocardiogram (ECG, EKG) shows sinus tachycardia with a heart rate of 120 beats per minute. An occasional premature ventricular contraction (PVC), T wave inversion, and ST segment elevation are noted. A chest X-ray is within normal limits with no signs of pulmonary edema. Mrs. Darsana's laboratory results include potassium (K^+) 4.0 mEq/L, magnesium (Mg) 1.9 mg/dL, total creatine kinase (CK) 157 μ/L, CK-MB 7.6 ng/ml, relative index 4.8%, and troponin I 2.8 ng/ml. Her stool tests negative for occult blood.

Questions

1. What are the components of the initial nursing assessment of Mrs. Darsana when she arrives in the emergency department?

2. Mrs. Darsana has a history of unstable angina. Explain what this is.

3. Briefly discuss what causes an MI. Include in the discussion the other terms used for this diagnosis.

4. The nurse listens to Mrs. Darsana's heart sounds to see if S_3, S_4, or a murmur can be heard. What would the nurse suspect if these heart sounds were heard?

Questions (continued)

5. What factors are considered when diagnosing an acute myocardial infarction?

6. Briefly define the terms *depolarization*, *repolarization*, and *isoelectric line*.

7. Describe what T wave inversion and ST segment elevation look like on an ECG monitor strip and what causes each in a client with an MI.

8. Besides her unstable angina, what factors increased Mrs. Darsana's risk for an MI?

9. Identify which of Mrs. Darsana's presenting symptoms are consistent with the profile of a client who is having an MI.

10. The nurse overhears Mrs. Darsana's son asking his mother sternly "Mom. Why didn't you tell me that you were having chest pain sooner? You should have never ignored this. You could have died right there at my house." How might the nurse explain Mrs. Darsana's actions to the son?

11. Provide a rationale for why Mrs. Darsana was given sublingual nitroglycerin and aspirin en route to the hospital.

12. Briefly discuss the laboratory tests that are significant in the determination of an acute myocardial infarction (AMI).

13. Laboratory results in the emergency department on

April 1 at 1645:

Total CK = 216 μ/L CK-MB = 5.6 ng/ml relative index = 2.2% Troponin I = 2.8 ng/ml

April 2 at 0045:

Total CK = 242 μ/L CK-MB = 8.1 ng/ml relative index = 3.3% Troponin I = 5.2 ng/ml

April 2 at 0615:

Total CK = 298 μ/L CK-MB = 9.2 ng/ml relative index = 3.0% Troponin I = 4.1 ng/ml

April 3 at 0615:

Total CK = 203 μ/L CK-MB = 6.1 ng/ml relative index = 3.0% Troponin I = 1.7 ng/ml

Are Mrs. Darsana's laboratory results consistent with those expected for a client having an acute myocardial infarction?

14. Briefly describe four interventions you anticipate will be initiated/considered during the acute phase of Mrs. Darsana's MI.

15. Identify five criteria that could exclude an individual as a candidate for thrombolytic therapy with a tissue plasminogen activator (tPA).

16. An echocardiogram reveals that Mrs. Darsana has an ejection fraction of 50%. How could the nurse explain the meaning of this result to Mrs. Darsana?

17. Identify three appropriate nursing diagnoses for the client experiencing an AMI.

18. Rank the following five nursing diagnoses for Mrs. Darsana in priority order.

Acute pain related to (r/t) myocardial tissue damage from inadequate blood supply

Fear r/t threat to well-being

Decreased cardiac output r/t ineffective cardiac tissue perfusion secondary to ventricular damage, ischemia, dysrhythmia

Risk for injury r/t adverse effect of pharmacologic therapy

Deficient knowledge r/t condition, treatment, prognosis

Mrs. Yates

GENDER

Female

AGE

70

SETTING

- Home

ETHNICITY

- Black American

CULTURAL CONSIDERATIONS

- The impact of diet on heart failure.

PREEXISTING CONDITION

- Hypertension (HTN); heart failure (HF, CHF); coronary artery disease (CAD); myocardial infarction (MI) five years ago; ejection fraction (EF) of 55%.

COEXISTING CONDITION

COMMUNICATION

DISABILITY

SOCIOECONOMIC

- Widow. Lives alone. Able to care for self independently. Nonsmoker.

SPIRITUAL/RELIGIOUS

PHARMACOLOGIC

- Aspirin (acetylsalicylic acid, ASA); clopidogrel bisulfate (Plavix); lisinopril (Prinivil, Zestril); carvedilol (Coreg); furosemide (Lasix); potassium chloride (KCl)

LEGAL

ETHICAL

ALTERNATIVE THERAPY

PRIORITIZATION

DELEGATION

MODERATE

THE CARDIOVASCULAR SYSTEM & THE BLOOD

Level of difficulty: Moderate

Overview: This case requires the nurse to recognize the symptoms of heart failure and collaborate with the primary care provider to initiate treatment. The pathophysiology of heart failure is reviewed. Several heart failure classification systems are defined. Rationales for prescribed diagnostic tests and medications are provided. The nurse must consider the impact of the client's diet on the exacerbation of symptoms and provide teaching. Nursing diagnoses are prioritized to guide care.

Client Profile

Jeraldine Yates is a 70-year-old woman originally from Alabama. She lives alone and is able to manage herself independently. She is active in her community and church. Mrs. Yates was admitted to the hospital two months ago with heart failure. Since her discharge, a visiting nurse visits every other week to assess for symptoms of heart failure and see that Mrs. Yates is continuing to manage well on her own.

Case Study

The visiting nurse stops in to see Mrs. Yates today. The nurse immediately notices that Mrs. Yates's legs are very swollen. Mrs. Yates states, "I noticed they were getting a bit bigger. They are achy, too." The nurse asks Mrs. Yates if she has been weighing herself daily to which Mrs. Yates replies, "I got on that scale the last time you were here, remember?" The nurse weighs Mrs. Yates and she has gained 10 pounds. Additional assessment findings indicate that Mrs. Yates gets short of breath when ambulating from one room to the other (approximately 20 feet) and must sit down to catch her breath. Her oxygen saturation is 95% on room air. Bibasilar crackles are heard when auscultating her lung sounds. The nurse asks Mrs. Yates if she is currently or has in the past few days experienced any chest, arm, or jaw pain or become nauseous or sweaty. Mrs. Yates states, "No, I didn't have any of that. I would know another heart attack. I didn't have one of those." The nurse asks about any back pain, stomach pain, confusion, dizziness, or a feeling that Mrs. Yates might faint. Mrs. Yates denies these symptoms stating, "No. None of that. Just a little more tired than usual lately." Her vital signs are temperature 97.6°F (36.4°C), blood pressure 140/70, pulse 93, and respirations 22. The nurse reviews Mrs. Yates's list of current medications. Mrs. Yates is taking aspirin, clopidogrel bisulfate, lisinopril, and carvedilol. The nurse calls the health care provider who asks the nurse to draw blood for a complete blood count (CBC), basic metabolic panel (BMP), brain natriuretic peptide (B-type natriuretic peptide assay or BNP), troponin, creatine kinase (CPK), creatine kinase-MB (CKMB), and albumin. The health care provider also prescribes oral (PO) furosemide and asks the nurse to arrange an outpatient electrocardiogram (ECG, EKG), chest X-ray, and echocardiogram.

Questions

1. Which assessment findings during the nurse's visit are consistent with heart failure?

2. Why did the visiting nurse ask Mrs. Yates about back pain, stomach pain, confusion, dizziness, or a feeling that she might faint?

3. Discuss anything else the nurse should assess during her visit with Mrs. Yates.

4. Explain what the following terms indicate and include the normal values: *cardiac output, stroke volume, afterload, preload, ejection fraction,* and *central venous pressure.*

5. Discuss the body's compensatory mechanisms during heart failure. Include an explanation of the Frank-Starling law and the neurohormonal model in your discussion.

6. Heart failure can be classified as left or right ventricular failure, systolic versus diastolic, according to the New York Heart Association (NYHA) and using the ACC/AHA (American Heart Association) guidelines. Explain these four classification systems and the signs and symptoms that characterize each.

7. According to each classification system discussed above in question # 6, how would you label the type of heart failure Mrs. Yates is experiencing?

8. Discuss Mrs. Yates's predisposing risk factors for heart failure. Is her age, gender, or ethnicity significant?

9. Provide a rationale for why each of the following medications is included in Mrs. Yates's medication regimen: *aspirin, clopidogrel bisulfate, lisinopril,* and *carvedilol.*

Questions (continued)

10. The nurse is teaching Mrs. Yates about her newly prescribed furosemide. Explain the rationale for adding furosemide to Mrs. Yates's medication regimen, when she should expect to see the therapeutic results (urination), and instructions regarding the administration of furosemide.

11. The visiting nurses asks the primary health care provider if he/she will prescribe potassium chloride for Mrs. Yates. Why has the nurse suggested this?

12. What information will each of the following blood tests provide: *CBC, BMP, BNP, troponin, CPK, CKMB,* and *albumin?*

13. What will the health care provider look for on the electrocardiogram, chest X-ray and echocardiogram?

14. Mrs. Yates's son comes to stay with his mother so she will not be alone. What should the nurse tell Mr. Yates about when he should bring his mother to the hospital?

15. The visiting nurse returns the next day. Mrs. Yates does not seem to be diuresing as well as the nurse anticipated. The swelling in her legs is still considerable, and there is no change in her weight. When asked about her frequency of voiding, Mrs. Yates does not seem to have noticed much difference. While the nurse is unpacking her stethoscope to assess lung sounds, Mrs. Yates says, "Honey, I was just making myself a ham salad sandwich. Would you like one?" The nurse declines and becomes concerned because of this offer. Why is the nurse concerned?

16. The nurse asks Mrs. Yates to tell her more about how she cooks. Specifically, the nurse asks Mrs. Yates about the types of foods and food preparation. With great pride, Mrs. Yates leads the nurse to the kitchen and explains, "Honey. I'm from the South and we cook soul food. Today I am cooking my famous pea soup for the church dinner tonight. I use ham hocks. Have you ever had those? My son says they are not good for me. He has been trying to get me to eat healthier foods. Last week he brought me turkey sausage to try instead of my pork sausage in the morning. I know he means well but some foods are tradition and you don't break soul food tradition." What information has the nurse gathered that is of concern?

17. The nurse arranges for Mrs. Yates's son to be present at the next home visit so that the nurse can teach them both about proper dietary choices and fluid restrictions. List five points of information that the nurse should include in the teaching.

18. During the dietary teaching, the nurse asks Mrs. Yates to describe a typical day of meals and snacks. Mrs. Yates lists coffee with whole milk, eggs and sausage for breakfast, a sandwich or soup for lunch, fried chicken with vegetables for dinner, and fruit, pretzels, or rice pudding for snacks. Which of these foods will the nurse instruct Mrs. Yates to limit, and are there alternatives that the nurse can suggest?

19. Since changing her diet, Mrs. Yates has responded to her outpatient treatment plan and has noticed marked improvement in how she feels. The nurse wants to make sure that Mrs. Yates understands the importance of monitoring her weight. What instructions should the nurse give Mrs. Yates regarding how often to weigh herself and what weight change should be reported to her health care provider or the nurse?

20. Prioritize five nursing diagnoses that the visiting nurse should consider for the recent events regarding Mrs. Yates's care.

GENDER

Female

AGE

20

SETTING

■ Hospital

ETHNICITY

■ Black American

CULTURAL CONSIDERATIONS

■ Increased risk for sickle cell disease

PREEXISTING CONDITION

■ Sickle cell disease

COEXISTING CONDITION

COMMUNICATION

DISABILITY

SOCIOECONOMIC

■ Risk for substance abuse

SPIRITUAL/RELIGIOUS

PHARMACOLOGIC

■ Acetaminophen (Tylenol); hydroxyurea (Droxia); morphine sulfate (MS contin); ibuprofen (Advil; Motrin); acetaminophen 300 mg/codeine 30 mg (Tylenol with codeine No. 3); meperidine hydrochloride (Demerol); hydromorphone hydrochloride (Dilaudid)

LEGAL

ETHICAL

ALTERNATIVE THERAPY

■ Breathing techniques; relaxation; distraction; transcutaneous nerve stimulation (TENS)

PRIORITIZATION

DELEGATION

THE CARDIOVASCULAR SYSTEM & THE BLOOD

Level of difficulty: Difficult

Overview: This case requires the nurse to define different types of anemia, recognize the symptoms of a sickle cell crisis, and discuss short- and long-term management of sickle cell disease. Nursing diagnoses appropriate for the client are prioritized.

DIFFICULT

Client Profile

Ms. Fox is a 20-year-old black American who presents to the emergency department with complaints of chest pain and some shortness of breath. Ms. Fox indicates that she has had a nonproductive cough and low-grade fever for the past two days. She recognizes these symptoms as typical of her sickle cell crisis episodes and knew it was important she come in to get treatment.

Case Study

Ms. Fox was diagnosed with sickle cell anemia as a child and has had multiple crises requiring hospitalization. Ms. Fox states that the pain in her chest is an "8" on a 0 to 10 pain scale. She describes the pain as a "constant burning pain." Her vital signs are temperature of 100.8°F (38.2°C), blood pressure 120/76, pulse 96, and respiratory rate of 22. Her oxygen saturation on room air is 94%. She is having some difficulty breathing and is placed on 2 liters of oxygen by nasal cannula. Ms. Fox explains that she took Extra Strength Tylenol for the past two days in an effort to manage the pain, but when this did not work and the pain got worse, she came in for a stronger pain medication. She explains that in the past she has been given morphine for the pain and prefers to use the patient-controlled analgesia (PCA) pump. Blood work reveals the following values: white blood cell count (WBC) 18,000 cells/mm^3, red blood cell count (RBC) 3×10^6, mean corpuscular volume (MCV) 70 μm^3, red cell distribution width (RDW) 20.4%, hemoglobin (Hgb) 7.5 g/dL, hematocrit (Hct) 21.8%, and reticulocyte count 23%. Ms. Fox is admitted for pain management, antibiotic treatment, and respiratory support.

Questions

1. Three types of anemia are *hypoproliferative, bleeding,* and *hemolytic.* Provide a basic definition of the etiology of each type and one example of each type.

2. Discuss how Ms. Fox's laboratory results are consistent with clients who have sickle cell anemia.

3. Describe the structure and function of normal red blood cells in the body.

4. Describe the structure and effects of red blood cells (RBCs) that contain sickle cell hemoglobin molecules.

5. Is sickle cell anemia an inherited anemia or an acquired anemia? Explain.

6. Discuss the relationship between sickle cell anemia and Ms. Fox's ethnicity.

7. Discuss the characteristic signs and symptoms of sickle cell anemia.

8. Discuss the potential complications associated with sickle cell anemia.

9. Describe the pharmacologic management for a client with sickle cell anemia. Include a discussion of the potential adverse effects of the medication.

10. Describe the use of transfusion therapy for management of sickle cell anemia. Include a discussion of the potential complications of chronic red blood cell transfusions.

11. Bone marrow transplantation (BMT) offers a potential cure for sickle cell disease. Why is BMT a treatment option available to only a small number of clients with sickle cell disease?

12. In the adult, three types of sickle cell crisis are possible: sickle crisis, aplastic crisis, and sequestration crisis. Briefly describe the pathophysiological changes that lead to each type.

13. There are four common patterns of an acute vaso-occlusive sickle cell crisis: *bone crisis, acute chest syndrome, abdominal crisis,* and *joint crisis.* Briefly

Questions (continued)

describe the characteristic symptoms of each pattern.

14. Which pattern discussed in question number 13 is most congruent with Ms. Fox's presenting signs and symptoms?

15. Discuss the symptoms the nurse should look for while completing an assessment of a client in potential sickle cell (vaso-occlusive) crisis.

16. Briefly discuss the factors that can trigger a sickle cell crisis.

17. Prioritize three potential nursing diagnoses appropriate for Ms. Fox.

18. Describe the nursing management goals during the acute phase of a sickle cell crisis.

19. Explain why individuals with sickle cell disease may be at risk for substance abuse.

20. Discuss the long-term prognosis for Ms. Fox.

Mrs. O'Grady

GENDER

Female

AGE

55

SETTING

- Hospital

ETHNICITY

- White American

CULTURAL CONSIDERATIONS

PREEXISTING CONDITION

- Hypertension (HTN); angina; total abdominal hysterectomy six months ago; allergy to shellfish

COEXISTING CONDITION

- Positive myocardial perfusion imaging study (stress test)

COMMUNICATION

DISABILITY

SOCIOECONOMIC

SPIRITUAL/RELIGIOUS

PHARMACOLOGIC

- Dipyridamole (Persantine); atenolol (Tenormin); atorvastatin calcium (Lipitor); conjugated estrogen, oral (Premarin)

LEGAL

- Informed consent

ETHICAL

ALTERNATIVE THERAPY

PRIORITIZATION

DELEGATION

THE CARDIOVASCULAR SYSTEM & THE BLOOD

Level of difficulty: Difficult

Overview: This case requires the nurse to convey an understanding of the cardiac catheterization procedure. Appropriate client care pre- and postcardiac catheterization is discussed. The client's current medications are reviewed. Discharge teaching is provided.

DIFFICULT

Client Profile

Mrs. O'Grady is a 55-year-old female with a history of angina and recent hospital admission for complaints of chest pain and shortness of breath. It is determined that she did not suffer a myocardial infarction. Mrs. O'Grady's health care provider has scheduled her for a cardiac catheterization after learning that the results of her dipyridamole (Persantine) myocardial perfusion imaging study (stress test) were abnormal.

Case Study

Mrs. O'Grady is having a cardiac catheterization today. The cardiac catheterization lab nurse assigned to care for Mrs. O'Grady will provide teaching, check to see that there are no contraindications for Mrs. O'Grady consenting to the procedure, and provide pre- and postprocedure care.

Questions

1. Why has Mrs. O'Grady's health care provider prescribed a cardiac catheterization? What information will this procedure provide?

2. What are the potential contraindications that can prevent someone from being able to have a cardiac catheterization? What is the contraindication that must be considered in Mrs. O'Grady's case? Why is this of concern?

3. Discuss the preprocedure assessments the nurse will complete prior to Mrs. O'Grady's cardiac catheterization.

4. Discuss interventions the nurse will complete prior to Mrs. O'Grady's cardiac catheterization.

5. Provide a brief rationale for why each of the following medications have been prescribed for Mrs. O'Grady: atenolol (Tenormin); atorvastatin calcium (Lipitor); conjugated estrogen, oral (Premarin).

6. What are two appropriate nursing diagnoses to consider for Mrs. O'Grady prior to her having the cardiac catheterization?

7. Mrs. O'Grady asks the nurse, "What are they going to do to me today?" Explain what a cardiac catheterization involves and how long Mrs. O'Grady can expect the procedure to last. Briefly describe the difference between a left-sided and right-sided catheterization.

8. What are the risks of having a cardiac catheterization? What are the two most common complications during the procedure?

9. List at least five manifestations of an adverse reaction to the contrast dye the nurse will watch for.

10. How should the nurse respond when Mrs. O'Grady asks, "How soon will I know if something is wrong with me?"

11. What is "informed consent"? Is consent required prior to a cardiac catheterization? Why or why not?

12. Immediately following the cardiac catheterization procedure, what is the nurse's responsibility to help minimize bleeding at the femoral puncture site, and what will be Mrs. O'Grady's prescribed activity?

13. Discuss the priorities of the nursing assessment following a femoral cardiac catheterization. Be sure to note in your discussion when the health care provider should be notified.

14. What are two nursing diagnoses to consider for Mrs. O'Grady following the cardiac catheterization?

15. Mrs. O'Grady has a left groin puncture site. She needs to go to the bathroom, but is still on bed rest. What is the proper way for the nurse to assist her?

16. The results of Mrs. O'Grady's cardiac catheterization indicate that she does not have any significant heart disease and her coronary arteries are patent. The health care provider discharges her. Her husband has been called to bring her home. What instructions should the nurse provide regarding activity, diet, and medications?

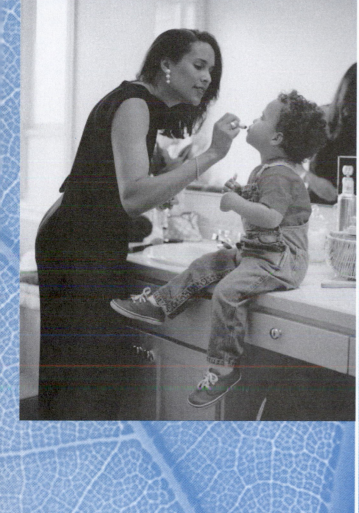

## PART FIVE

The Skeletal System

Mr. Mendes

GENDER

Male

AGE

81

SETTING

- Hospital

ETHNICITY

- Portuguese

CULTURAL CONSIDERATIONS

- Language barrier

PREEXISTING CONDITION

- Peripheral vascular disease (PVD); type 1 diabetes; below the knee amputation (BKA, B-K amputation) of left leg two weeks ago

COEXISTING CONDITION

- Left lower lobe pneumonia

COMMUNICATION

- Non-English speaking

DISABILITY

- Uses a wheelchair. Needs assistance with activities of daily living (ADLs).

SOCIOECONOMIC

- Admitted from a rehabilitation health care center.

SPIRITUAL/RELIGIOUS

PHARMACOLOGIC

LEGAL

- Use of a medical interpreter.

ETHICAL

- Use of a medical interpreter.

ALTERNATIVE THERAPY

PRIORITIZATION

DELEGATION

THE SKELETAL SYSTEM

Level of difficulty: Easy

Overview: This case challenges the nurse to identify strategies to help overcome a language barrier and form a therapeutic nurse–client relationship. Legal and ethical concerns regarding the use of an interpreter are considered. Stump care for the client with a recent amputation is discussed.

Client Profile

Mr. Mendes is an 81-year-old man who speaks only Portuguese. He is quite frail, weighing only 110 pounds. He had a below the knee amputation of his left leg two weeks ago. Mr. Mendes has been admitted to the hospital from a rehabilitation center with an acute change in mental status and diminished lung sounds in the left base. Mr. Mendes is diagnosed with left lower lobe pneumonia and antibiotic therapy is prescribed. The nurse assigned to care for Mr. Mendes does not speak Portuguese.

Case Study

Mr. Mendes requires complete assistance with activities of daily living (ADLs). A medical interpreter is not assigned to the nursing unit. If needed, the nurse can ask a Portuguese-speaking nursing staff member to help interpret what Mr. Mendes is trying to express. However, the nurse must develop a way of communicating with Mr. Mendes so the nurse can assess Mr. Mendes's level of comfort, provide care, and identify any needs.

Questions

1. Briefly discuss the challenges of developing a nurse–client relationship when a language barrier exists between the client and nurse.

2. Explain the difference between a medical "interpreter" and a medical "translator."

3. Family members are often willing to interpret for the client and are more readily available. Discuss the use of medical interpreters and why, legally and ethically, family members (or friends of the client) are not the preferred interpreter(s).

4. Describe a therapeutic nurse–client relationship.

5. The nurse does not speak Portuguese. Discuss nonverbal strategies the nurse can implement to help develop a therapeutic relationship with Mr. Mendes.

6. Provide the most likely explanation for why Mr. Mendes presented with an acute change in mental status.

7. Briefly discuss how Mr. Mendes's past medical history relates to his below the knee leg amputation.

What is the benefit of having a below the knee (B-K) amputation versus an above the knee (A-K) amputation?

8. The interpreter tells the nurse that Mr. Mendes would like the nurse to remove the bed linens from his left foot and raise his leg on pillows. He states, "My foot aches and maybe if you put it up it on some pillows will feel better." Provide a rationale for Mr. Mendes's request. Should the nurse elevate his stump on pillows as requested? Why or why not?

9. Mr. Mendes has not yet been fit for a prosthesis. The nurse provides care of his stump. Briefly discuss the nursing interventions involved in stump care. What outcome goals does the nurse hope to achieve through proper stump care?

10. List five nursing diagnoses appropriate to consider for Mr. Mendes's plan of care.

GENDER

Female

AGE

77

SETTING

- Hospital

ETHNICITY

- Black American

CULTURAL CONSIDERATIONS

- Age-related complications.

PREEXISTING CONDITION

- Osteoporosis

COEXISTING CONDITION

- Recent fall.

COMMUNICATION

DISABILITY

- Potential impact of a hip fracture on quality of life.

SOCIOECONOMIC

- Lives at home.

SPIRITUAL/RELIGIOUS

PHARMACOLOGIC

- Alendronate sodium (Fosamax)

LEGAL

ETHICAL

ALTERNATIVE THERAPY

PRIORITIZATION

DELEGATION

- Home safety assessment by the visiting nurse.

THE SKELETAL SYSTEM

Level of difficulty: Easy

Overview: This case requires that the nurse consider appropriate pre- and postoperative nursing interventions for a client with a hip fracture. A new medication is prescribed and teaching is needed. Considerations for recovery related to the client's age as well as the safety of her home environment are discussed. The nurse is asked to prioritize appropriate nursing diagnoses for the client's postoperative plan of care.

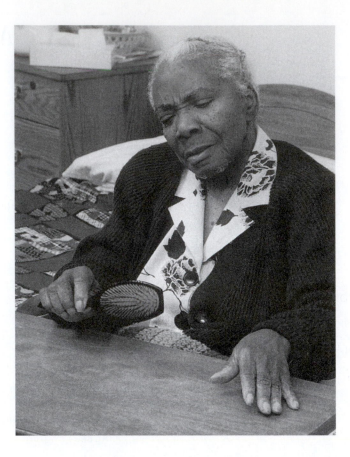

Client Profile

Mrs. Damerae is a 77-year-old woman who was transported to the emergency department following a fall onto her right hip on a snowy morning. "I just wanted to check the mail. I was making my way down my front walk slowly. I had my good boots on. But there must have been ice under the snow and I slipped. It all happened so fast. I was up. I was down. And here I am."

Case Study

Physical exam reveals that Mrs. Damerae's right leg is shorter than her left leg and her right leg is externally rotated. There is bruising of her right hip. An X-ray confirms that Mrs. Damerae has an extracapsular fracture of the trochanter region of her right hip. Mrs. Damerae will have an open reduction of the fracture and internal fixation (ORIF) surgery the next morning.

Questions

1. Prior to surgery, the health care provider chooses to place Mrs. Damerae's right leg in Buck's extension (traction). Why is this intervention prescribed prior to surgery?

2. A trochanter roll is another option for Mrs. Damerae. What is a trochanter roll and how would it be useful?

3. How might Mrs. Damerae's age affect her hospitalization and recovery?

4. Briefly discuss how Mrs. Damerae's past medical history played a role in her injury.

5. Mrs. Damerae's surgeon informs her of the potential complications of hip surgery. Identify at least three complications the surgeon will address.

Questions (continued)

6. Prioritize five nursing diagnoses appropriate for Mrs. Damerae following surgery.

7. Explain how the nurse should move Mrs. Damerae in order to position her safely on her side to wash her back.

8. The nurse applies graduated compression stockings (TEDs) and sequential compression devices (SCDs) as prescribed. What is the rationale for these interventions?

9. Mrs. Damerae asks for assistance to the bathroom. The nurse checks to see that the appropriate equipment is available in the bathroom before assisting the client to ambulate. What is the nurse looking for in the bathroom?

10. Mrs. Damerae is assisted back to bed. She asks that the head of her bed be raised so she can read. How high should the head of the bed be raised and why?

11. Mrs. Damerae is seated in a reclining chair. What reminders will the nurse give Mrs. Damerae regarding positioning while sitting and why is positioning so important?

12. Identify the indications of a possible hip dislocation that the nurse should watch for.

13. If the nurse notices any of the above signs, discuss the appropriate action for the nurse to take.

14. Alendronate sodium is prescribed for Mr. Damerae. What is the rationale for the use of alendronate sodium? Discuss the client education regarding proper administration to maximize the benefits of alendronate sodium and adverse effects.

15. Following discharge from a rehabilitation unit, a visiting nurse will provide follow-up care for Mrs. Damerae. On the first home visit, the nurse conducts a home safety assessment. Identify at least five components of a safe home environment.

Mr. Lourde

GENDER

Male

AGE

73

SETTING

■ Hospital

ETHNICITY

■ White American

CULTURAL CONSIDERATIONS

PREEXISTING CONDITION

■ Left hip replacement two years ago. Septic shock with left hip osteomyelitis last year with subsequent removal of the hip replacement prosthesis. Allergies to meperidine hydrochloride (Demerol), morphine sulfate (MS Contin), and vancomycin hydrochloride (Vancocin).

COEXISTING CONDITION

COMMUNICATION

DISABILITY

SOCIOECONOMIC

SPIRITUAL/RELIGIOUS

PHARMACOLOGIC

■ Linezolid (Zyvox), fondaparinux (Arixtra), hydrocodone bitartrate/acetaminophen (Vicodin), acetaminophen (Tylenol), docusate sodium (Colace)

LEGAL

ETHICAL

ALTERNATIVE THERAPY

PRIORITIZATION

DELEGATION

MODERATE

THE SKELETAL SYSTEM

Level of difficulty: Moderate

Overview: This case requires that the nurse understand the risk associated with postoperative wound infection following a hip replacement. The manifestations characteristic of osteomyelitis are discussed. The nurse must care for the surgical incision site with a daily dressing change and maintenance of a HemoVac drainage system. The client's prescribed medications are reviewed for purpose and potential adverse effects. The purpose and potential complications of a peripherally inserted central catheter (PICC) are explained.

Client Profile

Mr. Lourde is a 73-year-old man whose wife noticed a lump on his left hip that has increased in size over the past two weeks. The skin around the lump is red and swollen. Mr. Lourde complains of increasing discomfort in his left hip. His wife became concerned when he felt warm and his temperature was 101°F (38.3°C) so she brought him to the hospital. Mr. Lourde is diagnosed with an abscess of his left hip. A needle aspiration of the abscess reveals 30 cc of purulent exudate. Mr. Lourde is admitted for surgical incision and drainage of a suspected recurrence of osteomyelitis and for intravenous antibiotic therapy.

Case Study

A surgical incision and drainage is performed to remove necrotic tissue, sequestrum, and surrounding granulation tissue. A bacterial infection is identified as *Enterococcus faecalis*. The nurse reviews the client's kardex and notes the dressing change prescribed is a dry sterile dressing to the left hip daily with reinforcement as needed.

The nurse medicates Mr. Lourde with hydrocodone/acetaminophen (Vicodin) thirty minutes prior to the dressing change. While changing the hip dressing, the nurse notes there are seven intact sutures along the incision line, and a HemoVac drain is in place. Minimal drainage is noted at the incision site. The site is slightly swollen, but there are no signs of infection. The HemoVac has drained 30 cc of dark red blood. Mr. Lourde tolerates the dressing change with minimal discomfort. He is afebrile at 98°F (36.7°C).

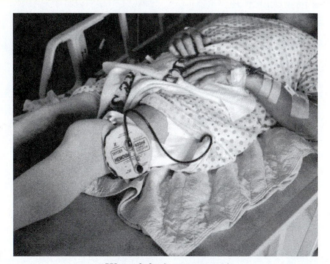

Wound drainage reservoir

Questions

1. Discuss the time frame within which signs of an infection at the site of a hip replacement usually occur. What possible complications are of concern when a client develops an infection at the site of a hip replacement?

2. Discuss the pathophysiology of osteomyelitis. Include an explanation of a sequestrum, involucrum, and Brodie's abscess.

3. Discuss the clinical manifestations of osteomyelitis.

Questions (continued)

4. The health care provider suspects a recurrence of Mr. Lourde's osteomyelitis. How will the health care provider confirm this diagnosis?

5. Discuss the treatment options if Mr. Lourde has osteomyelitis of his left hip.

6. Mr. Lourde will require at least three to eight weeks of high-dose intravenous antibiotic therapy. The health care provider has requested that a PICC be inserted. Explain what a PICC is and the potential complications associated with this device.

7. What information should be included in the nurse's documentation of the dressing change?

8. Explain why the nurse does not document the stage of the left hip wound.

9. Write two expected outcomes for the duration of time that a HemoVac drainage reservoir system is in place. How often should the nurse empty the drain and how will the nurse ensure that the system is working correctly to drain the incision site?

10. Each of the medications below is prescribed for Mr. Lourde. For each, provide the therapeutic drug classification and discuss the purpose of the medication for Mr. Lourde and potential adverse effect(s) that the nurse should monitor.

    1. Linezolid (Zyvox)

    2. Fondaparinux (Arixtra)

    3. Hydrocodone bitartrate/acetaminophen (Vicodin)

    4. Acetaminophen (Tylenol)

    5. Docusate sodium (Colace)

11. Help the nurse generate three appropriate nursing diagnoses for Mr. Lourde.

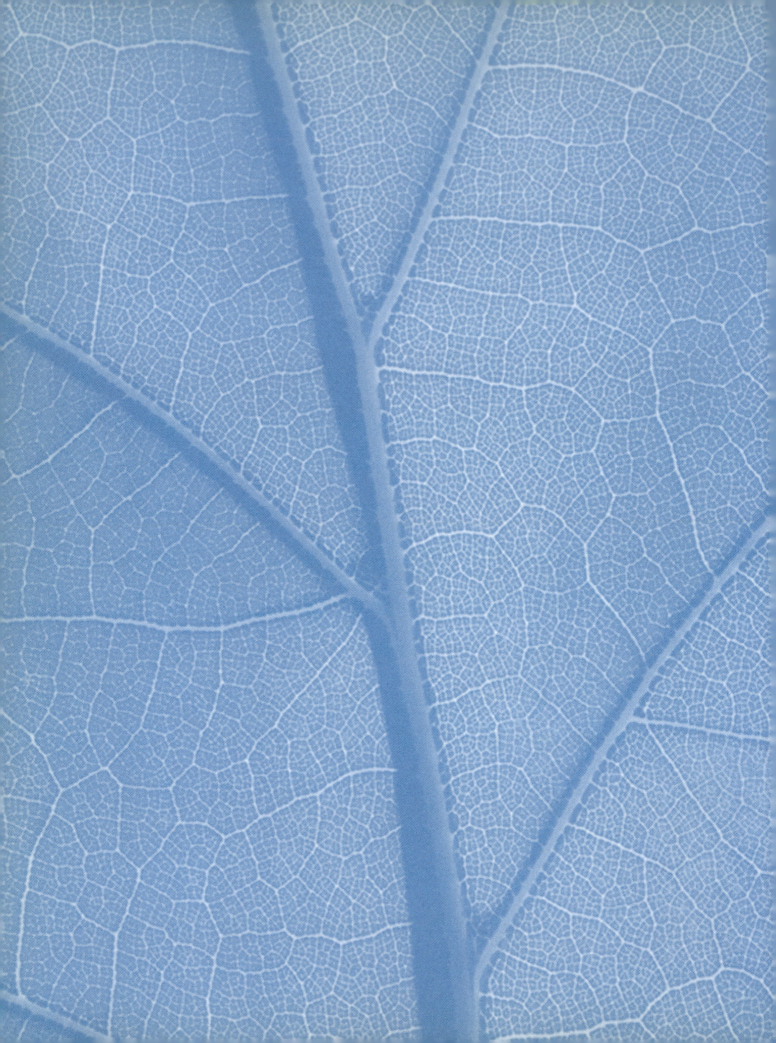

PART SIX

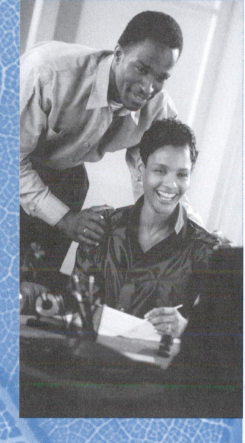

The Muscular System

Mr. O'Brien

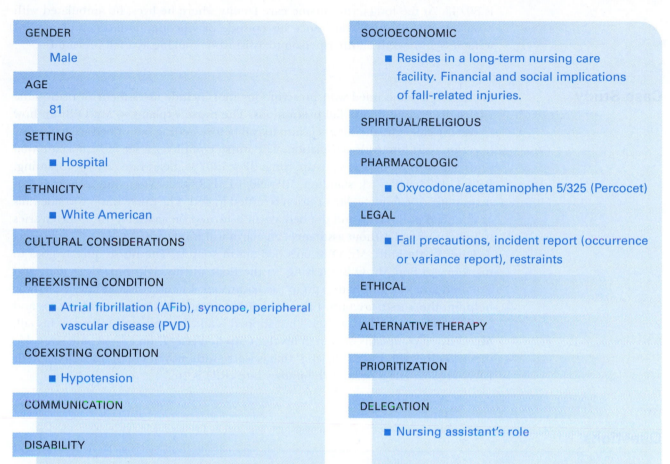

GENDER

Male

AGE

81

SETTING

■ Hospital

ETHNICITY

■ White American

CULTURAL CONSIDERATIONS

PREEXISTING CONDITION

■ Atrial fibrillation (AFib), syncope, peripheral vascular disease (PVD)

COEXISTING CONDITION

■ Hypotension

COMMUNICATION

DISABILITY

■ Ambulates with a walker and one assist

SOCIOECONOMIC

■ Resides in a long-term nursing care facility. Financial and social implications of fall-related injuries.

SPIRITUAL/RELIGIOUS

PHARMACOLOGIC

■ Oxycodone/acetaminophen 5/325 (Percocet)

LEGAL

■ Fall precautions, incident report (occurrence or variance report), restraints

ETHICAL

ALTERNATIVE THERAPY

PRIORITIZATION

DELEGATION

■ Nursing assistant's role

THE MUSCULAR SYSTEM

Level of difficulty: Easy

Overview: This case requires the nurse to identify appropriate interventions upon learning that a client has fallen. The nurse is asked to discuss fall precautions and proper documentation of a client safety incident. The use of a restraint is considered. The nurse must also assess the client for orthostatic (postural) hypotension. The incidence of falls, injuries resulting, fall-related deaths, financial and social implications, and need for long-term care following a fall are reviewed.

Client Profile

Mr. O'Brien is an alert and oriented 81-year-old man admitted to the hospital with complaints of dizziness and syncope. His blood pressure (BP) on admission is 80/43. At the long-term nursing care facility where he lives, he ambulated with a walker independently but, since his episode of syncope, he has complained of weakness and needs another person to assist while walking as a fall precaution.

Case Study

Mr. O'Brien is admitted with prescriptions that include assessment of orthostatic vital signs every shift and fall precautions. The nurse explains to Mr. O'Brien how to use the call light and instructs him to call before getting out of bed so that someone can assist him with ambulation. The nurse completes a set of orthostatic vital signs. His orthostatic vital signs are lying: BP = 120/84, heart rate (HR) = 73; sitting: BP = 114/73, HR = 83; standing: BP = 96/61, HR = 92. When the assessment of orthostatics is complete, Mr. O'Brien is settled in bed. The nurse raises two side rails at the head of the bed, and the bed alarm is turned on so that if Mr. O'Brien tries to get out of bed without assistance, an alarm will notify staff.

Later in the shift, Mr. O'Brien's bed alarm sounds. The nurse quickly goes to his room to find Mr. O'Brien lying on the floor on his right hip. He is alert and oriented and states, "I had to go to the bathroom. I know I should have called for help but the nurses are busy. I figured I could go myself. Only two more steps and I could have reached my walker. I just slipped is all." Immediately following his fall, Mr. O'Brien complains of pain in his right hip that is a "7" on a 0–10 pain scale. He describes the pain as a "dull ache" that is worse with movement of his right leg. His BP is 110/62, HR is 88, and respiratory rate (RR) is 16.

Questions

1. Which clients are at greatest risk for falls in the acute care setting? Consider physiological and environmental risk factors for falls.

2. Identify seven areas of a fall risk appraisal assessment.

3. Discuss the initial nursing interventions when the nurse enters Mr. O'Brien's room and finds him lying on the floor.

4. Discuss who should be notified about Mr. O'Brien's fall and what type of documentation is needed regarding the incident.

5. What test(s) will the health care provider most likely prescribe since Mr. O'Brien is complaining of pain in his right hip?

6. The nurse double checks to see that appropriate fall precautions are in place. Identify ten measures to help prevent falls in older adults.

7. What can the nursing assistant do to assist in maintaining Mr. O'Brien's safety?

8. The nurse must complete an incident report. Discuss the purpose of an incident report and list the elements/type of data to address when completing this report.

9. Mr. O'Brien was assisted back to bed with a Hoyer lift and two assists. His vital signs remained within his baseline throughout the remainder of the shift and he is afebrile. An X-ray of his right hip was negative for a fracture. There is no physical deformity of the right hip or other injuries apparent, but a moderate amount of ecchymosis of his right hip that extends around to his lower back and right upper buttock is noted. His health care provider, Dr. Sutton, prescribed one tablet of oxycodone/acetaminophen 5/325 by mouth (PO) that decreased Mr. O'Brien's pain to a "2/10" within forty minutes of administration. He remains alert and oriented, continues on bed rest, and used the urinal once for 200 cc of clear yellow urine. The bed alarm is on, the call bell is in reach, and

Questions (continued)

there are two side rails up. Mr. O'Brien has verbalized an understanding of how and when to use the call bell.

Write a nursing progress note regarding the fall to enter into Mr. O'Brien's chart. Use the S.O.A.P.I.E. or Focus/D.A.R. method for writing a nursing note.

10. Provide a brief explanation of what orthostatic (postural) hypotension is and identify the blood pressure and heart rate values that define orthostatic (postural) hypotension.

11. Explain the steps of assessing orthostatic vital signs. From a lying to standing position, is Mr. O'Brien exhibiting signs of orthostatic hypotension based on the vital signs the nurse collected?

12. Identify Mr. O'Brien's predisposing risk factors for a fall.

13. The use of a vest restraint could be considered for Mr. O'Brien to prevent another fall. Define a "restraint" and provide examples of physical restraints and chemical restraints.

14. Discuss the risk of client injury associated with the use of restraints and the prescription requirements to implement restraints.

15. Identify five alternatives to using restraints.

16. Discuss the incidence of and mortality associated with falls in the older adult population. In your discussion, address the incidence of falls in general, injuries resulting, fall-related deaths, financial and social implications, and the need for long-term care as a result. Finally, is there a difference in the incidence and mortality between men and women? If so, explain.

17. The most common fracture resulting from a fall is a hip fracture. Discuss the incidence of and mortality associated with a hip fracture, as well as the difference in the incidence of hip fractures between men and women.

18. What is a "HipSaver"?

19. Write an appropriate three-part nursing diagnosis to include in Mr. O'Brien's plan of care regarding his fall.

GENDER

Female

AGE

48

SETTING

■ Primary Care

ETHNICITY

■ White American

CULTURAL CONSIDERATIONS

PREEXISTING CONDITION

■ Gastroesophogeal reflux disease (GERD), irritable bowel syndrome (IBS)

COEXISTING CONDITION

COMMUNICATION

DISABILITY

■ Potential disability resulting from chronic illness.

SOCIOECONOMIC

■ Wife; mother of three children (ages 21, 19, and 16 years); employed as an elementary school teacher.

SPIRITUAL/RELIGIOUS

PHARMACOLOGIC

■ Pantoprazole sodium (Protonix); acetaminophen (Tylenol); lidocaine hydrochloride

LEGAL

ETHICAL

ALTERNATIVE THERAPY

■ Complementary therapies for managing symptoms of fibromyalgia.

PRIORITIZATION

DELEGATION

MODERATE

FIBROMYALGIA

Level of difficulty: Moderate

Overview: The client has been recently diagnosed with fibromyalgia. This case requires the nurse to provide the client with information about her diagnosis. The impact of a chronic illness on the client's quality of life is considered.

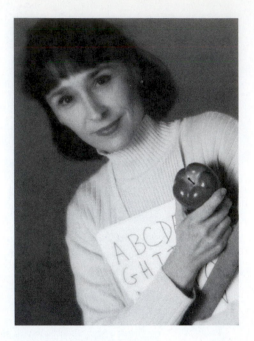

Client Profile

Mrs. Roberts is a 48-year-old elementary school teacher and mother of three children. Her past medical history includes GERD, which is well controlled with daily pantoprazole (Protonix). She also has a history of irritable bowel syndrome. For the past three and a half years, she has experienced "incredible" exhaustion and arthritis-like symptoms that make her "hurt all over."

Case Study

Years of assessment and testing to rule out several diagnostic possibilities have finally resulted in the diagnosis of fibromyalgia. A follow-up appointment is scheduled at the primary care provider's office to discuss the diagnosis with Mrs. Roberts. Her husband accompanies her to the appointment.

Questions

1. How might the nurse explain what fibromyalgia is to Mr. and Mrs. Roberts? Include the prevalence of fibromyalgia in the United States and the diagnostic criteria.

2. What are the common manifestations of fibromyalgia?

3. Mrs. Roberts asks, "I live a healthy lifestyle. What caused me to get this?" How will the nurse respond?

4. Discuss the focus of care for the client with fibromyalgia.

5. Discuss interventions that may be suggested to help Mrs. Roberts manage her fibromyalgia. Consider medications, exercise, rest, and alternative therapies.

6. Mr. Roberts asks, "How will fibromyalgia affect my wife's everyday life?" What are the potential quality-of-life changes that Mrs. Roberts may experience because of this chronic condition?

7. How can the nurse support Mrs. Roberts as she begins to cope with the news of this new diagnosis?

8. Generate at least three possible nursing diagnoses appropriate for Mrs. Roberts.

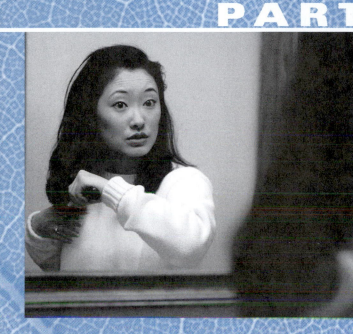

## PART SEVEN

The Integumentary System

GENDER

Female

AGE

70

SETTING

- Home

ETHNICITY

- White American

CULTURAL CONSIDERATIONS

PREEXISTING CONDITION

- Cerebral vascular accident (CVA) ten months ago with right-sided weakness

COEXISTING CONDITION

- Urinary incontinence; impaired mobility

COMMUNICATION

DISABILITY

- Right-sided weakness. Ambulates with a walker.

SOCIOECONOMIC

- Lives alone in a first-floor apartment.

SPIRITUAL/RELIGIOUS

PHARMACOLOGIC

LEGAL

ETHICAL

ALTERNATIVE THERAPY

PRIORITIZATION

- Educating client and caregiver to promote skin integrity.

DELEGATION

THE INTEGUMENTARY SYSTEM

Level of difficulty: Easy

Overview: This case requires that the nurse understand the impact of incontinence on impaired skin integrity. The nurse teaches the client and primary caregiver ways to minimize episodes of incontinence and promote good skin care.

Client Profile

Mrs. Sweeney is a 70-year-old woman who had a stroke less than a year ago. Mrs. Sweeney is alert and oriented. She feels the sensation to void, but right-sided weakness prevents her from always being able to get to the bathroom in time. For this reason, she wears incontinence undergarments. Mrs. Sweeney's daughter, Adele, stops by twice each day to check on Mrs. Sweeney and prepare meals for her. There are times when Mrs. Sweeney is incontinent and remains in a wet undergarment until Adele comes to visit.

Case Study

While assisting Mrs. Sweeney in the bathroom, Adele notices that Mrs. Sweeney's coccyx and perineum area are reddened and excoriated. Adele learns that Mrs. Sweeney sometimes sits in a wet undergarment until she arrives. Mrs. Sweeney explains, "I know I am wet. It is just easier to wait for you to get here than to try and change the undergarment myself." Adele is concerned. She calls a local visiting nurses association to get some information about how to manage Mrs. Sweeney's incontinence and asks if there is any skin therapy to reduce the redness.

Questions

1. Describe at least three factors that affect voiding and may result in incontinence in an adult.

2. What is incontinence? Describe the characteristics of each of the six types of urinary incontinence: *stress, reflex, urge, functional, total* (chronic incontinence), and *transient* (acute incontinence).

3. Which type of incontinence does Mrs. Sweeney have and what data support the diagnosis?

4. Mrs. Sweeney tells the nurse, "I try to limit the amount of fluid I drink to one or two small glasses a day so that I do not have to go to the bathroom as much." What teaching should the nurse provide in response to Mrs. Sweeney's comment?

5. Explain at least three factors that are contributing to Mrs. Sweeney's impaired skin integrity.

6. What will the visiting nurse most likely tell Mrs. Sweeny and Adele to consider in an effort to minimize Mrs. Sweeney's incontinent episodes?

7. What are three suggestions the visiting nurse will include while teaching Adele to care for Mrs. Sweeney's skin?

8. List five nursing diagnoses that are appropriate for Mrs. Sweeney.

Mr. Dennis

GENDER

Male

AGE

57

SETTING

- Hospital

ETHNICITY

- White American

CULTURAL CONSIDERATIONS

PREEXISTING CONDITION

COEXISTING CONDITION

- Herpes zoster infection

COMMUNICATION

DISABILITY

SOCIOECONOMIC

SPIRITUAL/RELIGIOUS

PHARMACOLOGIC

- Oxycodone/acetaminophen (Percocet), acyclovir (Zovirax); hydrocortisone (Sarna HC); famciclovir (Famvir); valacyclovir hydrochloride (Valtrex); gabapentin (Neurontin); triamcinolone (Aristocort, Kenacort, Kenalog); aluminum sulfate (Domeboro)

LEGAL

ETHICAL

ALTERNATIVE THERAPY

- Cutaneous stimulation; distraction

PRIORITIZATION

- Pain management

DELEGATION

- Client assignment considerations to avoid client care by pregnant staff members.

THE INTEGUMENTARY SYSTEM

Level of difficulty: Easy

Overview: Although in pain, the client refuses medication for fear of becoming addicted. The nurse provides teaching to clarify the myths and facts of pain medication and provide alternatives to pharmacological pain management. Treatment options for herpes zoster are discussed. Client assignments are considered to reduce the risks of exposure for pregnant staff.

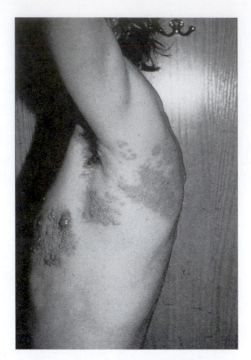

Herpes Zoster. *Courtesy of Robert A. Silverman, M.D., Clinical Associate Professor, Department of Pediatrics, Georgetown University*

Client Profile

Mr. Dennis is a 57-year-old man admitted with pain secondary to herpes zoster. He describes the pain as "agonizing" and states, "I feel like my skin is burning." The health care provider has prescribed acyclovir (Zovirax) and oxycodone/acetaminophen (Percocet) for Mr. Dennis. Mr. Dennis is reluctant to ask for the pain medication. He states, "I do not even want to start with that stuff. I have heard you can become addicted to pain medication very easily."

Case Study

The nurse sits with Mr. Dennis and discusses with him the common myths surrounding pain management and pain medications. Education regarding nonpharmacologic pain management strategies results in instruction on how to use distraction. The nurse also brings Mr. Dennis a cooling pad to facilitate pain management through cutaneous stimulation. Mr. Dennis feels better now about asking for his prescribed pain medication. Now that he is receiving (oxycodone/acetaminophen) Percocet on a regular basis in conjunction with alternative pain management strategies, he states his pain "has decreased considerably."

Questions

1. What is herpes zoster? Briefly discuss its cause and incidence.

2. Discuss the characteristic manifestations of herpes zoster and its typical progression and

healing time. What would a diagnosis of "ophthalmic herpes zoster" indicate?

3. Mr. Dennis describes his initial pain as "agonizing" and then states his pain has decreased

Questions (continued)

"considerably." Discuss the assessment tools that help quantify the subjective experience of pain.

4. Create two columns. In the first column, provide at least three myths about the pain experience and the use of pain medication. In the second column, provide a fact that dispels each myth.

5. Discuss how the nurse can facilitate effective pain management for Mr. Dennis.

6. Describe cutaneous stimulation as an alternative pain management strategy.

7. Describe the use of distraction as an alternative pain management strategy.

8. Discuss the focus of treatment and treatment options for herpes zoster. Consider acute treatment, as well as long-term treatment of postherpetic neuralgia.

9. Help the nurse generate two appropriate nursing diagnoses for Mr. Dennis's plan of care.

10. When creating the client assignment, the charge nurse purposely does not assign Mr. Dennis to a pregnant staff nurse. Discuss the potential risks associated with a pregnant woman's exposure to herpes zoster, and the method and time frame during which the infected client can transmit the virus to others.

Mrs. Sims

GENDER

Female

AGE

72

SETTING

- Hospital

ETHNICITY

- White American

CULTURAL CONSIDERATIONS

PREEXISTING CONDITION

- Heart failure (HF, CHF), cerebral vascular accident (CVA) with subsequent right-sided hemiplegia

COEXISTING CONDITION

- MRSA (methicillin-resistant *Staphylococcus aureus*); receiving nutrition via a g-tube

COMMUNICATION

DISABILITY

- Needs complete assistance with ADLs and turning and repositioning.

SOCIOECONOMIC

- Cost containment to decrease financial burden on health care system.

SPIRITUAL/RELIGIOUS

PHARMACOLOGIC

- Mupirocin (Bactroban); vancomycin (Vancocin)

LEGAL

OSHA guidelines

ETHICAL

- Noncompliance with contact precaution policies.

ALTERNATIVE THERAPY

PRIORITIZATION

- Nursing organization and time management.

DELEGATION

- Delegating retrieval of equipment and supplies.

MODERATE

THE INTEGUMENTARY SYSTEM

Level of difficulty: Moderate

Overview: This case requires that the student nurse understand the transmission of nosocomial infections and initiate appropriate isolation precautions for MRSA. Treatment options for MRSA are explored. The student nurse serves as a client advocate by recognizing the importance of compliance with proper contact precautions by visitors and health care personnel. The importance of developing good time management and delegation skills is discussed. Finally, the financial burden of caring for a client with MRSA is considered with regard to the nurse's responsibility for cost containment.

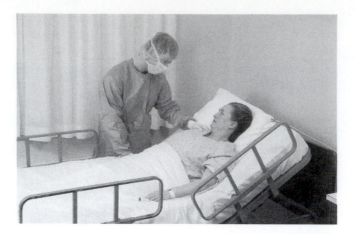

Client Profile

Mrs. Sims is a 72-year-old female admitted with heart failure. Her heart failure has been resolved. Mrs. Sims needs complete care with her activities of daily living (ADLs) and with repositioning. Arrangements were being made for her discharge back to the long-term care facility when lab results revealed she is positive for MRSA in her urine. The long-term care facility will not readmit her until her MRSA is resolved. Mrs. Sims is in a private room and has been placed on contact precautions. Vancomycin is prescribed with peak and trough labs.

Case Study

The student nurse caring for Mrs. Sims follows the contact precaution guidelines as indicated by a sign outside of Mrs. Sims's door. The student nurse dons the personal protective equipment (PPE) located in a precaution cart outside the room. Once in the room to take a set of morning vital signs, the student nurse notices that there is not a separate blood pressure cuff or stethoscope assigned to the client. The student nurse removes the PPE and finds the staff nurse assigned to the client to ask for a blood pressure cuff and stethoscope. The staff nurse is able to locate a disposable stethoscope to remain in the client's room, but not a blood pressure cuff. The staff nurse instructs the student to use the unit's electronic blood pressure machine and to wash it thoroughly with antibacterial wipes after each use.

Throughout the day, the student realizes how much additional time is necessary to complete each care need for Mrs. Sims since before entering the room, the student must don the PPE. The student also makes note of several precaution carts lining the hallway and realizes how prevalent infectious diseases are on this one hospital unit alone.

The student is pleased to see that when family members come to visit, they take the time to put on the proper PPE and remind new visitors to do the same. However, the student nurse notices that other nursing staff, housekeeping personnel, and the health care provider enter the room on several occasions without putting on the required equipment.

Questions

1. What is MRSA?

2. How is MRSA transmitted?

3. Which individuals are at the greatest risk for becoming infected with MRSA?

4. What are five nursing interventions that will help minimize the spread of MRSA while caring for Mrs. Sims?

5. Was it appropriate for the staff nurse to instruct the student nurse to use the unit's electronic blood pressure machine and wash it thoroughly with antibacterial wipes after each use? Explain why or why not.

6. Discuss the importance of efficiency in gathering needed supplies and time management when caring for a client on contact precautions.

7. Discuss appropriate delegation to others when the student nurse requires additional supplies or equipment once in the client's room.

8. What treatment options are there to help resolve Mrs. Sims's MRSA?

9. Mrs. Sims is taking vancomycin (Vancocin). A peak and trough is ordered. Explain peak and trough levels and the purpose of these laboratory tests.

10. What diagnostic test(s) will be done to confirm negative or positive MRSA infection prior to Mrs. Sims's discharge to the long-term care facility?

11. Discuss the ethical considerations regarding the lack of compliance by hospital personnel with the indicated contact precautions?

12. What could the nursing student do to help facilitate greater compliance with the contact precautions by hospital staff caring for and entering Mrs. Sims's room?

13. Discuss the financial considerations of caring for a client with MRSA.

14. List two nursing diagnoses appropriate for the plan of care for a client with MRSA.

Mr. Vincent

GENDER

Male

AGE

32

SETTING

- Primary Care

ETHNICITY

- White American

CULTURAL CONSIDERATIONS

PREEXISTING CONDITION

COEXISTING CONDITION

COMMUNICATION

DISABILITY

SOCIOECONOMIC

- Married for five years. Physical education teacher for ten years.

SPIRITUAL/RELIGIOUS

PHARMACOLOGIC

- Oxycodone and acetaminophen 5/325 (Percocet), bacitracin ointment, interferon alpha-2b recombinant (INF-alpha 2b, Intron A)

LEGAL

ETHICAL

ALTERNATIVE THERAPY

PRIORITIZATION

DELEGATION

THE INTEGUMENTARY SYSTEM

Level of difficulty: Difficult

Overview: This case requires the nurse to recognize the risk factors and characteristics of melanoma. The diagnostic process and treatment options for a malignant skin lesion are discussed. The nurse considers the client's need for emotional support.

DIFFICULT

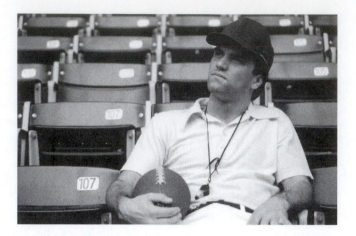

Client Profile

Mr. Vincent is a 32-year-old man who has scheduled an appointment with a dermatologist to have a black spot on his right ear assessed. Mr. Vincent states, "My wife noticed a jet-black circular area on my ear about two weeks ago and she suggested I get it looked at since she did not remember the dark spot being there before. I know that too much time in the sun is not very good for your skin. I'm a physical education teacher so I am out in the sun a lot, and I admit that I do not always remember to apply sunscreen."

Case Study

There is a dark area on Mr. Vincent's right ear approximately 0.4 cm by 0.4 cm round in size. The color of the surrounding skin is normal. Mr. Vincent says that he noticed the spot about four months earlier but did not think much of it. "I figured it was a mole. Since it did not hurt, I really didn't give it much thought."

Questions

1. You are the nurse working with the dermatologist. Make a list of questions you could ask regarding the area of concern to help determine if the site on Mr. Vincent's ear could be melanoma.

2. Explain the ABCD criteria for assessing a skin lesion.

3. The dermatologist examines the area under a dermoscope and then performs a punch biopsy. What is a punch biopsy and what will this test help to determine?

4. The pathology report from the punch biopsy states, "deep penetrating nevi with atypical features worrisome for melanoma." The dermatologist suggests that Mr. Vincent have a sentinel lymph node mapping and biopsy procedure. How might the nurse explain what this procedure is, why it is done, and potential common and serious adverse effects/complications?

5. Mrs. Vincent says, "How did this happen? My husband has dark hair and olive skin. I thought only fair-skinned redheads got skin cancer." Is there any truth to Mrs. Vincent's assumption? List 5 risk factors the nurse should include in an explanation of what puts individuals at greater risk for skin cancer.

6. Discuss the incidence of dark-skinned individuals diagnosed with melanoma.

7. The results of the sentinel lymph node mapping and biopsy reveal that the most proximal lymph

Questions (continued)

node near Mr. Vincent's parotid gland is positive with a 0.1 mm micrometastasis. Given that the punch biopsy was suspicious for melanoma and that there is a positive sentinel lymph node, the dermatologist prescribes a CT scan of the head, chest, neck, abdomen, thorax, and pelvis, a MRI of the brain, and a PET scan of the body to determine the extent of Mr. Vincent's melanoma. Mr. Vincent asks "What gland is it near?" and then states, "I know what a CT scan and MRI are but what is a PET scan?" What function does the parotid gland serve? Explain a PET scan to Mr. Vincent.

8. What does it mean to explain cancer according to its "stage" using the tumor, lymph nodes, metastasis (TNM) system? Melanoma may be staged according to a "clinical stage" and a "pathological stage." Briefly discuss the difference.

9. It has been six weeks since his initial visit to the dermatologist, and Mr. and Mrs. Vincent are meeting with the dermatologist today to get results of the diagnostic tests. They learn that Mr. Vincent has been diagnosed with "Stage IIIA T1a, N1a, M0" malignant melanoma. What does this stage mean?

10. Mr. Vincent asks the dermatologist "What is my prognosis?" What is Mr. Vincent's five-year survival rate?

11. Identify two nursing diagnoses the nurse should consider for Mr. Vincent when he learns of his diagnosis of melanoma.

12. Discuss what the nurse can do to reduce the fear and anxiety that Mr. Vincent may feel upon learning that he has melanoma.

13. Results of Mr. Vincent's CT scan, MRI, and PET scan are negative. The suggested intervention is a curative lymph node dissection. There are no postoperative complications and Mr. Vincent is being discharged home. He is given a prescription for oxycodone and acetaminophen 5/325 one to two tablets every four to six hours as needed for postsurgical incisional pain. He has staples at his surgical incision site to which Bacitracin is applied

and the site covered with a sterile dressing. He will return to the surgeon's office two days after discharge to have the dressing removed and a postoperative incision check. The nurse is providing discharge teaching. What are the common adverse effects of oxycodone and acetaminophen 5/325 and instructions for safe administration? What warning signs indicate that Mr. Vincent should call his surgeon?

14. Identify two nursing diagnoses the nurse should consider for Mr. Vincent following his lymph node dissection.

15. Four weeks later, Mr. Vincent sees an oncologist to discuss recommendations regarding adjunct treatment. The oncologist explains that the only FDA-approved therapy for stage III melanoma is high-dose interferon (INF)-alpha 2b, which offers a modest survival benefit with the risk of adverse effects. What are the adverse effects of high-dose interferon (INF)-alpha 2b?

16. The oncologist suggests Mr. Vincent also consider treatment offered through participation in a clinical trial. What is a clinical trial and what are the three phases of a clinical trial?

17. Mr. Vincent does some research and takes some time to consider the treatment options and discuss them with his wife. He decides that presented with only the possibility, and not a guarantee, of an increase in survival rate with the interferon therapy, the benefit does not outweigh the risk of the adverse effects. He declines interferon treatment and is going to explore clinical trials. As Mr. Vincent's nurse, how should you respond to Mr. Vincent's decision?

18. What will Mr. Vincent require in terms of follow-up care? Discuss how often Mr. Vincent will need to see the dermatologist, the symptoms to report, precautions to take, and the need for emotional support.

19. How likely is it that someone else Mr. and Mrs. Vincent know will have skin cancer?

Mr. Lee

GENDER

Male

AGE

55

SETTING

- Hospital

ETHNICITY

- Black American

CULTURAL CONSIDERATIONS

PREEXISTING CONDITION

- Head trauma three months ago.

COEXISTING CONDITION

- Recent seizure.

COMMUNICATION

DISABILITY

- Potential long-term complications.

SOCIOECONOMIC

SPIRITUAL/RELIGIOUS

PHARMACOLOGIC

- Phenytoin (Dilantin)

LEGAL

ETHICAL

ALTERNATIVE THERAPY

PRIORITIZATION

- Adverse medication reaction.

DELEGATION

THE INTEGUMENTARY SYSTEM

Level of difficulty: Difficult

Overview: This case requires the nurse to implement strategies to maintain the client's safety in the event of a seizure. The nurse also must recognize the signs and symptoms of an adverse reaction to a medication. The client must be transferred to the appropriate level of care. Treatment goals and priority nursing diagnoses are reviewed.

Client Profile

Mr. Lee is a 55-year-old man with a history of head trauma three months ago after falling from a ladder. He is seen in the emergency department today after experiencing a seizure at work. Mr. Lee received a loading dose of phenytoin in the emergency department and admitted for a thorough work-up.

Case Study

Upon arrival to the nursing unit, Mr. Lee is alert and oriented but lethargic. The following day, Mr. Lee has received two doses of phenytoin, and he has not had a seizure since admission. His lethargy has resolved. Midafternoon, Mr. Lee calls for the nurse. He shows the nurse his arms and hands and asks, "Look at these red splotches and blisters. What do you think this is from?" The nurse asks Mr. Lee if he has any other symptoms. He replies, "My eyes are itchy and burning and my throat is a little sore. Maybe I am allergic to the laundry detergent the hospital uses to wash the bed sheets." Assessment reveals symmetric reddish-purple macules and bullae on his arms, hands, chest, and back. Mr. Lee's vital signs are within normal limits except his temperature, which is 102.1°F (38.9°C).

Questions

1. Should the nurse be concerned that upon arrival to the nursing unit Mr. Lee is lethargic?

2. What is the rationale for prescribing phenytoin for Mr. Lee?

3. Mr. Lee's plan of care includes seizure precautions. Explain how the nurse implements these precautions.

4. What do you believe is the cause of Mr. Lee's skin condition?

5. Discuss three critical interventions upon diagnosing Mr. Lee's reaction.

6. Mr. Lee is transferred to the burn unit. Explain the rationale for this transfer.

7. Identify four treatment goals the nurse will include while documenting Mr. Lee's plan of care.

8. Mr. Lee's wife notices that the nurse checked the thermostat in Mr. Lee's room even though Mr. Lee did not express discomfort with the room temperature. Why was the nurse checking the temperature in the room?

9. Mr. Lee's laboratory results are: hemoglobin (Hgb) 18 g/dL, hematocrit (Hct) 57%, potassium (K^+) 6.5 mEq/L, sodium (Na^{2+}) level is 126 mEq/L, and his bicarbonate (HCO_3^-) is 15 mEq/L. Are these results within normal limits? If not, explain what is causing any abnormal result.

10. The nurse dons a protective gown, mask, gloves, and cap prior to changing Mr. Lee's dressings. Why is this precaution necessary?

11. Is Stevens Johnson Syndrome self-limiting or life threatening? Explain your answer.

12. Briefly discuss three potential complications the nurse will watch for as Stevens Johnson Syndrome progresses.

13. Mr. Lee's coworker comes to visit and brings a beautiful vase full of flowers from her garden. The nurse asks that the visitor not bring the floral arrangement into Mr. Lee's room. What is the rationale for the nurse's request?

14. Clients with Stevens Johnson Syndrome sometimes suffer long-term effects. Briefly discuss three long-term complications that may result.

15. Identify five nursing diagnoses appropriate for Mr. Lee's plan of care while being cared for on the burn unit. Prioritize the diagnoses you have identified.

16. While providing discharge teaching, what should the nurse tell Mr. Lee (and his family) about preventing a recurrence of this adverse medication reaction in the future?

17. What resource can the nurse suggest to help provide support once Mr. Lee is discharged from the hospital?

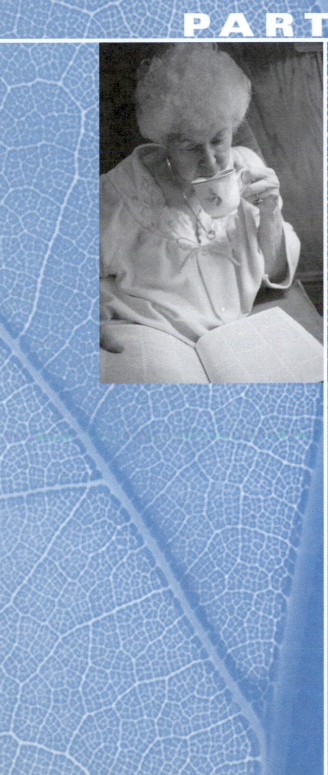

The Nervous/ Neurological System

Mrs. Giammo

GENDER

Female

AGE

59

SETTING

■ Hospital

ETHNICITY

■ Black American

CULTURAL CONSIDERATIONS

PREEXISTING CONDITION

■ Hypertension (HTN)

COEXISTING CONDITION

■ Hypercholesterolemia

COMMUNICATION

DISABILITY

SOCIOECONOMIC

■ History of tobacco use for twenty-five years; quit ten years ago. Husband smokes one pack per day. Positive family history of heart disease. Occasionally takes walks in the neighborhood with friends but does not have a regular exercise regimen.

SPIRITUAL/RELIGIOUS

PHARMACOLOGIC

■ Atenolol (Tenormin); heparin (Heparin Sodium); atorvastatin (Lipitor)

LEGAL

ETHICAL

ALTERNATIVE THERAPY

■ Lifestyle modification

PRIORITIZATION

DELEGATION

THE NERVOUS/NEUROLOGICAL SYSTEM

Level of difficulty: Easy

Overview: This case requires the nurse to recognize the signs and symptoms of a transient ischemic attack (TIA) and define the difference between a cerebrovascular accident (CVA, stroke) and a TIA. The nurse must recognize the risk factors for a possible stroke and suggest lifestyle modifications to decrease risk. Explanations of test results and physical assessment findings are offered. Appropriate nursing diagnoses for this client are prioritized.

Client Profile

Mrs. Giammo is a 59-year-old woman who was brought to the emergency department by her husband. Mr. Giammo noticed that all of a sudden his wife "was slurring her speech and her face was drooping on one side." Mrs. Giammo told her husband that she felt some numbness on the right side of her face and in her right arm. Mr. Giammo was afraid his wife was having a stroke so he brought her to the hospital.

Case Study

In the emergency department, Mrs. Giammo is alert and oriented. Her vital signs are temperature 98.2°F (36.7°C), blood pressure 148/97, pulse 81, and respiratory rate 14. An electrocardiogram (ECG, EKG) monitor shows a normal sinus rhythm. Mrs. Giammo is still complaining of "numbness" of the right side of her face and down her right arm. Her mouth is noted to divert to the right side with a slight facial droop when she smiles. Her speech is clear. She is able to move all of her extremities and follow commands. Her pupils are round, equal, and reactive to light (4 mm to 2 mm) and accommodation. There is no nystagmus noted. Her right hand grasp is weaker than her left. Mrs. Giammo does not have a headache and denies any nausea, vomiting, chest pain, diaphoresis, or visual complaints. She is not experiencing any significant weakness, has a steady gait, and is able to swallow without difficulty. Laboratory blood test results are as follows: white blood cell count (WBC) 8,000 cells/mm^3, hemoglobin (Hgb) 14 g/dL, hematocrit (Hct) 44%, platelets = 294,000 mm^3, erythrocyte sedimentation rate (ESR) 15 mm/hr, prothrombin time (PT) 12.9 seconds, international normalized ratio (INR) 1.10, sodium (Na^{2+}) 149 mEq/L, potassium (K$^+$) 4.5 mEq/L, glucose 105 mg/dL, calcium (Ca^{2+}) 9.5 mg/dL, blood urea nitrogen (BUN) 15 mg/dL, and creatinine (creat) 0.8 mg/dL. A head computed tomography (CT) scan is done which shows no acute intracranial change and a magnetic resonance imagery (MRI) is within normal limits. Mrs. Giammo is started on an intravenous heparin drip of 25,000 units in 500 cc of D5W at 18 ml per hour (900 units per hour). Mrs. Giammo is admitted for a neurology evaluation, magnetic resonance angiography (MRA) of the brain, a fasting serum cholesterol, and blood pressure monitoring. Upon admission to the nursing unit, her symptoms have resolved. There is no facial asymmetry and her complaint of numbness has subsided.

Questions

1. The neurologist's consult report states, "At no time during the episode of numbness did the client ever develop any scotoma, amaurosis, ataxia, or diplopia." Explain what these terms mean.

2. The neurology consult report includes the following statement: "Client's diet is notable for moderate amounts of aspartame and no significant glutamate." What are *aspartame* and *glutamate*? Why did the neurologist assess Mrs. Giammo's intake of aspartame and glutamate?

3. Discuss the pathophysiology of a transient ischemic attack (TIA). Include in your discussion what causes a TIA and the natural course of a TIA.

4. Mrs. Giammo asks, "How is what I had different from a stroke?" Provide a simple explanation of how a transient ischemic attack (TIA) differs from a cerebrovascular accident (CVA, stroke).

5. Discuss the defining characteristics of a transient ischemic attack (TIA).

6. How does Mrs. Giammo's case fit the profile of the "typical" client with a TIA?

7. Mrs. Giammo has her fasting cholesterol levels checked. How long must Mrs. Giammo fast before the test?

8. Mrs. Giammo's cholesterol lab work reveals total cholesterol = 242 mg/dL, low-density lipoprotein

Questions (continued)

(LDL) = 165 mg/dL, high-density lipoprotein (HDL) = 30 mg/dL. Discuss the normal values of each and which of her results are of concern and why.

9. When told that her cholesterol levels are elevated, Mrs. Giammo asks, "I always see commercials on television saying you should lower your cholesterol. What is cholesterol anyway?" How could the nurse explain what cholesterol is and why it increases the risk of heart disease and stroke?

10. Identify Mrs. Giammo's predisposing risk factors for a TIA and possible stroke. Which factors can she change and which factors are beyond her control?

11. Mrs. Giammo takes atenolol at home. What is the most likely reason why she has been prescribed this medication?

12. The nurse hears a carotid bruit on physical assessment. What is a bruit and why is this of concern to the nurse? What would be likely diagnostic procedures ordered by the health care provider because of this assessment finding?

13. If a carotid ultrasound, carotid duplex, and/or MRA reveal carotid artery stenosis, what surgical procedure can resolve the stenosis?

14. Provide a simple rationale for including intravenous heparin in Mrs. Giammo's treatment plan.

15. Identify the potential life-threatening adverse effects/complications of heparin therapy and the treatment of heparin toxicity or overdose.

16. To assess for bleeding and possible hemorrhage, explain what the nurse monitors while Mrs. Giammo is on heparin therapy.

17. What is the major complication associated with a TIA?

18. Identify six nursing diagnoses in order of priority appropriate for Mrs. Giammo.

19. Atorvastatin 10 mg PO per day is prescribed for Mrs. Giammo. Explain the therapeutic effects of atorvastatin.

20. What type of lifestyle modifications should the nurse discuss with Mrs. Giammo (and her husband) prior to discharge?

Mr. Aponi

GENDER

Male

AGE

85

SETTING

- Long-term care

ETHNICITY

- Native American

CULTURAL CONSIDERATIONS

- Touch; nonverbal behavior

PREEXISTING CONDITION

- Progressive dementia over the past seven years.

COEXISTING CONDITION

- Urinary incontinence

COMMUNICATION

- Impaired communication secondary to altered mental status.

DISABILITY

- Unable to care for himself independently due to cognitive decline.

SOCIOECONOMIC

- Lives in a long-term care facility. Wife passed away five years ago. He has no children.

SPIRITUAL/RELIGIOUS

PHARMACOLOGIC

LEGAL

ETHICAL

ALTERNATIVE THERAPY

PRIORITIZATION

DELEGATION

THE NERVOUS/NEUROLOGICAL SYSTEM

Level of difficulty: Easy

Overview: This case requires the nurse to distinguish the difference between dementia and delirium and plan nursing care accordingly. How the client's cultural beliefs impact care is considered.

Client Profile

Mr. Aponi has a history of dementia. His dementia limits his ability to respond appropriately to questions and at times Mr. Aponi is easily agitated and resistant to nursing care. He refuses to take his medications, spitting them back out, gripping the bedside rail when the nurse tries to turn him, and yelling out for his wife to save him.

Case Study

Mr. Aponi is an 85-year-old man with a history of dementia. He is a resident of a long-term facility. Mr. Aponi's frequent incontinence necessitates the development of therapeutic communication to facilitate activities of daily living (ADL) care and frequent skin hygiene. The nurse caring for Mr. Aponi for the first time soon learns that talking slowly and softly is the most effective way of focusing the client's attention and prompting him to follow basic instructions such as turning side to side. The nurse feels uneasy about speaking to Mr. Aponi as if he were a child in some ways. However, the nurse finds that this manner of speech keeps Mr. Aponi calm and that he responds well to praise and compliments and that he is very helpful to the nurse in assisting with his own care.

On the second day of caring for him, the nurse notes that Mr. Aponi is more agitated and needs frequent reorientation regarding where he is. The nurse needs the assistance of another person to hold Mr. Aponi's arm steady while assessing his blood pressure since Mr. Aponi keeps pulling his arm away yelling "no." At one point in the day, Mr. Aponi tells the nurse, "There was a little boy in the room a minute ago. Where did he go?" The nurse knows there was not a little boy in the room, but does not know how to respond. The nurse ignores Mr. Aponi's comment and redirects his attention to what is on television.

When saying good-bye to Mr. Aponi at the end of the second day, the nurse is disappointed that Mr. Aponi does not seem to recognize the nurse nor remember that the nurse has been caring for him for the past two days. The nurse is saddened to see him so confused and is emotionally exhausted after two days of responding to his frequent labile changes in behavior.

Questions

1. The nurse caring for Mr. Aponi overhears another nurse state, "Well of course he is confused. He is 85 years old." How should Mr. Aponi's nurse respond?

2. Discuss the characteristics that define *delirium* and *dementia*. What is the principal difference between the diagnoses of delirium and dementia?

3. Describe the following strategies for caring for a confused client: validation, reality orientation, redirection, and reminiscence.

4. Explain why Mr. Aponi may state, "There was a little boy in the room a minute ago. Where did he go?" Which of the above strategies (in question 3) would be most effective in responding to his statement?

5. What are three nursing diagnoses appropriate for Mr. Aponi's plan of care?

6. Discuss the importance of nonverbal communication when communicating with a person who is confused and agitated. Consider Mr. Aponi's ethnicity.

Mrs. Greene

GENDER

Female

AGE

92

SETTING

■ Hospital

ETHNICITY

■ White American

CULTURAL CONSIDERATIONS

PREEXISTING CONDITION

COEXISTING CONDITION

■ Urinary tract infection (UTI)

COMMUNICATION

■ Impaired communication secondary to altered mental status.

DISABILITY

SOCIOECONOMIC

SPIRITUAL/RELIGIOUS

PHARMACOLOGIC

■ Levofloxacin (Levaquin)

LEGAL

■ Restraints

ETHICAL

ALTERNATIVE THERAPY

PRIORITIZATION

DELEGATION

THE NERVOUS/NEUROLOGICAL SYSTEM

Level of difficulty: Easy

Overview: This case requires the nurse to recognize the most likely etiology of an acute change in mental status. Appropriate nursing interventions for a client requiring a physical restraint are considered.

Client Profile

Mrs. Greene is a 92-year-old woman who presents to the emergency room with an acute change in mental status and generalized weakness. Her past medical history is unremarkable. She has not had episodes of confusion in the past.

Case Study

It is determined that Mrs. Greene has a urinary tract infection (UTI) for which she is started on intravenous (IV) levofloxacin (Levaquin). Mrs. Greene's confusion escalates to visual hallucinations, pulling out two IV sites, and restless nights of little sleep. Bilateral soft wrist restraints are prescribed to maintain her safety, the integrity of the IV site, and the Foley catheter.

While the nurse is providing care for Mrs. Greene, Mrs. Greene's son visits. He is very distraught over Mrs. Greene's state of confusion and her inability to recognize him. Mrs. Greene is unable to answer her son's questions appropriately and frequently states, "I told you I do not want to cook today." Visibly upset and tearful, Mr. Greene states, "I don't understand. She was perfectly normal three days ago. I stopped by to visit and she was outside working in her garden and her conversation with me made perfect sense."

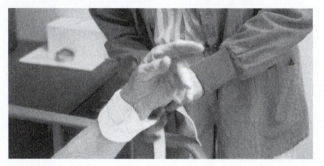

Soft wrist restraint

Questions

1. What do you suspect is the reason for Mrs. Greene's confusion?

2. Would you describe Mrs. Greene's confusion as delirium or dementia? Provide a rationale for your decision and explain the difference between delirium and dementia.

3. What are three appropriate nursing diagnoses that address Mrs. Greene's change in mental status?

4. State at least three outcome goals that should be included in the plan of care for Mrs. Greene's diagnosis of acute confusion.

5. Provide five nursing interventions to include in the plan of care for Mrs. Greene's diagnosis of acute confusion.

6. Briefly discuss strategies that help prevent the need for restraints. List five nursing interventions to include in Mrs. Greene's plan of care now that she needs bilateral soft wrist restraints for her safety.

Mrs. Perry

GENDER

Female

AGE

35

SETTING

■ Hospital

ETHNICITY

■ White American

CULTURAL CONSIDERATIONS

PREEXISTING CONDITION

■ Alcohol abuse for four years.

COEXISTING CONDITION

■ Pancreatitis

COMMUNICATION

DISABILITY

SOCIOECONOMIC

■ Married. Stay-at-home mother of two children (ages 8 and 5 years old).

SPIRITUAL/RELIGIOUS

PHARMACOLOGIC

■ Ethyl alcohol (alcohol, ethanol); lorazepam (Ativan); folic acid (folate, vitamin B); thiamine (vitamin B_1)

LEGAL

ETHICAL

ALTERNATIVE THERAPY

PRIORITIZATION

■ Client safety during alcohol withdrawal.

DELEGATION

THE NERVOUS/NEUROLOGICAL SYSTEM

Level of difficulty: Moderate

Overview: The nurse in this case is asked to define terminology associated with alcohol abuse and discuss the effects alcohol has on the body. This case requires that the nurse recognize the initial manifestations of alcohol withdrawal and anticipate the symptoms the client may exhibit while hospitalized. The use of lorazepam (Ativan) and rationale for folic acid (folate, vitamin B) and thiamine (vitamin B_1) supplementation in the treatment of alcohol withdrawal is reviewed. The pertinent Healthy People 2010 health promotion considerations for the client are identified.

Client Profile

Mrs. Perry is a 35-year-old woman admitted to the hospital with pancreatitis. During her stay, Mrs. Perry experiences alcohol withdrawal.

Case Study

Mrs. Perry arrives at the emergency department with complaints of severe abdominal pain. She is admitted to the nursing unit at noon with a diagnosis of pancreatitis. While completing the nursing admission assessment, Mrs. Perry tells the day shift nurse that she drinks "a couple of cases of beer each week." She states her last drink was this morning. While doing rounds, the evening shift nurse notices that Mrs. Perry has tremors and is very anxious and restless. Her vital signs are blood pressure 130/82, heart rate 88, respiratory rate 16, and temperature 99.6°F (37.5°C). The health care provider is notified. Daily folic acid and thiamine, and lorazepam as needed, are prescribed.

Questions

1. Briefly discuss the classification, metabolism, and excretion of alcohol.

2. Provide a definition for each of the following terms associated with alcohol use: *psychoactive substance, addiction, blackout, detoxification, intoxication, overdose, recidivism, sobriety, substance abuse, substance dependence, tolerance,* and *withdrawal.*

3. What are the characteristic effects of alcohol on the body?

4. What is considered the legal blood alcohol intoxication level in most of the United States?

5. Discuss the potential life-threatening complications associated with acute alcohol intoxication. What causes these complications?

6. When should the nurse expect the manifestations of alcohol withdrawal to begin and what symptoms will the nurse anticipate in the next few days?

7. What are delirium tremens (DTs)? Discuss the life-threatening complications of DTs.

8 Why is Lorazepam (Ativan) prescribed as part of the management of Mrs. Perry's alcohol withdrawal? Discuss the most effective administration schedule of Lorazepam (Ativan) for Mrs. Perry.

9. Provide a rationale for the prescription of folic acid (folate, vitamin B) and thiamine (vitamin B_1) in the management of alcohol withdrawal.

10. Generate five possible nursing diagnoses to address Mrs. Perry's alcohol withdrawal.

11. Discuss the Healthy People 2010 goal pertinent in Mrs. Perry's case and Mrs. Perry's health promotion priorities.

Mr. Cooper

GENDER

Male

AGE

73

SETTING

- Home

ETHNICITY

- White American

CULTURAL CONSIDERATIONS

PREEXISTING CONDITION

COEXISTING CONDITION

COMMUNICATION

- No answering machine. Slurred speech.

DISABILITY

- Progressive, degenerative disease.

SOCIOECONOMIC

- Lives alone. Non-smoker.

SPIRITUAL/RELIGIOUS

PHARMACOLOGIC

- Ibuprofen (Motrin); riluzole (Rilutek)

LEGAL

- Advance directive.

ETHICAL

ALTERNATIVE THERAPY

- Palliative Care.

PRIORITIZATION

- End-of-life planning.

DELEGATION

- Collaboration between health care provider, home care nurse, home care physical therapist (PT), home care occupational therapist (OT), speech-language pathologist (SLP).

THE NERVOUS/NEUROLOGICAL SYSTEM

Level of difficulty: Difficult

Overview: This case explores the onset and diagnosis of ALS. Management of ALS with regard to medication and an interdisciplinary team approach is discussed. The nurse must consider how the prognosis of ALS will affect the client and his family. End-of-life issues are addressed.

DIFFICULT

Client Profile

Mr. Cooper is a 73-year-old man with no significant past medical history. He lives alone and is very independent in function and spirit. He was seen in the emergency department six weeks ago for complaints of "arthritis in his right knee." He was examined, given a prescription for ibuprofen, provided with a cane, and instructed to follow up with his health care provider. When Mr. Cooper sees his health care provider for his follow-up visit, the health care provider notices that as Mr. Cooper enters the examination room, he has right footdrop. When the health care provider asks Mr. Cooper what has brought him in today Mr. Cooper states "I have arthritis in this right knee." Mr. Cooper explains that he has had this "arthritis" for three months. However, when asked about pain in the knee, Mr. Cooper denies any pain and states "well, maybe it's a nerve problem." On physical exam, his vital signs are within normal limits and consistent with Mr. Cooper's baseline. The health care provider notes that Mr. Cooper has no strength or power in his right lower extremity from the knee down. There is increased tone in his upper right extremity, indicating that those muscles are tighter than they should be. The health care provider also notices hyperreflexia. The health care provider prescribes a head computed tomography (CT) scan and multiple blood tests. The results of the CT scan and blood tests are all within normal limits. An urgent referral to a neurologist is made, and the health care provider asks the nurse to arrange for Mr. Cooper to have magnetic resonance imagery (MRI) of his head and neck and an electromyelogram (EMG). The nurse plans to arrange dates for these tests and to call Mr. Cooper with instructions. Mr. Cooper is fitted for an ankle-foot orthosis (AFO) brace and home physical therapy is arranged as prescribed by the health care provider.

Case Study

The nurse attempts to notify Mr. Cooper of the dates, times, and instructions regarding his MRI and EMG. However, Mr. Cooper does not have an answering machine. The health care provider is notified and she decides to call Mr. Cooper from home to see if she can reach him at home and give him the information. When the health care provider calls Mr. Cooper, he is speaking with slurred speech. The health care provider asks Mr. Cooper how long he has had difficulty speaking clearly to which Mr. Cooper replies, "I just have a touch of laryngitis is all." Mr. Cooper denies a cough, runny nose, fever, discomfort in his throat, and dysphagia. Concerned, the health care provider suggests that Mr. Cooper go to the emergency department for an evaluation. Despite the health care provider's repeated suggestions, Mr. Cooper refuses.

The next day, the health care provider calls Mr. Cooper's home physical therapist and asks the therapist to call her during the visit and let her know if Mr. Cooper is still exhibiting slurred speech. Later that morning, the physical therapist notifies the health care provider that indeed Mr. Cooper continues to have slurred speech. Per the health care provider's request, Mr. Cooper is transported to the emergency department. An MRI is unrevealing. However, an EMG is consistent with amyotrophic lateral sclerosis (ALS).

Questions

1. What is footdrop and why does it occur in a person with ALS?

2. An AFO brace is prescribed for Mr. Cooper. What does this brace do?

3. An EMG is prescribed for Mr. Cooper. Does this test require his consent? Explain this test to Mr. Cooper and provide instruction regarding anything he should do to prepare for this test.

4. Mr. Cooper who is with his daughter, asks the nurse, "What is ALS? Is it a type of arthritis like I thought?" It can be a sad and emotionally difficult explanation to give, but how would you explain the diagnosis to Mr. Cooper? Include in your discussion the symptoms, cause, incidence, and usual age of onset.

5. What is the prognosis for Mr. Cooper?

6. Riluzole is prescribed for Mr. Cooper. Explain how this medication works. What are the benefits of its use in clients with ALS?

7. Mr. Cooper is prescribed riluzole 50 mg PO every twelve hours. The nurse is teaching Mr. Cooper about his new medication. What should the nurse tell him about how to take riluzole with regard to timing and missed doses? Offer dietary suggestions to maximize the effects of riluzole.

8. Mr. Cooper lives alone, but his daughter and family live close by. The nurse is pleased to learn that the daughter (and family) will be involved in Mr. Cooper's care and be a support system for him as he copes with his disease. Discuss the issues and arrangements the nurse should address with Mr. Cooper and his daughter, considering Mr. Cooper's prognosis.

9. Describe the purpose of the following advance directive alternatives: living will, health care proxy or durable power of attorney, and an advance care medical directive.

10. Discuss the concerns regarding Mr. Cooper's slurred speech. With whom should the nurse collaborate to help Mr. Cooper?

11. The nurse will collaborate with the home care physical therapist to develop an exercise and mobility program and ensure Mr. Cooper's safety in his home. Create a list of at least five components of a safe home environment.

12. An occupational therapist will work with Mr. Cooper to help him with strategies to maintain his independence with activities of daily living (ADLs) for as long as possible. Discuss at least five pieces of equipment available to assist Mr. Cooper with his ADLs.

13. Identify five nursing diagnoses appropriate for Mr. Cooper's plan of care following his diagnosis of ALS.

14. Identify three nursing diagnoses appropriate for Mr. Cooper's plan of care as his ALS progresses.

15. What is palliative care?

16. Why do you think Mr. Cooper self-diagnosed himself with "arthritis" and "laryngitis"?

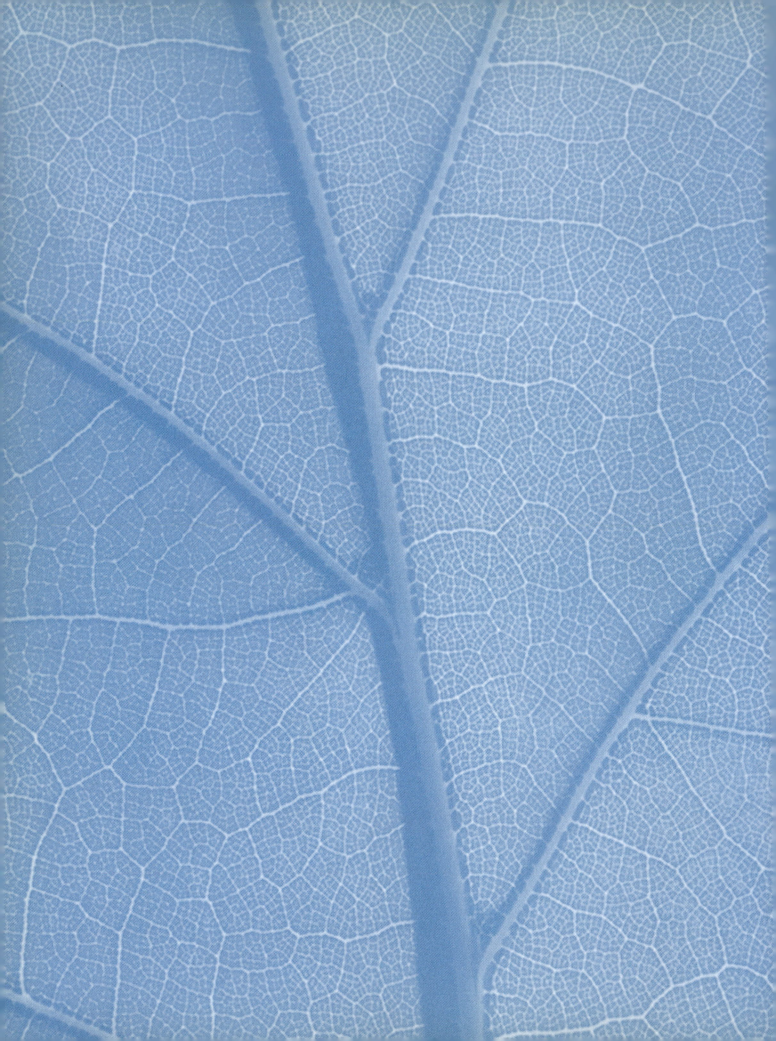

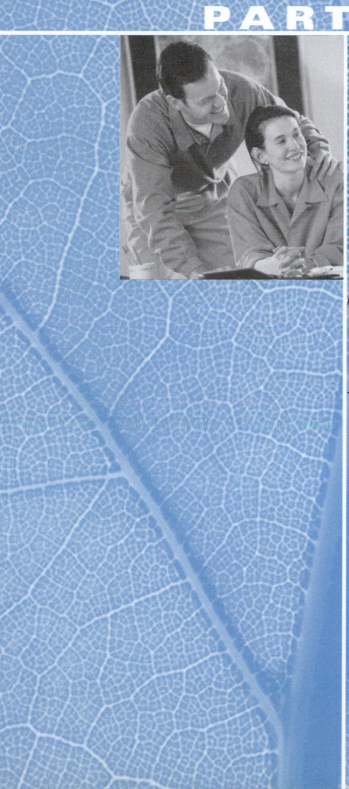

## PART NINE

The Endocrine/ Metabolic System

Mr. Rogers

GENDER

Male

AGE

81

SETTING

- Long-term care

ETHNICITY

- White American

CULTURAL CONSIDERATIONS

PREEXISTING CONDITION

- Benign prostatic hypertrophy (BPH); Gout

COEXISTING CONDITION

COMMUNICATION

- Alert and oriented x 3

DISABILITY

SOCIOECONOMIC

- Long-term care resident for past nine years.

SPIRITUAL/RELIGIOUS

PHARMACOLOGIC

- Colchicine; allopurinol (Alloprim); probenecid (Benemid); sulfinpyrazone (Anturane)

LEGAL

ETHICAL

ALTERNATIVE THERAPY

PRIORITIZATION

DELEGATION

- Nursing collaboration with the dietician.

THE ENDOCRINE/METABOLIC SYSTEM

Level of difficulty: Easy

Overview: The client's symptoms are consistent with cellulitis. His history, however, necessitates consideration of the possibility of a recurrence of gout. The case requires the nurse to consider the defining characteristics of cellulitis and gout. Treatment options are discussed for the two possible diagnoses. Nursing priorities are considered following a definitive medical diagnosis.

Client Profile

Mr. Rogers is an 81-year-old resident of a long-term care facility who tells the nurse, "I have an ache in my right foot." He offers an explanation, suggesting, "I must have stepped on something or twisted my ankle. Maybe I got bit by a bug when I was outside yesterday." The nurse notes the medial aspect of Mr. Rogers' right ankle is reddened, slightly swollen, and warm. His temperature is within normal limits. He has a strong pedal pulse bilaterally.

Case Study

Mr. Rogers's ankle is X-rayed and there is no fracture noted. He has full range-of-motion of his right ankle and lower extremity, although the pain in his ankle increases with movement. A Doppler ultrasound rules out a deep vein thrombosis.

Questions

1. Prior to the Doppler ultrasound, how could the nurse explain this diagnostic procedure to prepare Mr. Rogers?

2. Define cellulitis and discuss its common manifestations.

3. Briefly explain what gout is and describe the causes of primary and secondary gout.

4. What are the common characteristics of each of the four stages of gout?

5. Explain what will facilitate a definitive diagnosis (cellulitis or gout) in Mr. Rogers's case.

6. If it is determined that Mr. Rogers has cellulitis, what treatments will the health care provider most likely prescribe?

7. If Mr. Roger's symptoms are diagnosed as a recurrence of gout, what treatments will the health care provider most likely prescribe? Consider short- and long-term treatment.

8. The nurse collaborates with the dietician to adjust Mr. Rogers's diet to decrease his uric acid levels. Provide at least two examples of purine-containing foods and discuss appropriate fluid and alcohol intake to promote uric acid secretion.

9. Write a nursing diagnosis the nurse will consider adding to Mr. Rogers's plan of care upon learning the definitive diagnosis is gout.

Mr. Jenaro

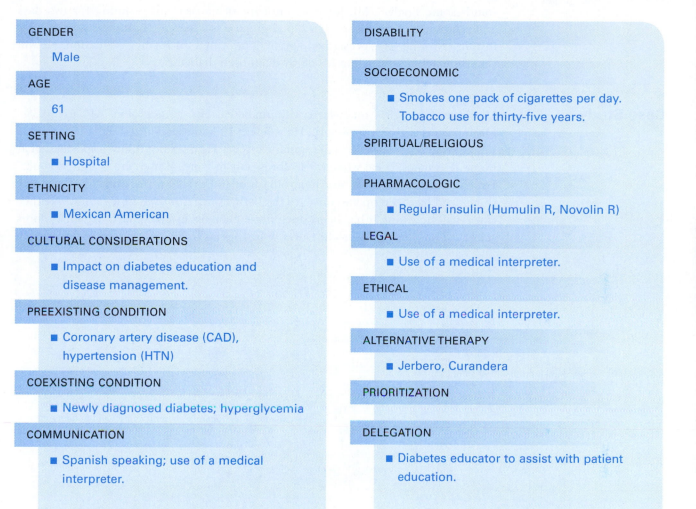

GENDER

Male

AGE

61

SETTING

- Hospital

ETHNICITY

- Mexican American

CULTURAL CONSIDERATIONS

- Impact on diabetes education and disease management.

PREEXISTING CONDITION

- Coronary artery disease (CAD), hypertension (HTN)

COEXISTING CONDITION

- Newly diagnosed diabetes; hyperglycemia

COMMUNICATION

- Spanish speaking; use of a medical interpreter.

DISABILITY

SOCIOECONOMIC

- Smokes one pack of cigarettes per day. Tobacco use for thirty-five years.

SPIRITUAL/RELIGIOUS

PHARMACOLOGIC

- Regular insulin (Humulin R, Novolin R)

LEGAL

- Use of a medical interpreter.

ETHICAL

- Use of a medical interpreter.

ALTERNATIVE THERAPY

- Jerbero, Curandera

PRIORITIZATION

DELEGATION

- Diabetes educator to assist with patient education.

MODERATE

THE ENDOCRINE/METABOLIC SYSTEM

Level of difficulty: Moderate

Overview: This case requires the nurse to recognize the signs of hyperglycemia and convey an understanding of diabetes-related lab values. Type 1 and type 2 diabetes, complications of diabetes, and dietary guidelines are discussed. The nurse must consider the impact that culture may have on diabetes management. The nurse works with a diabetes educator to educate this newly diagnosed diabetic about blood glucose monitoring, medication administration, foot care, sick day management, and proper diet and exercise. The ethical and legal considerations of using an interpreter are addressed.

Client Profile

Mr. Jenaro is a 61-year-old Spanish-speaking man who presents to the emergency room with his wife Dolores. Mrs. Jenaro is also Spanish speaking, but understands some English. Mr. Jenaro complains of nausea and vomiting for two days and symptoms of confusion. His blood glucose is 796 mg/dL. Intravenous regular insulin (Novolin R) is prescribed and he is admitted for further evaluation. He will require teaching regarding his newly diagnosed diabetes.

Case Study

Mr. Jenaro is newly diagnosed with diabetes. His hemoglobin A1C is 10.3%. Mr. Jenaro is slightly overweight. He is 5 feet 10 inches tall and weighs 174 pounds (79 kg). He reports no form of regular exercise. He does not follow a special diet at home. He states, "I eat whatever Dolores puts in front of me. She is a good cook." For the past few months, Mrs. Jenaro has noticed that her husband "has been very thirsty and has been up and down to the bathroom a hundred times a day." Neither can recall how long it has been since these changes in Mr. Jenaro began. Dolores states, "It has been quite a while now. It just seems to be getting worse and worse."

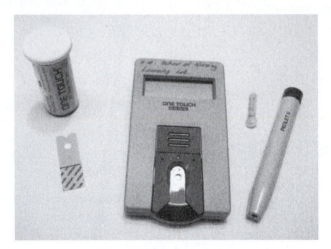

Test strips, blood-glucose meter, and penlette

Questions

1. The nurse does not speak Spanish. Discuss what the nurse should keep in mind to facilitate effective communication using an interpreter. What is the difference between the role of a medical "interpreter" and that of a medical "translator"?

2. Describe the following serum glucose tests used to help confirm the diagnosis of diabetes mellitus: casual, fasting, postprandial, and oral glucose tolerance test.

3. When evaluating Mr. Jenaro's postprandial result, what is important to consider regarding his age and tobacco use?

4. Explain what a hemoglobin A1C (HbA$_{1C}$) lab test tells the health care provider.

5. How might the nurse briefly explain what diabetes is in lay terms to Mr. and Mrs. Jenaro?

6. Explain the difference between type 1 diabetes and type 2 diabetes and who is at increased risk for developing each type. Based on this understanding, which type of diabetes does Mr. Jenaro have?

7. Discuss the prevalence of diabetes and the potential long-term complications of diabetes.

8. List five nursing diagnoses appropriate to consider for Mr. Jenaro.

Questions (continued)

9. Discuss Mr. and Mrs. Jenaro's learning needs. Consider the communication preferences of Mexican Americans.

10. Discuss the dietary recommendations for a diabetic based on the Diabetes Food Pyramid.

11. Discuss how culture may influence Mr. Jenaro's diabetes management in terms of food choices, diet and exercise, and use of an alternative health care provider.

12. Discuss the information the nurse and/or diabetes educator should include when teaching Mr. Jenaro about proper foot care.

13. Discuss the lifestyle considerations the nurse and/or diabetes educator should discuss with Mr. Jenaro and his wife.

14. Discuss what Mr. Jenaro should be taught about how to manage his diabetes on days that he is ill (e.g., if he were to have a stomach virus).

15. Mr. Jenaro meets his friends at a local bar once a week for a beer or two. What impact does alcohol have on a diabetic? Should he discontinue this social activity?

GENDER

Female

AGE

88

SETTING

- Hospital

ETHNICITY

- White American

CULTURAL CONSIDERATIONS

PREEXISTING CONDITION

- Heart failure (HF, CHF); hypothyroidism; gastroesophageal reflux disease (GERD); allergy to penicillin (PCN)

COEXISTING CONDITION

COMMUNICATION

DISABILITY

SOCIOECONOMIC

SPIRITUAL/RELIGIOUS

PHARMACOLOGIC

- Potassium chloride (KCl); pantoprazole sodium (Protonix); levothyroxine sodium (Synthroid); spironolactone (Aldactone); metoclopramide (Reglan); morphine sulfate (MS Contin)

LEGAL

ETHICAL

ALTERNATIVE THERAPY

PRIORITIZATION

DELEGATION

THE ENDOCRINE/METABOLIC SYSTEM

Level of difficulty: Difficult

Overview: This case discusses the diagnostic characteristics and treatment of acute pancreatitis. Use of the Ranson and Glasgow criteria assessment tools to determine disease severity is explained. Potential complications of acute pancreatitis are considered. The nurse educates the client about a scheduled diagnostic procedure to help reduce the client's anxiety. Safe administration of a medication via a nasogastric tube is ensured.

DIFFICULT

Client Profile

Mrs. Miller is an 88-year-old woman who presented with complaints of nausea, vomiting, and abdominal pain. Her vital signs on admission are temperature 99.6°F (37.6°C), blood pressure 113/82, pulse 84, and respiratory rate 20. Her laboratory tests reveal white blood cell count (WBC) 13,000/mm^3, potassium (K$^+$) 3.2 mEq/L, lipase 449 units/L, amylase 306 units/L, total bilirubin 3.4 mg/dL, direct bilirubin 2.2 mg/dL, aspartate aminotransferase (AST) 142 U/L, and alanine aminotransferase (ALT) 390 U/L. Physical examination reveals a distended abdomen that is very tender on palpation. Bowel sounds are present in all four quadrants, but hypoactive. Mrs. Miller is admitted with a diagnosis of acute pancreatitis. She will be kept nothing by mouth (NPO). Intravenous (IV) fluid of D5½ NS with 40 mEq of potassium chloride (KCl) per liter at 100 cc per hour is prescribed. The health care provider prescribes continued administration of her preadmission medications, that is, pantoprazole sodium and levothyroxine sodium (in IV form since the client is NPO) and spironolactone (available in oral form), and adds the prescription of IV metoclopramide and morphine sulfate. A nasogastric (NG) tube is inserted and attached to low wall suction. She is scheduled to have a kidneys, ureters, and bladder (KUB) abdominal X-ray in the morning.

Case Study

Mrs. Miller's NG tube is draining yellow-brown drainage. Her pain is being managed effectively with IV morphine 4 mg every four hours. She is NPO and awaiting transport to radiology for a KUB. Mrs. Miller is anxious and has many questions for the nurse: "What is the test I am having done today? What is pancreatitis? Will I need to have surgery? Why did they put this tube in my nose? When will I be able to eat real food?"

Questions

1. Briefly explain acute pancreatitis and discuss its incidence.

2. Mrs. Miller's admitting diagnosis is acute pancreatitis. Can a person have chronic pancreatitis? If so, what is the incidence, and how would you define chronic pancreatitis?

3. Discuss the common clinical manifestations of acute pancreatitis.

4. Briefly discuss the diagnostic tests that help confirm the diagnosis of pancreatitis.

5. Identify the assessment findings in Mrs. Miller's case that are consistent with acute pancreatitis.

6. Mrs. Miller asks, "What is the test I am having done today?" How would the nurse describe a KUB to Mrs. Miller?

7. Identify the possible causes of acute pancreatitis. Discuss the physiology of the two major causes of acute pancreatitis in the United States, and note which individuals are at greatest risk.

8. The severity of an acute pancreatitis episode can be assessed using two tools: (1) Ranson/Imrie criteria and (2) modified Glasgow criteria. Describe each of these tools.

9. Briefly discuss the treatment options for pancreatitis, and explain why Mrs. Miller has an NG tube to low wall suction.

10. Discuss the complications that can arise if pancreatitis is not treated.

11. Evaluate Mrs. Miller's potassium level. Should the nurse question the health care provider's prescription for the diuretic spironolactone? Why or why not?

12. Because Mrs. Miller is NPO, the nurse must administer the oral spironolactone via the NG tube. Is it appropriate to crush this medication? Why or why not? What intervention should the nurse take following administration of the medication to facilitate absorption?

Questions (continued)

13. Which type of diet will Mrs. Miller advance to when her NPO status is discontinued? What types of liquids are allowed on this diet?

14. Identify the priority nursing diagnosis for Mrs. Miller's plan of care and two additional nursing diagnoses that the nurse should consider.

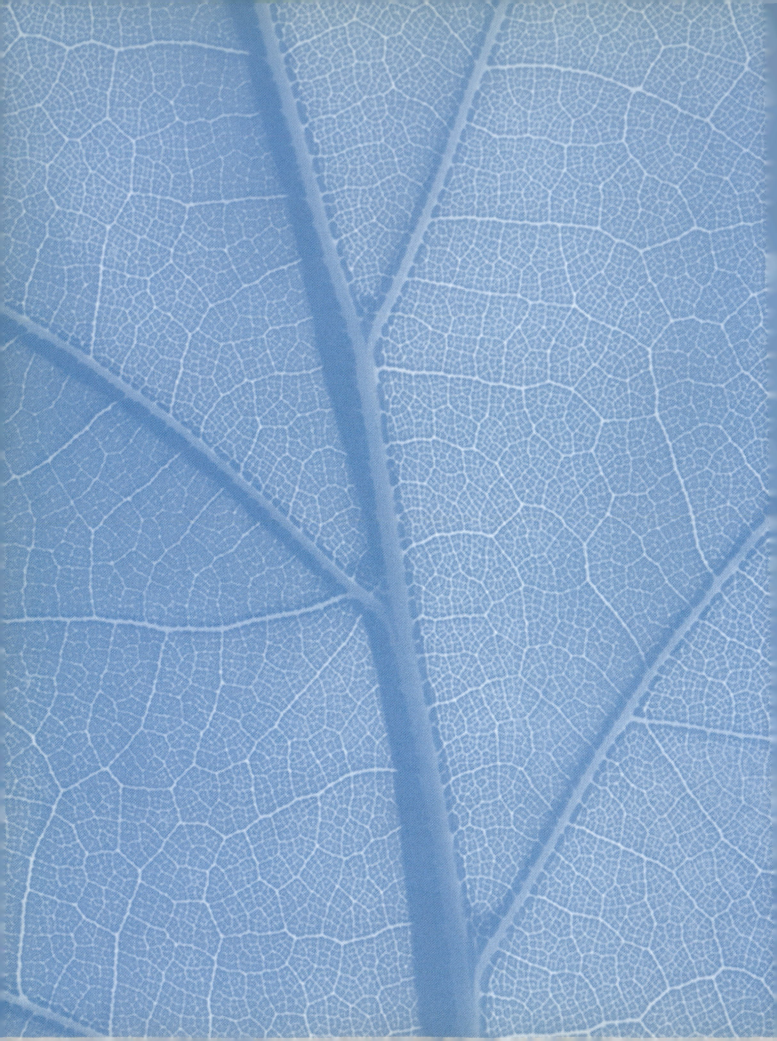

PART TEN

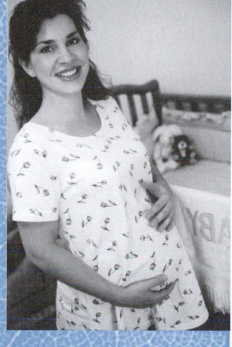

The Reproductive System

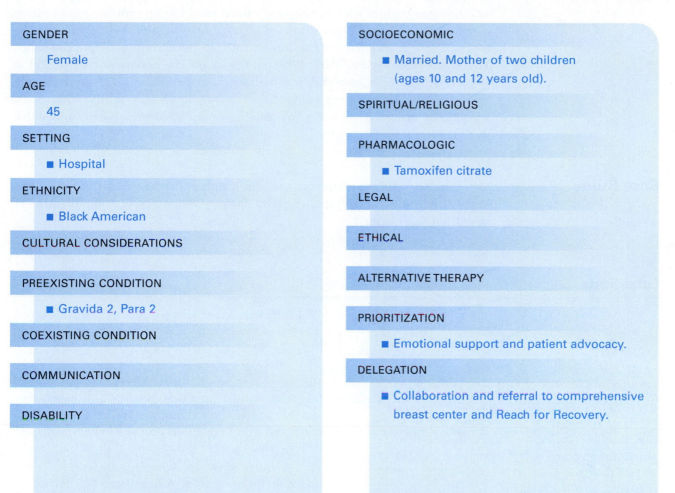

GENDER

Female

AGE

45

SETTING

■ Hospital

ETHNICITY

■ Black American

CULTURAL CONSIDERATIONS

PREEXISTING CONDITION

■ Gravida 2, Para 2

COEXISTING CONDITION

COMMUNICATION

DISABILITY

SOCIOECONOMIC

■ Married. Mother of two children (ages 10 and 12 years old).

SPIRITUAL/RELIGIOUS

PHARMACOLOGIC

■ Tamoxifen citrate

LEGAL

ETHICAL

ALTERNATIVE THERAPY

PRIORITIZATION

■ Emotional support and patient advocacy.

DELEGATION

■ Collaboration and referral to comprehensive breast center and Reach for Recovery.

THE REPRODUCTIVE SYSTEM

Level of difficulty: Easy

Overview: The client in this case requires nursing support during the diagnostic phase of breast cancer. Nursing care for the pre- and postoperative client is discussed. Priority nursing diagnoses in the postoperative period are identified. The use of tamoxifen after surgery is explained and the purpose of a port-a-cath device is reviewed. The nurse must provide discharge instructions and referral for ongoing rehabilitation and support.

Client Profile

Mrs. Whitney is a 45-year-old woman who noticed a lump in her left breast during her monthly breast self-exam two weeks ago. She made an appointment with her gynecologist who documents "a fixed round lump with irregular borders palpated in the upper outer quadrant of left breast at 2:00. Left axillary edema noted. There is symmetry of the breasts with no puckering or nipple discharge. The client denies pain." Mrs. Whitney began having her menstrual period at 10 years of age. She has two children, both of whom she breastfed for approximately twelve months. Mrs. Whitney's oldest sister died of breast cancer. Mrs. Whitney has a diagnostic mammogram and a fine-needle aspiration biopsy. It is determined that she has stage II breast cancer.

Case Study

Mrs. Whitney will have a lumpectomy with lymph node dissection (partial mastectomy). A Jackson-Pratt (JP) drain will be in place postoperatively. Following surgery, tamoxifen is prescribed.

Questions

1. Discuss the best time of the month to perform breast self-examination (BSE).

2. What factors placed Mrs. Whitney at greater risk for the development of breast cancer? Discuss the risk factors associated with Mrs. Whitney's ethnicity.

3. Mrs. Whitney's past medical history is "gravida 2, para 2." Explain what these terms indicate.

4. Briefly discuss the relationship between breastfeeding and Mrs. Whitney's risk of breast cancer.

5. Discuss the priority nursing intervention prior to Mrs. Whitney's biopsy and immediately following diagnosis.

6. The nurse is teaching Mrs. Whitney how to use an incentive spirometer (IS). How will the nurse tell Mrs. Whitney to use the IS and what will the nurse explain as the rationale for IS use postoperatively?

7. Mrs. Whitney is discharged from the post-anesthesia care unit (PACU) following her lumpectomy and lymph node dissection. Now that she is in your care on the nursing unit, discuss what you will assess.

8. Identify five postoperative nursing diagnoses to consider for Mrs. Whitney. List the diagnoses in order of priority.

9. In the immediate postoperative period prior to removal of the Jackson-Pratt (JP) drain, how should the nurse assist Mrs. Whitney to position her left arm?

10. The nurse hangs a sign above Mrs. Whitney's bed to alert other members of the health care team about interventions to maintain Mrs. Whitney's safety and prevent complications of her surgery. Discuss what the sign should say.

11. The nurse gives Mrs. Whitney contact information for "Reach for Recovery." Discuss the support services available through this program.

12. Mrs. Whitney is going home today. The nurse is teaching her about possible complications of her surgery. Explain what lymphedema is, the chances of developing lymphedema, and its manifestations. Identify at least two other complications the nurse will include in the discharge teaching.

13. Discuss why tamoxifen is prescribed as part of Mrs. Whitney's treatment plan.

14. Mrs. Whitney asks about the adverse effects of tamoxifen. Create a list of the possible common and potentially life-threatening adverse effects of this medication. What instructions should you include regarding sexual activity?

CLINICAL DECISION MAKING

Case Studies in Pharmacologic Nursing

Hyacinth Martin
BSN, MA, MSEd, MPS, RNBC

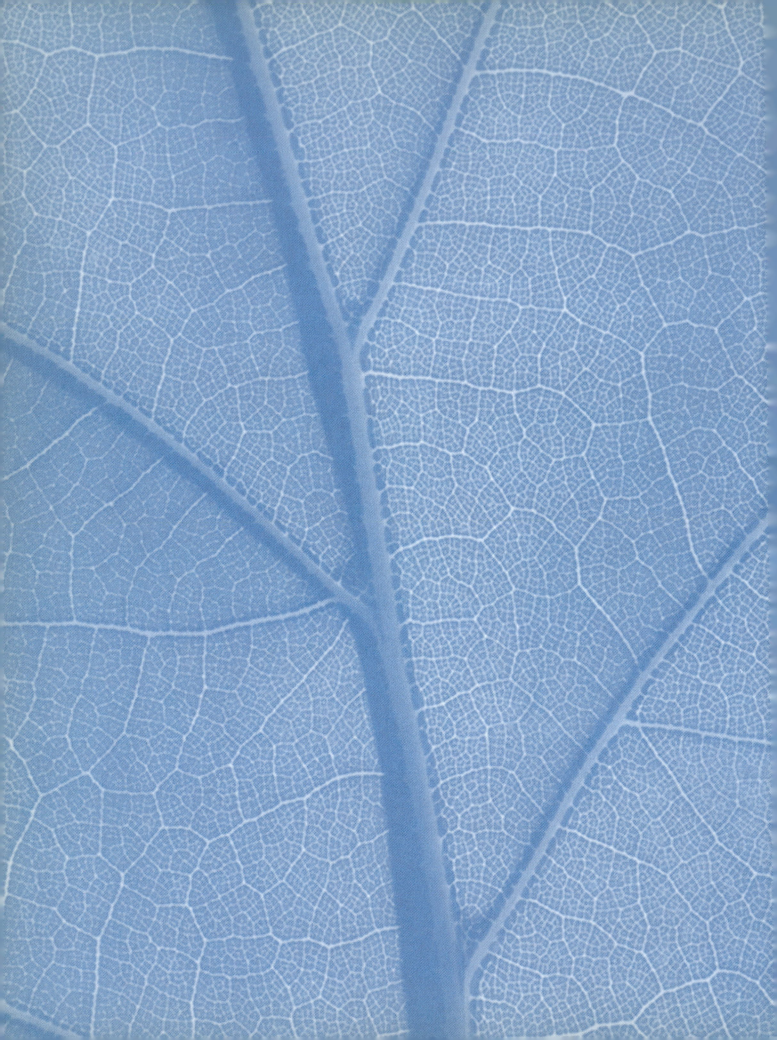

PART ONE

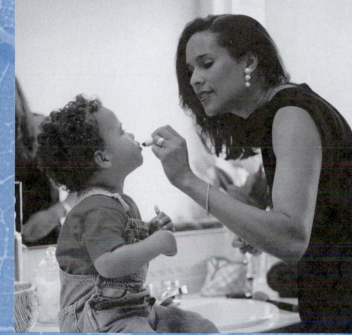

The Digestive and Urinary Systems

Cyanocobalamin (Vitamin B$_{12}$ Deficiency Anemia, Pernicious Anemia)

GENDER

M

AGE

64

SETTING

- Hospital

ETHNICITY/CULTURE

- White

PREEXISTING CONDITIONS

- Zollinger-Ellison syndrome

COEXISTING CONDITIONS

- Total gastrectomy

LIFESTYLE

- Retired

COMMUNICATION

DISABILITY

SOCIOECONOMIC STATUS

- Middle

SPIRITUAL/RELIGIOUS

- Catholic

PHARMACOLOGIC

- Vitamin B$_{12}$
- Folic acid (Apo-Folic)

PSYCHOSOCIAL

- Periods of irritability and depression

LEGAL

ETHICAL

ALTERNATIVE THERAPY

- Clams
- Frankfurters
- Red beans

PRIORITIZATION

- Monitor for signs of alteration in cognition or irritability

DELEGATION

- RN
- Client education

THE DIGESTIVE AND URINARY SYSTEMS

Level of difficulty: Easy

Overview: This case involves a thorough assessment of the past medical and surgical history. The nurse must observe the client for signs of impaired memory or irritability during the assessment.

Client Profile

Mr. L is a 64-year-old client who had a total gastrectomy of the small and large bowel resection including the ileum two years ago. Mr. L is referred to the hospital inpatient clinic by his primary health care provider for further evaluation after a routine annual examination.

Case Study

During the initial interview, Mr. L complains of having had anorexia, nausea, vomiting, and abdominal pain for the past two days. Physical assessment findings include paresthesia of the hands and feet, reduced vibratory and position senses, ataxia, and muscle weakness. Assessment data on his daily nutritional intake includes frankfurters, brewer's yeast, clams, dried beans, and carrots. Vital signs taken by the nursing assistant are:

Blood pressure: 120/78

Pulse: 78

Respirations: 18

Temperature: 98.4° F

Tentative diagnosis of pernicious anemia is made and the health care provider prescribes serum laboratory data: hematocrit, hemoglobin, methylmalonic acid and homocysteine level, platelet count, red blood cell count, folic acid level, and peripheral blood smear. Mr. L is to return to the clinic in two days for a follow-up on the results of the laboratory data, confirmation of the diagnosis, and prescription as required. Mr. L returns to the clinic as scheduled. His laboratory results are:

Hematocrit (Hct): 38%

Hemoglobin (Hgb): 16 g/dL

Methylmalonic acid and homocysteine levels: elevated

Platelet count: 200,000/mm^3

Red blood cell (RBC) count: 2,500,000/mm^3

Folic acid: 3 ng/mL

Also, the peripheral blood smear shows oval, macrocytic, and hyperchromic RBCs. The health care provider reviews the data, and a diagnosis of pernicious anemia is confirmed.

The following are prescribed:
- Cyanocobalamin (vitamin B$_{12}$) 2,000 mcg PO per day for two weeks, then 1,000 mcg PO per day
- Folic acid (Apo-Folic) 0.4 mg PO daily

Questions

1. Explain the pathophysiology of vitamin B_{12} deficiency and its relationship to pernicious anemia.

2. Why is vitamin B_{12} anemia called megaloblastic anemia?

3. Discuss classic manifestations of vitamin B_{12} deficiency anemia a nurse should expect to observe during assessment of this client.

4. Discuss the specific relationship of erythrocytes (RBCs) and vitamin B_{12} deficiency and nursing management.

5. Discuss common nursing diagnoses for vitamin B_{12} deficiency anemia.

6. What are the purposes for the prescribed medications?

7. What are the most common adverse reactions, drug-to-drug, drug-to-food/herbal interactions of cyanocobalamin (vitamin B_{12})?

8. Discuss factors that may inhibit folic acid absorption.

9. Discuss client education for vitamin B_{12} deficiency anemia.

10. Discuss nursing implications for clients with vitamin B_{12} deficiency anemia.

Renal Calculi

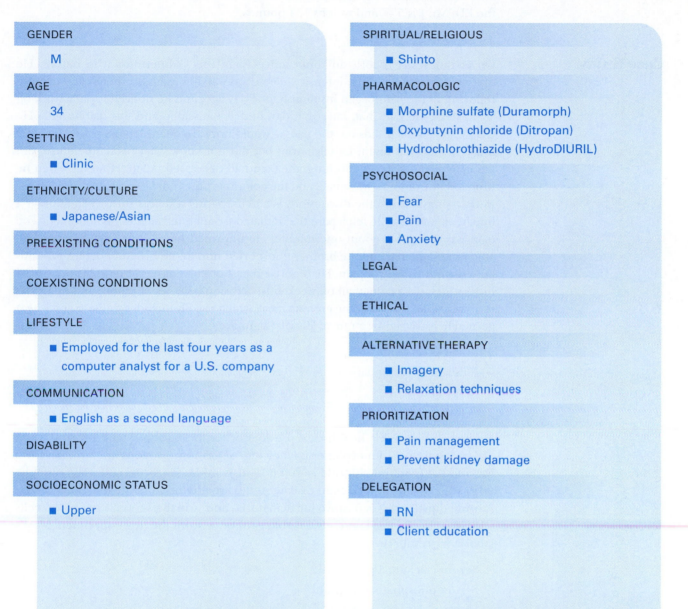

GENDER

M

AGE

34

SETTING

■ Clinic

ETHNICITY/CULTURE

■ Japanese/Asian

PREEXISTING CONDITIONS

COEXISTING CONDITIONS

LIFESTYLE

■ Employed for the last four years as a computer analyst for a U.S. company

COMMUNICATION

■ English as a second language

DISABILITY

SOCIOECONOMIC STATUS

■ Upper

SPIRITUAL/RELIGIOUS

■ Shinto

PHARMACOLOGIC

■ Morphine sulfate (Duramorph)
■ Oxybutynin chloride (Ditropan)
■ Hydrochlorothiazide (HydroDIURIL)

PSYCHOSOCIAL

■ Fear
■ Pain
■ Anxiety

LEGAL

ETHICAL

ALTERNATIVE THERAPY

■ Imagery
■ Relaxation techniques

PRIORITIZATION

■ Pain management
■ Prevent kidney damage

DELEGATION

■ RN
■ Client education

THE DIGESTIVE AND URINARY SYSTEMS

Level of difficulty: Easy

Overview: This case involves pain management as well as questioning the client about personal or family history of urologic stones, obtaining a diet history, including fluid intake patterns. If the client has a history of stone formation, it should be determined if chemical analysis of the stone(s) was performed in the past and what the preventive measures were.

Client Profile

Mr. J is a 34-year-old male who arrives at the emergency department (ED) of a busy urban hospital accompanied by his brother, who drove Mr. J from his office to the ED. Mr. J is 5′6″ and weighs 134 pounds.

Case Study

On arrival, Mr. J reports an "unbearable" pain that is intermittent in nature. He describes the pain as more intense while he was walking to his brother's car. Mr. J also reports that the pain began insidiously, one day ago, and he noticed it while working at his desk. He said that, later that day, he felt nauseated and was diaphoretic. He tried to take some fluids but the nausea would not subside, which decreased his fluid intake. Later that night, he felt warm, but did not know what his temperature was. Upon awakening in the morning, the pain had decreased much. However, when he urinated, the amount was small, and the color was pink-red. He prepared and left for work, trying to avoid the discomfort. While preparing a report for presentation at a luncheon meeting, he felt a pain that radiated from his left side to his abdomen. The pain was severe for about one minute. He informed his brother, who works in an adjoining building, and the brother transported him to the ED. Mr. J denies previous episodes of this type of pain. He reports no past or current medication history. Social history includes racquetball on weekends, occasional games of tennis, and he enjoys drinking white wine with the evening meal, which usually includes rhubarb and wheat germ. He is triaged by a nurse. His vital signs are:

> Blood pressure: 130/82
> Pulse: 94 and regular
> Respirations: 18
> Temperature: 101.0° F

He is seen by the ED health care provider, who does a history and physical, then orders a stat dose of morphine sulfate 5 mg/SQ. An intravenous line with dextrose 5% and 0.45 sodium chloride at 100 mL/hr is initiated. A computed tomography (CT) scan is done and calcium oxalate stones are identified in the left kidney calyx. A urine dipstick test is positive for hematuria, and urinalysis reveals red blood cells (RBCs) in the urine. There is no turbidity or odor from the urine specimen. Mr. J's laboratory results are:

> Serum calcium: 10.5 mg/dL
> Serum phosphate: 5 mg/dL
> Serum uric acid: 9 mg/dL
> Urine uric acid: 800 mg/24 hr
> Urine calcium: 260 mg/24 hr
> Urine phosphate: 1.3 g/24 hr
> Urine specific gravity: 1.026

After the health care provider reviews the laboratory data and diagnostic results, a diagnosis of renal calculi is confirmed. Mr. J's pain has subsided and he denies feeling nauseated. He has voided 100 mL of dusky-colored urine with trace elements of blood. The urine is strained and there is one visible stone. A sample of the urine is sent to the lab for microscopic analysis. Mr. J's vital signs are:

> Blood pressure: 110/70
> Pulse: 78 and regular

Respirations: 14

Temperature: 98.4° F

Mr. J will be discharged in the late evening. Mr. J is to return to his primary health care provider for follow-up care in two weeks.

The following are prescribed:

- Morphine sulfate (Astromorph PF) 1–2 mg IV q1–2h
- Oxybutynin chloride (Ditropan) 5 mg PO two times per day, today only
- Hydrochlorothiazide (HydroDIURIL) 50 mg PO two times per day
- IV D 5.45% NS at 100 mL/hr until 5:00 PM today and encourage fluid intake of two to three liters today
- Accurate intake and output, and strain all urine
- Discharge after 5:00 PM with follow-up appointment in two weeks

Questions

1. Discuss factors that contribute to urolithiasis.

2. Discuss the most common types of kidney stones.

3. Discuss common manifestations of urolithiasis.

4. Discuss common complications of urolithiasis.

5. What are the purposes for the prescribed orders?

6. What are the most common adverse reactions, drug-to-drug, drug-to-food/herbal interactions of the prescribed medications?

7. Discuss other diagnostic tests used to identify urolithiasis.

8. Discuss endourologic procedures used to remove or crush urolithiasis.

9. Discuss the difference between a ureterolithotomy and a pyelolithotomy.

10. Discuss client education for urolithiasis.

Stage IIC Cancer of the Prostate

GENDER

Male

AGE

52

SETTING

- Urology outpatient clinic of a medical center

ETHNICITY/CULTURE

- Mexican American

PREEXISTING CONDITIONS

COEXISTING CONDITIONS

- Strong familial predisposition; two brothers with colon cancer

LIFESTYLE

- Utility employee
- Worked with asbestos for 28 years

COMMUNICATION

- English as a second language

DISABILITY

SOCIOECONOMIC STATUS

- Middle

SPIRITUAL/RELIGIOUS

- Catholic

PHARMACOLOGIC

PSYCHOSOCIAL

- Anxiety
- Depression
- Fatigue

LEGAL

- Work-related factor may result in compensation

ETHICAL

- Possibility of early retirement

ALTERNATIVE THERAPY

- St. John's Wort

PRIORITIZATION

- Initial interview
- Questions about genitourinary history

DELEGATION

- RN
- Client education

MODERATE

THE DIGESTIVE AND URINARY SYSTEMS

Level of difficulty: Moderate

Overview: This case involves the use of the nursing process, systems assessment, and critical thinking skills to provide optimum care while monitoring fluid and electrolyte status. Focus will be on family history, knowledge of the disease process, and the importance of compliance with treatment regimens.

Client Profile

Mr. G is a 52-year-old married male who is 5′10″ and weighs 190 pounds. He is employed by a major utility gas company. Mr. G is scheduled for an office visit with his family health care provider due to results of prior laboratory and diagnostic tests.

Case Study

Mr. G reports frequency of urination with reduction in urinary stream, dysuria, nocturia, change in bowel habits (constipation and occasional diarrhea), and a feeling of incomplete bowel emptying. He is concerned about the symptoms because of his family history of colon cancer. He also reports having had a history of gastric ulcers for five years and a family history cancer in both of his brothers. When questioned about his dietary habits, Mr. G reports maintaining a diet low in fiber, and high in fat, protein, and refined carbohydrates. However, every year since he turned 40, he has undergone an annual physical exam with his primary health care provider that includes digital/rectal examination His most recent digital/rectal examination was "abnormal;" his stools have been negative guaiac annually. At age 50, he had a proctosigmoidoscopy because of unusual constipation. His vital signs are:

Blood pressure: 140/78

Pulse: 80

Respirations: 18

Temperature: 98.4° F

During a rectal assessment at the clinic, a colon mass is located and will be staged as needed after further examination. The health care provider does a complete history and physical examination, then the client is scheduled for the following diagnostic tests: colonoscopy, serum for prostatic-specific antigen, acid phosphatase, alkaline phosphatase, and a transurethral ultrasonography (TRUS). Mr. G returns to the medical center on different dates to have the tests done. The tests are done as scheduled, and the results are received and reviewed by an oncologist and the medical team. Mr. G's laboratory results are:

Prostatic-specific antigen (PSA): 3.8 ng/mL

Acid phosphatase: 0.53 I/L

Serum alkaline phosphatase: 128 U/L

The TRUS reveals small tumors in the prostate gland. The oncologist, surgeon, and health care provider explain the results to Mr. G and make a diagnosis of prostate cancer Stage IIC. Plans for treatment are explained to the client and the decision is made for treatment. Mr. G remains in the Same Day Care oncology unit of the hospital for further instructions but will be sent home today.

The following are prescribed:

- External-beam irradiation with 175 rads × one week. Start first dose today then discharge to home.
- Oxybutynin chloride (Ditropan) 5 mg PO two times per day
- Return to Same Day Care oncology unit × six more days

Questions

1. Discuss the risk factors and pathophysiology of prostate cancer.

2. Discuss clinical manifestations of prostate cancer.

3. Discuss cultural and ethnic considerations for the male reproductive system.

4. Discuss diagnostic studies used to aid the confirmation of prostate cancer.

5. What are the purposes of the prescribed treatment and medication?

6. What are common adverse reactions to the prescribed treatment and medication?

7. Discuss other therapies that may be prescribed to treat prostate cancer.

8. Discuss surgical procedures used for Stage IIC prostate cancer.

9. Discuss postoperative complications of prostate surgeries.

10. Discuss client education for prostate cancer.

Ulcerative Colitis

GENDER

F

AGE

35

SETTING

- Hospital

ETHNICITY/CULTURE

- White American

PREEXISTING CONDITIONS

- Stress

COEXISTING CONDITIONS

- Recurrent respiratory infection
- Emotional stress

LIFESTYLE

- Phlebotomy supervisor for a large private, nonprofit medical organization

COMMUNICATION

DISABILITY

SOCIOECONOMIC STATUS

- Middle

SPIRITUAL/RELIGIOUS

- Episcopalian

PHARMACOLOGIC

- Mesalamine (Asacol)
- Sulfasalazine (Azulfidine)
- Metronidazole (Flagyl)

PSYCHOSOCIAL

- Anxiety

LEGAL

ETHICAL

- Is the quality of life optimal for a 35-year-old client with ulcerative colitis disease?

ALTERNATE THERAPY

- Flaxseed
- Vitamin C
- Aloe vera

PRIORITIZATION

- Assess pain
- Maintain fluid and electrolyte balance

DELEGATION

- RN
- Client education

MODERATE

THE DIGESTIVE AND URINARY SYSTEMS

Level of difficulty: Moderate

Overview: This case involves accurate assessment of fluid loss, monitoring for signs of dehydration, and critical assessment of the abdomen for characteristics of bowel sounds, distention, and tenderness. It also involves prioritization in a triage situation to prevent serious complications.

Client Profile

Ms. V is a 35-year-old, unmarried phlebotomy supervisor for a large medical team. Ms. V is 5′10″ and weighs 120 pounds. She has a two-year history of inflammatory bowel disease and has been hospitalized twice for exacerbations of intermittent diarrhea and colicky pain in the right lower quadrant. She appears anxious upon arrival at the emergency department (ED) and verbalizes frustration with the recurring problems. Ms. V also reports occasional periods of depression, which she relates to the disease.

Case Study

Ms. V's fiancé accompanies her to the ED. Her vital signs on admission are:

Blood pressure: 110/68

Pulse: 104 and regular

Respirations: 20

Temperature: 101.2° F

Ms. V experienced ten bloody bowel movements of moderate amounts accompanied by localized abdominal pain prior to arriving in the ED. An intravenous line with IV fluid of D_5LR at 150 cc/hr is initiated via a peripheral venous access. Ms. V is later seen by the ED health care provider and a gastroenterologist for initial assessment and data collection to help determine her diagnosis. Ms. V is placed on "nothing by mouth" (NPO) status, except ice chips. Plans to insert a nasogastric tube if she vomits are discussed with the health care provider and nurse. Serum labs prescribed prior to invasive diagnostic work-up include: hematocrit, hemoglobin, white blood cell count, erythrocyte sedimentation rate, serum sodium, serum potassium, serum chloride, albumin, stool for occult blood, ova, parasites, culture, and sensitivity. Results of the serum labs are:

White blood cell (WBC) count: 12,000/mm³

Erythrocyte sedimentation rate (ESR): 24 mm/hr

Hemoglobin (Hgb): 15.2 g/dL

Hematocrit (Hct): 30.5%

Potassium (K+): 2.6 mEq/L

Blood urea nitrogen (BUN): 18 mg/dL

Sodium (Na): 134 mEq/L

Chloride (Cl⁻): 98 mEq/L

Creatinine: 0.09 mg/dL

A double-contrast barium enema with air contrast and colonoscopy with biopsies are discussed with Ms. V and will be scheduled for the next day if the vomiting and diarrhea subsides. The vomiting and diarrhea subside and the double-contrast barium enema and biopsies are done, which provide the definitive diagnosis of ulcerative colitis (UC). The results are reviewed by the radiologist, followed by discussion with the multidisciplinary team and the client, and the plan of care is initiated.

The following are prescribed:

- Mesalamine (Asacol) 800 mg PO three times per day
- Sulfasalazine (Azulfidine) 250 mg PO four times per day
- Metronidazole (Flagyl) 7.5 mg/kg IV q6h

- Loperamide (Imodium) 4 mg PO followed by 2 mg after each formed stool
- Potassium chloride (K-chloride) 10 mEq/100 mL IV × four doses, repeat serum potassium after last dose

Questions

1. What are common nursing diagnoses for the client with UC?

2. What are the expected findings of the barium enema with air contrast and endoscopy?

3. What is the purpose of intestinal biopsies in diagnosing UC?

4. What type of psychotherapy would be most effective for Ms. V at this time?

5. Discuss a serious cardiac complication that may develop due to Ms. V's low serum potassium level.

6. What are the purposes for the prescribed orders?

7. What are the most common adverse reactions, drug-to-drug, drug-to-food/herbal interactions of the prescribed medications?

8. Identify complementary and alternative therapies for clients with UC.

9. Discuss specific nursing intervention activities for clients receiving intravenous potassium replacement for hypokalemia.

10. Discuss community-based nursing care for clients with risk for hypokalemia being discharged to home.

Acute Renal Failure

GENDER

F

AGE

60

SETTING

- Hospital

ETHNICITY/CULTURE

- Black American

PREEXISTING CONDITIONS

- Hypertension
- Diabetes mellitus type 2

COEXISTING CONDITIONS

- Diabetes
- Hypertension

LIFESTYLE

- Housewife

COMMUNICATION

- Spanish and English

DISABILITY

- Yes

SOCIOECONOMIC STATUS

- Low

SPIRITUAL/RELIGIOUS

- Catholic

PHARMACOLOGIC

- Dopamine HcL
- Lantus (Insuline glargine)
- Human regular insulin (Humulin R)
- Nifedipine (Procardia)
- Furosemide (Lasix)
- Calcium carbonate (Os-cal)
- Digoxin (Lanoxin)
- Sodium polystyrene sulfonate (Kayexelate)

PSYCHOSOCIAL

- Depression

LEGAL

ETHICAL

- Is there an ethical dilemma of randomizing clients with ARF to a certain dialysis modality?

ALTERNATIVE THERAPY

- Prayer

PRIORITIZATION

- Determine risk factors for ARF
- Assess fluid balance
- Monitor serum potassium levels

DELEGATION

- RN
- Client education

MODERATE

THE DIGESTIVE AND URINARY SYSTEMS

Level of difficulty: Moderate

Overview: This case involves critical assessment of the client. The nurse must question the client about decrease in urinary output; history of hypertension; use of prescribed medications/herbals taken independently; history of constipation or diarrhea, anorexia, nausea or vomiting, and unusual fatigue. The case involves prioritization in a triage situation with other clients experiencing acute onset of other diseases. The nurse must use critical thinking in triaging clients in order of highest priority to avoid or manage complications that could develop. The nurse must be knowledgeable about sites of drug metabolism and must constantly monitor for unintended effects of prescribed drugs.

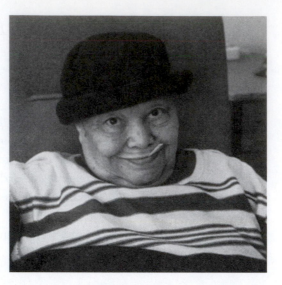

Client Profile

Ms. D is a 60-year-old client who lives in an apartment building in a "comfortable" two-bedroom apartment. Her significant others include her parents, who are alive and reside in a nursing home; and four younger brothers and one sister, all of whom are alive and well and have frequent contact with Ms. D. Her family history includes both parents having hypertension and a younger brother having type I diabetes for five years. Ms. D is 5′5″ and weighs 190 pounds.

Case Study

Ms. D is admitted to the hospital with complaints of increased fatigue, lethargy, and occasional confusion. After the initial interview, history, and physical examination by a registered nurse (RN) and a physician's assistant (PA), Ms. D is transferred from the triage area to a medical care unit. Vital signs in the emergency department (ED) are:

Blood pressure:160/98

Pulse: 78

Respirations: 16

Temperature: 98.5° F

Ms. D informs the receiving nurse in the medical unit that she is on lantus (Insulin glargine) ten units daily at bedtime, and does fingerstick glucose monitoring every four hours during the day. She admits being anxious because during the past two weeks she has experienced unusual dryness of the skin, which requires scratching. Ms. D decided to come to the hospital and goes to the ED because she believes she will get attention faster. When Ms. D is asked about the amount of urine voided since she awoke, she informs the receiving nurse and PA that since she has awakened, she has urinated a smaller amount within a seven-hour period when compared to other times. However, Ms. D believes the decrease in urinary output is related to her decrease in appetite, including fluids. Ms. D is currently taking furosemide 40 mg PO daily, captopril 50 mg PO two times per day for high blood pressure, and ibuprofen or naproxen occasionally for joint pains. She is also taking insulin for diabetes and ibuprofen PRN joint pain prescribed by her primary health care provider. Ms. D also reports a noted decrease in urinary output and unusual irritation frequently. She is admitted to the unit and placed on a cardiac monitor.

A peripheral intravenous line is inserted, and IV fluid of NaCL 0.45% at 75 mL/hr is initiated. The nurse continues with the physical assessment and auscultation of her heart sounds. There is S_3 gallop and bilateral rales over lung fields, especially at the bases, and +1 pedal edema at the ankles. Ms. D is placed in a semi-Fowler's position, and the nurse assigns a certified nursing assistant to remain with Ms. D, while she documents her findings. A chest X-ray is done and signs of congested heart failure are evident. Furosemide 40 mg IV is administered stat. Ms. D is seen by a health care provider and a history and physical examination are done, the history and assessment done by the nurse are reviewed, and the following diagnostic and laboratory tests are ordered: X-ray of the kidneys, ureters, and bladder (KUB); renal ultrasonography; and a cystoscopy. Ms. D's laboratory values are:

Blood urea nitrogen (BUN): 25 mg/dL

Creatinine: 2.8 mg/dL

Sodium (Na): 130 mEq/L

Potassium (K+): 6.8 mEq/L

Calcium: 8 mg/dL

Magnesium: 3 mEq/L

Phosphorous: 6 mg/dL

Glucose: 118 mg/dL

Urine specific gravity: 1.002

Urine sodium concentration: 48 mEq/L.

A consent is signed for a cystoscopy and central venous pressure catheter insertion. The catheter is inserted and an X-ray is negative for malposition of the catheter. Intravenous fluid is changed to Lactated Ringers at 75 mL/hr, and a foley catheter is inserted and attached to a urometer collecting bag. The results of the diagnostic and labs tests are received and reviewed by the health care provider: the KUB is negative for stones obstructing the renal pelvis, ureters or bladder; the renal ultrasonography is negative for urinary obstruction, but the renal calyces and collecting ducts are dilated, and tissue perfusion is impaired. The cystoscopy is negative for obstruction of the lower urinary tract. The medical doctor, the PA, the RN, an endocrinologist, and a cardiologist review the results of the diagnostic studies. A primary diagnosis of ARF is made, and secondary diagnosis of congested heart failure. The health care provider discusses the plan of care, including hemodialysis, with Ms. D. She is transferred to the medical intensive care unit (MICU), an electrocardiogram (EKG) is done, and the client is placed on continuous telemetry to monitor for life-threatening arrhythmias. Because of the current elevated serum potassium level, the EKG reveals tall, peaked T waves, widening of the QRS complex, and ST segment depression. Dopamine HcL (Intropin) infusion 2 microgram/kg is initiated.

The following are prescribed:
- Furosemide (Lasix) 40 mg IV q6h × 24 hours
- Nifedipine (Procardia) 20 mg PO three times per day
- Lantus (Insulin gargline) 10 units SC at bedtime
- Human regular insulin (Humulin R): Fingerstick sliding scale (FSS) q4h PRN for:

  Glucose less than 100 mg/dL, no insulin coverage; 100–140, two units SC; 141–180, four units SC; 181–220, six units SC; 221–260, eight units SC; 261–300, ten units SC; 301–340, twelve units SC; greater than 341, call the MD.

- Calcium carbonate (Os-cal) 4 g PO with meals
- Digoxin (Lanoxin) 125 mg PO every morning
- Sodium polystyrene sulfonate (Kayexalate) 15 g PO daily for potassium level greater than 5 mEq/L
- Monitor serum creatinine, BUN, serum sodium, potassium, glucose, hematocrit and hemoglobin, urine protein, and urine specific gravity daily.
- Dietary consultation, strict intake and output, record daily weight

Questions

1. Discuss your understanding of the medical diagnosis of ARF, considering all of the information provided in the case study, and the pathophysiology of ARF.

2. Discuss some of the common causes of ARF.

3. Discuss the phases that ARF progresses through.

4. What are the primary strategies of treatment for ARF?

5. What are common nursing diagnoses for ARF?

6. Briefly discuss the types and purpose of hemodialysis use to eliminate toxic factors from the blood to prevent fatal complications.

7. Including dopamine HcL, which was administered in the MICU, what are the purposes for the prescribed orders?

8. What are the most common adverse reactions to the prescribed medications?

9. Discuss the drug-to-drug and drug-to-food/herbal interactions for the prescribed medications.

10. Discuss the gerontologic considerations of ARF.

11. Discuss client education for ARF.

Appendicitis

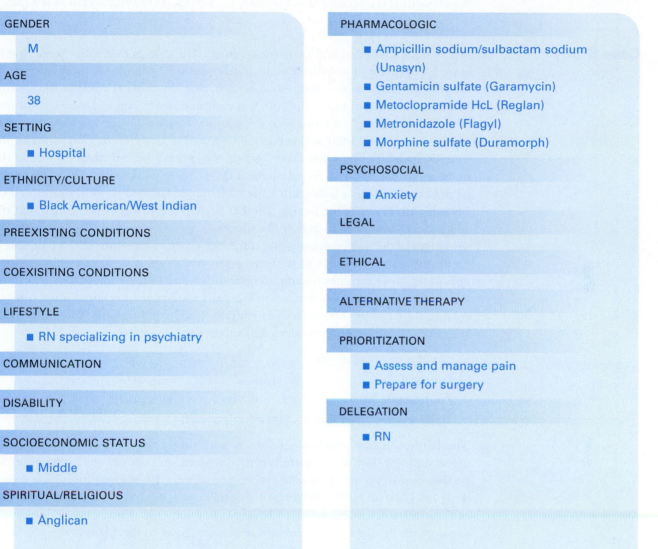

GENDER

M

AGE

38

SETTING

■ Hospital

ETHNICITY/CULTURE

■ Black American/West Indian

PREEXISTING CONDITIONS

COEXISITING CONDITIONS

LIFESTYLE

■ RN specializing in psychiatry

COMMUNICATION

DISABILITY

SOCIOECONOMIC STATUS

■ Middle

SPIRITUAL/RELIGIOUS

■ Anglican

PHARMACOLOGIC

■ Ampicillin sodium/sulbactam sodium (Unasyn)
■ Gentamicin sulfate (Garamycin)
■ Metoclopramide HcL (Reglan)
■ Metronidazole (Flagyl)
■ Morphine sulfate (Duramorph)

PSYCHOSOCIAL

■ Anxiety

LEGAL

ETHICAL

ALTERNATIVE THERAPY

PRIORITIZATION

■ Assess and manage pain
■ Prepare for surgery

DELEGATION

■ RN

MODERATE

THE DIGESTIVE AND URINARY SYSTEMS

Level of difficulty: Moderate

Overview: This case involves critical thinking and focused assessment skills to prioritize care for a client with appendicitis with peritonitis. It involves accurate assessment of pain with specific identification of location of pain and thorough assessment and auscultation of the chest to rule out lower lobe pneumonia. The triage nurse should be skilled at detecting signs of septic shock that could occur with the client with ruptured appendix.

Client Profile

Mr. W is a 38-year-old registered nurse who has specialized in psychiatric nursing. He is 5′4″ and weighs 210 pounds. Mr. W is brought by a neighbor to the emergency department (ED), accompanied by his wife. The mode of transportation is a car.

Case Study

Mr. W denies past medical or surgical history. He reports that while preparing to leave for his place of employment, he had an unusually sharp pain in his abdomen. He tells the triage nurse that he had been having "on and off" pain in the abdominal area and that, at times, the pain was continuous. He said today he felt "unusually cool" but thought it was due to the weather. However, when the pain shifted to his right lower quadrant and remained localized at the area halfway between the umbilicus and the right iliac crest (McBurney's point), he informed his wife of the need to go the ED. On arrival at the ED, Mr. W is complaining of nausea, and begins vomiting. He is assisted to a stretcher, and immediately positions himself on his side with his right leg flexed. The ED health care provider is notified and the triage nurse continues to gather the history by focusing on Mr. W's description of the origin of the pain, intensity, and duration. Upon completion of the pain assessment, the nurse proceeds to perform a physical examination, using the system's approach, then examines the most tender quadrant of the abdomen last. The lungs are clear on auscultation and normal breath sounds are present, ruling out any relationship with the abdominal pain and lower lobe pneumonia. The ED nursing technician monitors the vital signs and reports:

Blood pressure: 110/70

Pulse: 80

Respirations: 18

Temperature: 100.0° F

The ED health care provider sees Mr. W and history and assessment examination are completed. Mr. W is transferred to a medical surgical unit in preparation for further evaluation and probable emergency surgery. He is given morphine sulfate 4 mg IM. He is on NPO ("nothing by mouth") status but has intravenous fluid 0.9% sodium chloride at 125 mL/hr. Electrocardiogram (EKG) and chest X-ray results are normal. Results from serum labs drawn on arrival to the ED reveal:

White blood cell (WBC) count: 20,000/mm³

Hematocrit (Hct): 30%

Hemoglobin (Hgb): 15 mg/dL

Urinalysis reveals hematuria, albuminuria, and pyuria. Blood culture reveals gram-negative anaerobic bacilli. Ultrasound study shows the presence of appendicitis. Diagnostic tests and lab results done in the ED are reviewed, and a diagnosis of appendicitis is confirmed. Mr. W is informed of the need for surgery, an order for type and cross match for two units of packed red blood cells (PRBCs) is placed, an informed consent is signed, and the operating room staff is notified. Ampicillin sodium/sulbactam sodium (Unasyn) 1 g IV is administered stat, and the client is waiting "on call" to the operating room for an appendectomy.

The following are prescribed:

- NPO, start IV fluid D %.45% NaCL at 125 mL per hour
- Metoclopramide HcL (Reglan) 10 mg IV q6h PRN. Dilute in 50 mL normal saline and infuse over 30 minutes.

- Morphine sulfate (Duramorph) 8 mg q4h PRN pain
- Ampicillin sodium/sulbactam sodium (Unasyn) 1.5 g IV × one before surgery
- Gentamicin sulfate (Garamycin) 80 mg loading dose IV × one before surgery
- Metronidazole (Flagyl) 15 mg/kg IV before surgery

Questions

1. Define appendicitis.

2. Discuss the etiology and pathophysiology of appendicitis.

3. Discuss the classic manifestations of appendicitis and some diseases that mimic appendicitis.

4. Discuss the complications associated with acute appendicitis.

5. Discuss the collaborative management for appendicitis.

6. What are common nursing diagnoses for appendicitis?

7. If the client starts to vomit, what interventions should be carried out by the nurse, in order of priority?

8. What are the purposes for the prescribed medications?

9. What are the most common adverse reactions to the prescribed medications?

10. Discuss the drug-to-drug and drug-to-food/herbal interactions for the prescribed medications.

Lower Gastrointestinal Bleeding

GENDER

M

AGE

40

SETTING

- Hospital

ETHNICITY/CULTURE

- Jewish

PREEXISTING CONDITIONS

COEXISTING CONDITIONS

LIFESTYLE

- Criminal trial attorney

COMMUNICATION

DISABILITY

SOCIOECONOMIC STATUS

- Upper middle

SPIRITUAL/RELIGIOUS

- Judaism

PHARMACOLOGIC

- Diphenoxylate hydrochloride with Atropine sulfate (Lomotil)
- Mesalamine (5-Aminosalicylic acid) (Asacol)
- Alprazolam (Xanax)

PSYCHOSOCIAL

- Anxiety

LEGAL

ETHICAL

ALTERNATIVE THERAPY

PRIORITIZATION

- Stop the bleeding and diarrhea
- Decrease inflammation
- Rest the inflamed bowel
- Decrease stressful situations
- Correct nutritional deficiencies

DELEGATION

- RN
- Client education

MODERATE

THE DIGESTIVE AND URINARY SYSTEMS

Level of difficulty: Moderate

Overview: This case involves a thorough account of the current problem, symptoms, and any treatments related to the current problem; exploration of characteristics associated with reported or overt symptoms and factors that may be the cause of symptoms, assessment for pain, a common problem with gastrointestinal (GI) tract disorders. Observation of the skin in the rectal area for irritation or breakdown should be included in the assessment.

Client Profile

Mr. G is a 40-year-old male who is traveling with his wife for a holiday family reunion. However, upon arriving at the city of destination, he is taken from the airport to the emergency department (ED) of a city hospital because he is experiencing acute abdominal cramping. Also, upon going to the men's room at the airport, Mr. G reports developing severe bloody diarrhea. Mr. G is 5'9" and weighs 155 pounds.

Case Study

Mr. G is brought from the airport by emergency medical services (EMS) to the ED, accompanied by his wife. On arrival, Mr. G is alert and oriented to all stimuli. His vital signs are:

Blood pressure: 106/60

Pulse: 108

Respirations: 20

Temperature: 98.4° F

A nurse practitioner (NP) initiates the assessment. Mr.G reports loss of appetite and a recent increase in bowel movements, with up to 20 stools per day. In the past, Mr.G had only one bowel movement daily. He denies past medical or surgical history. However, Mr. G informs the nurse that he is worried, because recently his bowel movements look like they contain blood, mucous, and even pus. His heart sounds are normal, bilateral breath sounds are clear, and respirations are normal. His abdomen is distended and bowel sounds are hyperactive. Mr. G reports left lower quadrant abdominal pain. Rectal exam reveals bloody stools with presence of mucous. Stool laboratory exam is positive for blood, mucous, and pus. There are no other abnormalities on rectal examination. A specimen is drawn and sent to the lab for hematocrit, hemoglobin, red blood cell count, pANCA (perinuclear anti-neutrophil cytoplasmic antibody), anti-glycan antibody, serum iron, transferrin, and blood for type and cross match. Mr. G reports that he is allergic to "sulfas" and experiences breathing problems if he takes a sulfa drug. A 12-lead electrocardio-gram (EKG) is done and reveals normal sinus rhythm. A health care provider continues with the assessment after discussing the initial findings with the NP. An 18-gauge intravenous catheter is inserted and 0.9% NaCL is initiated at 100 mL per hour. Results of the labs reveal:

Hematocrit (Hct): 34%

Hemoglobin (Hgb): 10 mg/dL

Red blood cell (RBC) count: 4.5/mm³

pANCA (perinuclear antineutrophil cytoplasmic antibody): Elevated

Anti-glycan antibody: Elevated

Serum iron: 50 mg/dL

Transferrin: 230 mg/dL

Mr. G is transferred to the surgical unit where he receives two units of packed red blood cells (PRBCs). After the transfusion, Mr.G reports he is "feeling better." Mr. G prepares for a virtual colonoscopy by taking Fleet Prep Kit 1 (phospho-soda and Bisacodyl) and NuLytely® the night before the procedure. The colonoscopy is done, and it reveals diffuse inflammation of the mucosa and submucosa of the colon. Mr.G receives a medical diagnosis of ulcerative colitis. The multidisciplinary team discusses the findings of the diagnostic studies and his diagnosis of ulcerative colitis with Mr. G. Post transfusion labs reveal:

Hct: 40%

Hgb: 14 mg/dL

Post-transfusion vital signs are:

Blood pressure: 118/72

Pulse: 86

Respirations: 16

Temperature: 98.4 F

Because Mr. G is not from the state where he is hospitalized, he is discharged to home with a referral to a gastrointestinal specialist for a proctosigmoidoscopy, further evaluation to rule out diverticular diseases and benign anorectal diseases, and for reevaluation of his hematologic and GI status. A diagnosis of lower GI bleeding and ulcerative colitis is confirmed by clinical symptoms and the colonoscopy.

The following are prescribed on discharge:

- Diphenoxylate hydrochloride with atropine sulfate (Lomotil) 5 mg PO 3 to 4 times daily
- Mesalamine (5-Aminosalicylic acid) (Asacol) 400 mg PO three times daily
- Alprazolam (Xanax) 0.5 mg PO 3 times daily

Questions

1. Discuss common causes for lower GI bleeding in adults.

2. Discuss the potentially severe transfusion-related complications and the nursing implications.

3. What are common nursing diagnoses directly related to Mr. G's situation?

4. What are the purposes for the prescribed orders?

5. What are the most common adverse reactions, drug-to-drug, drug-to-food interactions of the prescribed medications?

6. Discuss other diagnostic tests the health care provider could have ordered to locate the source of bleeding.

7. Discuss the similarity and differences between invasive colonoscopy and virtual colonoscopy.

8. Discuss the nursing responsibilities for the client experiencing a proctosigmoidoscopy.

9. Discuss client education for lower GI bleeding.

Chronic Renal Failure (End-Stage Renal Disease)

GENDER

F

AGE

64

SETTING

- Hospital

ETHNICITY/CULTURE

- White American

PREEXISTING CONDITIONS

COEXISTING CONDITIONS

LIFESTYLE

- Retired interior decorator

COMMUNICATION

DISABILITY

SOCIOECONOMIC STATUS

- Middle

SPIRITUAL/RELIGIOUS

- Presbyterian

PHARMACOLOGIC

- Epoetin alfa recombinant (Epogen)
- Calcium carbonate (Os-cal)
- Aluminum hydroxide (Amphogel)
- Nifedipine (Procardia)
- Folic acid (Apo-Folic)
- Ferrous sulfate (Feosol)
- Ducosate sodium (Colace)
- Furosemide (Lasix)

PSYCHOSOCIAL

- Anxiety

LEGAL

ETHICAL

- Do all clients with renal failure have an unconditional right to dialysis, given the cost of dialysis and the relative few who benefit from it?

ALTERNATIVE THERAPY

PRIORITIZATION

- Complete history, including nutritional habits and current medications
- Discuss urinary elimination in detail

DELEGATION

- RN
- CNA
- Client education

THE DIGESTIVE AND URINARY SYSTEMS

Level of difficulty: Difficult

Overview: This case involves a thorough assessment of the client's condition, including current medications as well as careful systems assessment to prioritize care and prevent further complications and maintain kidney function and homeostasis for as long as possible. Accurate monitoring of blood pressure and serum potassium are critical since hypertension and hyperkalemia are common complications of end-stage renal disease (ESRD). Critical assessment of fluid status to identify imbalance is needed.

DIFFICULT

Client Profile

Mr. P, a 64-year-old retiree, is 4'10" and weighs 170 pounds. He shares a private home with his younger brother, who transported him to the emergency department (ED) of the hospital. On arrival, he complains of having had a headache for the past two hours. His vital signs are:

Blood pressure: 200/150

Pulse: 110

Respirations: 30

Temperature: 98.6° F

He is alert and oriented but is slow to respond to questions. He denies chest pain but reports nausea and feels he will vomit at anytime.

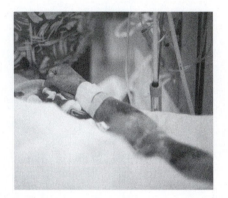

Case Study

Mr. P was diagnosed a year ago with end-stage renal failure secondary to hypertension, requiring treatment with hemodialysis. He is dialyzed at the clinic three times per week and is restricted to 1000 mL of fluid each day. He has a primary arteriovenous (AV) fistula in his left forearm (he is right handed). He reports current medications as:

Folic acid: 0.1 mg PO daily

Ferrous sulfate: 325 mg three times per day

Aluminum hydroxide: gel 500 mg PO twice

Erythropoietin alpha: self medicates with 50 units SC three times per week

Nifedipine: 30 mg PO three times per day

Mr. P reports not feeling his usual self, feeling tired on awakening this morning, and having difficulty getting out of bed. He is triaged and transferred to the medical intensive care (MICU), where an electrocardiogram (EKG) is done and shows sinus tachycardia and occasional unifocal premature ventricular contractions. Physical assessment reveals rales at the bases of the lungs and pitting edema of the lower extremities. Serum laboratory reports reveal:

Creatinine: 12 mg/dL

Blood urea nitrogen (BUN): 40 mg/dL

Sodium (Na): 150 mEq/L

Chloride: 100 mEq/L

Potassium (K+): 7.8 mEq/L

Phosphorous: 6.5 mg/dL

Calcium: 6 mg/dL

Hemoglobin (Hgb): 19 g/dL

Hematocrit (Hct): 28%

Glucose: 98 mg/dL

Arterial blood gas (ABG):

pH: 7.32

$PaCO_2$: 18 mm Hg

HCO_3: 8 mEq/L

PaO_2: 54

Mr. P is transferred to the dialysis unit soon after being transferred to the MICU and is dialyzed. A multidisciplinary team will participate in the overall plan of care, and the social worker, dietitian, and case manager will plan and coordinate home-care management.

The following are prescribed after the dialysis is completed:

- Folic acid (Apo-Folic) 0.1 mg PO daily
- Ferrous sulfate (Feosol) 325 mg PO three times per day
- Epoetin alfa (Epogen) 100 units/kg/dose SC three times per week
- Aluminum hydroxide gel (Amphogel) 500 mg PO four times per day
- Nifedipine (Procardia) 30mg PO three times per day
- Docusate sodium (Colace) 300 mg PO three times per day
- Calcium carbonate (Os-cal) 500 mg PO three times per day
- Furosemide (Lasix) 40 mg IV now and again in 4 hours

Questions

1. Discuss the pathophysiology of chronic renal failure, or ESRD.

2. Discuss the incidence, prevalence, and etiologies of ESRD in the United States.

3. Discuss why Mr. P was dialyzed soon after he was transferred to the MICU.

4. Discuss Mr. P's AV fistula and the purpose for it.

5. Discuss why the client is in metabolic acidosis.

6. What is the relationship between calcium, phosphorous, and chronic renal failure?

7. What are common nursing diagnoses for clients with ESRD?

8. Discuss hemodialysis (HD) versus peritoneal dialysis and why Mr. P was given hemodialysis instead of peritoneal dialysis.

9. What are the purposes for the prescribed medications?

10. What are the most common adverse reactions of the prescribed medications?

11. Discuss the drug-to-drug and drug-to-food/herbal interactions for the prescribed medications.

12. Discuss client education for ESRD.

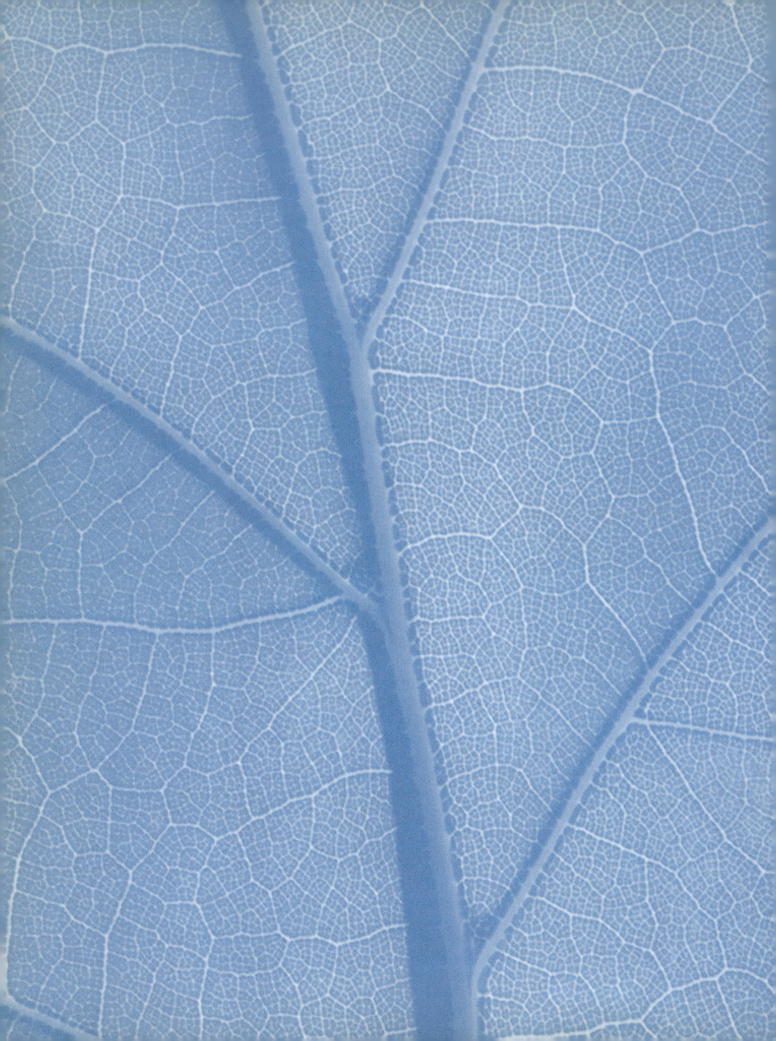

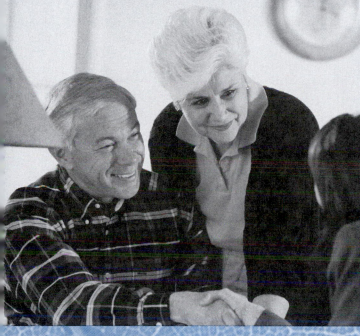

PART TWO

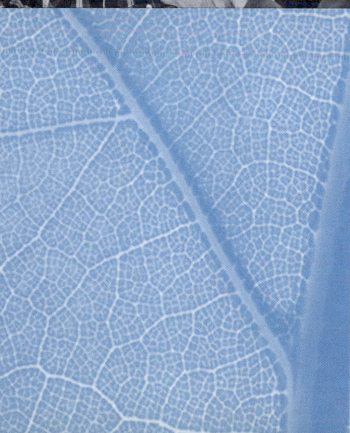

The Respiratory and Immune Systems

Chronic Bronchitis

GENDER

M

AGE

76

SETTING

- Skilled nursing facility

ETHNICITY/CULTURE

- White American

PREEXISTING CONDITIONS

COEXISTING CONDITIONS

- Viral infection
- Bacterial infection

LIFESTYLE

- Apartment building supervisor

COMMUNICATION

DISABILITY

- Decreased exercise tolerance

SOCIOECONOMIC STATUS

- Middle

SPIRITUAL/RELIGIOUS

- Protestant

PHARMACOLOGIC

- Albuterol (Proventil)
- Guaifenesin (Robitussin)
- Amoxicillin (Amoxil)
- Cefepime HcL (Maxipime)
- Ipratropium bromide (Atrovent)
- Acetaminophen (Tylenol)
- Oxygen

PSYCHOSOCIAL

- Anxiety
- Depression

LEGAL

ETHICAL

ALTERNATIVE THERAPY

PRIORITIZATION

- Maintain patent airway

DELEGATION

- RN
- Client education

THE RESPIRATORY AND IMMUNE SYSTEMS

Level of difficulty: Easy

Overview: This case involves prioritization of care to identify client's immediate needs and effective planning to have these needs met. The case also involves competence in identifying subtlety of grave changes with the client, such as absence of wheezing.

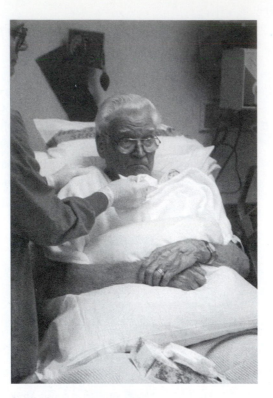

Client Profile

Mr. K, a 76-year-old male, is readmitted to the hospital's emergency department (ED) from a skilled nursing facility via an ambulette. On arrival, Mr. K shows signs of respiratory compromise as manifested by use of accessory muscles of the neck. The report from the nursing facility indicates that prior to this episode of respiratory impairment, Mr. K had been capable of carrying out basic activities of daily living such as combing his hair, mouth care, and dressing himself with only minimal assistance.

Case Study

During the past two weeks, Mr. K has been complaining of "stuffy" nose and has gradually begun to expectorate moderate amounts of respiratory secretions. The facility's health care provider is called because Mr. K has a temperature of 101° F and complains of chills even though the window of his room is closed and the air conditioning is off. His vital signs are:

Blood pressure: 124/86

Pulse: 80 and regular

Respirations: 20

Temperature: 101.0° F

Mr. K has a long history of cigarette smoking. On admission, he has thick, productive cough. The licensed practical nurse accompanying him informs the triage nurse that the cough has been unusually productive for more than one month, and Mr. K has had elevation of temperature of 101° F in the past that responded to Tylenol suppository. On auscultation, the ED nurse elicits loud rhonchi and wheezes. A complete history and physical is done, with physical findings that include clubbing of the fingers but no cyanosis or peripheral edema. A chest X-ray done on arrival to the ED reveals increased pulmonary congestion in the right lower lobe but no filtration or pleural effusion. Spirometry reveals airflow limitation with forced expiratory volume and forced vital capacity (FEV_1/FVC) 80%. Arterial blood gas (ABG) test reveals:

pH: 7.35
PO_2: 80
PCO_2: 47
HCO_3: 27

Mr. K is placed on two liters of oxygen via nasal cannula and is transferred to a respiratory unit of the hospital. On arrival at the unit, he continues to cough and, at times, coughs up blood-tinged sputum. A lab specimen is ordered, and results reveal sputum for culture and gram stain positive for Staphylococcus aureus and gram negative bacilli, white blood cell (WBC) with differential: WBC 14,000/mm^3 and eosinophils 600/mm^3. After the physical and laboratory data are reviewed, an admitting diagnosis of chronic bronchitis is confirmed.

The following are prescribed:

- Albuterol (Proventil) 2 puffs q4h and Ipratropium bromide (Atrovent) Soln, Inhl, 2.5 mL nebulization q4h
- Acetaminophen (Tylenol) 650 mg PO PRN temp greater than 100°
- Cefepime HcL (Maxipime) 1.5 g IV q12h
- Guaifenesin (Robitussin) 200 mg PRN q4h for cough
- D 5.45% NS IV infusion at 125 mL per hour

Questions

1. Discuss the cultural considerations for clients with chronic bronchitis related to history of cigarette smoking.

2. Discuss specific criteria used to diagnose chronic bronchitis.

3. Discuss the classic findings of clients with chronic bronchitis.

4. What are common nursing diagnoses for clients with chronic bronchitis?

5. What are the key features of cor pulmonale (right-sided heart failure), a complication of chronic bronchitis?

6. Discuss the breathing patterns commonly seen in clients with respiratory muscle fatigue.

7. What are the purposes for the prescribed orders?

8. What are the most common adverse reactions to the prescribed medications?

9. Discuss the drug-to-drug and drug-to-food/herbal interactions for the prescribed medications.

10. Discuss the key elements of stepped therapy for clients with chronic bronchitis.

11. What are the complementary and alternative therapies that help clients control dyspneic episodes?

Human Immunodeficiency Virus Infection (CDC Category A)

GENDER

F

AGE

32

SETTING

- Community clinic, a tertiary care center of a medical center

ETHNICITY/CULTURE

- Black South African

PREEXISTING CONDITIONS

COEXISTING CONDITIONS

LIFESTYLE

- Elementary school teacher

COMMUNICATION

- Xhosa and English as a second language

DISABILITY

SOCIOECONOMIC STATUS

- Middle

SPIRITUAL/RELIGIOUS

- Catholic

PHARMACOLOGIC

- Abacavir sulfate (Ziagen)
- Ritonavir (Norvir)
- Lamivudine/Zidovudine (Combivir)

PSYCHOSOCIAL

- Anxiety

LEGAL

- Client does not have the right not to release the names of those who may have contracted the disease from her.

ETHICAL

- Confidentiality—HIV is a reportable disease that carries a stigma.

ALTERNATIVE THERAPY

- Prayer
- Herbal medicines

PRIORITIZATION

- Maintain confidentiality
- Prepare for diagnostic tests

DELEGATION

- RN
- Client education

THE RESPIRATORY AND IMMUNE SYSTEMS

Level of difficulty: Easy

Overview: This case involves a thorough psychosocial and systems assessment and the use of optimum therapeutic communication to develop a sense of trust between client and health care providers. Room assignment is important due to the stigma of human immunodeficiency virus (HIV) and the client's lack of awareness of varying cultural views of the disease.

Client Profile

Ms. J is a 32-year-old female from Johannesburg, South Africa. She is vacationing with relatives who have resided in the United States for the past 40 years. Ms. J is accompanied by a cousin, a registered nurse, to the community center of a major city.

Case Study

On arrival at the clinic, Ms. J is restless as she waits for the next available nurse. During the initial interview, Ms. J informs the nurse that she is sexually active, practicing unprotected sex because she has been dating only her high-school sweetheart for years. Her reasons for seeking medical assistance are related to recent flu-like symptoms, including headache, fatigue, and occasional night sweats. Her report of unprotected sex and country of origin suggests the possibility of an early stage of human immunodeficiency virus (HIV). Her vital signs are:

Blood pressure: 150/98

Pulse: 120

Respirations: 22 and shallow

Temperature: 98.4° F

Ms. A is initially seen in the triage area of the ED by a nurse practitioner (NP), who notifies the ED physician of Ms. A's arrival and presenting symptoms. After the NP completes the history and physical, it is determined that Ms. J will need to return to the hospital for further evaluation. The NP, in collaboration with the clinic physician, assigns a tentative diagnosis of HIV to Ms. J, who is seen by a counselor and will return to the clinic in three weeks for a follow-up report on lab tests, then will see the primary health care provider at the hospital for a conclusive diagnosis. Lab results reveal CD4+/CD8 cell count 400 CD4+ cells/mm^3 of blood. Enzyme linked immunosorbent assay (ELISA) and Western Blot tests are positive for HIV, chest X-ray reveals normal lung field, and structures within the thorax are normal. Purified protein derivative (PPD) injection is administered, is read in 72 hours, and is negative for tuberculosis. The health care provider and NP review the diagnostic reports and the laboratory data and confirm the diagnosis of HIV. The findings are discussed with the client, after which the health care provider and NP spend much time listening to the client and allowing verbalization of feelings about the diagnosis. Request for consultation with a psychiatrist and social worker is submitted. The HIPPA (Health Insurance Portability and Accountability Act of 1996) form is discussed with and signed by the client. A copy of the form is given to the client.

The following are prescribed:

- Abacavir sulfate (Ziagen) 300 mg PO two times per day
- Ritonavir (Norvir) 600 mg PO two times per day
- Lamivudine/zidovudine (Combivir) one combination tablet (150 mg lamivudine/300 mg zidovudine) PO two times per day
- Epzicom (Abacavir) 300 mg PO two times per day

Questions

1. Discuss the pathophysiology of HIV infection.

2. Discuss the modes of transmission that have remained constant throughout the course of the HIV pandemic.

3. Discuss the protozoal infections detected in persons with HIV.

4. Discuss how HIV is classified.

5. Discuss the clinical manifestations of HIV and how the infection is diagnosed.

6. List common nursing diagnoses for clients with HIV infection diseases.

7. Discuss highly active antiretroviral therapy (HAART) and whether the prescribed medications meet its criteria.

8. What are the purposes for the prescribed medications?

9. What are the most common adverse reactions of the prescribed medications?

10. Discuss the drug-to-drug and drug-to-food/ herbal interactions for the prescribed medications.

11. Discuss the importance of the client seeing an HIV social worker before leaving the clinic.

12. Discuss dietary management for the person with HIV.

Pulmonary Tuberculosis

GENDER

M

AGE

50

SETTING

- Hospital

ETHNICITY/CULTURE

- White American

PREEXISTING CONDITIONS

COEXISTING CONDITIONS

LIFESTYLE

- Unemployed for five years
- Consumes beer or vodka daily

COMMUNICATION

DISABILITY

SOCIOECONOMIC STATUS

- Low

SPIRITUAL/RELIGIOUS

- Catholic

PHARMACOLOGIC

- Isoniazid (Nydrazid)
- Pyridoxine HcL (Aminoxin)
- Pyrazinamide (Tebrazid)
- Rifampin (Rifadin)
- Streptomycin sulfate (Streptomycin)
- Megestrol acetate (Megace)

PSYCHOSOCIAL

- Anxiety

LEGAL

- The client does not have the right to refuse providing names of persons who may have contracted the disease.

ETHICAL

- Cases of TB must be reported.
- Client's concern for confidentiality must still be addressed appropriately.

ALTERNATIVE THERAPY

PRIORITIZATION

- Private room
- Respiratory isolation
- Arrest TB process

DELEGATION

- RN
- Client education

THE RESPIRATORY AND IMMUNE SYSTEMS

Level of difficulty: Easy

Overview: This case involves a thorough assessment of the client's respiratory status, including social history and past exposure to tuberculosis (TB); the client's native country; and travel to foreign countries prior to migrating to the United States.

Client Profile

Mr. B is a 50-year-old male who is brought to the hospital emergency department (ED) by emergency medical service (EMS) from a community clinic after having bouts of vomiting while waiting to be seen by a health care provider.

Case Study

Mr. B's vital signs on arrival to the ED are:

> Blood pressure: 130/78
>
> Pulse: 78
>
> Respirations: 20
>
> Temperature: 99.0° F

He is known at the hospital; he frequently comes to the hospital's ED in a state of stupor or is taken by EMS because he has fallen while walking in the street. Today, he is coherent, responding to questions appropriately. Mr. B is 5′8″ and weighs 110 pounds. Social history reveals he is a high school graduate who worked as a bookkeeper for a trucking company. He has been unemployed for the past five years. His social history reveals cigarette smoking for 40 years; he has smoked two packs per day for 20 years. He is an undiagnosed alcoholic, a former cocaine and marijuana user, and was "detoxed" from the cocaine six years ago. He denies having used marijuana during the past eight years. Mr. B also reports infrequent feelings of depression and noted weight loss for the past two months. He has never been married but has a son whom he has not seen for several years. Mr. B is currently taking Megestrol acetate 200 mg PO every six hours as prescribed by a health care provider at the clinic he attends and reports compliance with the medication. The health care provider in the ED continues with the history and physical examination and gathers from Mr. B that he has been experiencing a dry cough and occasional night sweats. Mr. B is transferred from the ED to the respiratory unit, with written orders to place him on respiratory isolation. On arrival at the unit, he is placed in a single room, and respiratory precaution signs are initiated on the outside of the door that leads to his room. The pulmonologist meets with Mr. B on the unit and, after further gathering of data, orders: sputum for acid fast bacilli (AFB) X three sputum culture, Mantoux test with 0.1 ml of PPD intradermally, and chest X-ray. The results for the diagnostic tests are positive for the mycobacterium bacillus, and the diagnosis of pulmonary tuberculosis is confirmed.

The following are prescribed:

- Isoniazid (Nydrazid) (INH) 300 mg PO daily
- Rifampin (Rifadin) (RMP) 600 mg PO daily
- Pyrazinamide (PZA) (Tebrazid) 30 mg/kg PO daily
- Streptomycin sulfate (Streptomycin) 15 mg/kg IM single dose
- Pyridoxine HcL (Aminoxin) 100 mg PO daily
- Megestrol acetate (Megace) 200 mg PO q6h

Questions

1. Discuss the incidence and prevalence of pulmonary TB.

2. Discuss the etiology and pathophysiology of TB.

3. What are the risk factors for TB?

4. Discuss the Centers for Disease Control (CDC) recommendations for preventing transmission of TB in health care settings.

5. Discuss the common clinical manifestations of clients with TB and how they reflect the pathophysiology of TB.

6. Discuss the gerontologic considerations for TB.

7. Discuss the specific diagnostic studies used to confirm TB.

8. What are the purposes for the prescribed medications?

9. What are the most common adverse reactions of the prescribed medications?

10. Discuss the drug-to-drug and drug-to-food/herbal interactions for the prescribed medications.

11. Discuss the potential complications for the client with TB.

12. Discuss client education for TB.

Pulmonary Empyema

GENDER

M

AGE

55

SETTING

- Hospital

ETHNICITY/CULTURE

- Black American

PREEXISTING CONDITIONS

- Pericarditis

COEXISTING CONDITIONS

- Renal failure

LIFESTYLE

- Retired

COMMUNICATION

DISABILITY

SOCIOECONOMIC STATUS

- Low

SPIRITUAL/RELIGIOUS

- Baptist

PHARMACOLOGIC

- Cefuroxime sodium (Zinacef)
- Gentamicin sulfate (Garamycin)
- Morphine sulfate (Duramorph)
- Rabeprazole sodium (Aciphex)

PSYCHOSOCIAL

LEGAL

- Are there federal or state supplemental resources to cover hospital expenses for self-employed retired persons?

ETHICAL

- Insufficient Social Security income should not be a deterrent for quality health care.

ALTERNATIVE THERAPY

- Prayer

PRIORITIZATION

- Antibiotic therapy

DELEGATION

- RN
- Client education

THE RESPIRATORY AND IMMUNE SYSTEMS

Level of difficulty: Easy

Overview: This case involves the use of collaborative management and history assessment to determine recent febrile illness, chest pain, dyspnea, or unusual cough. The nurse must be skilled in managing clients in need of thoracic procedures and competent in respiratory assessment and caring for clients with chest tubes to underwater seal drainage.

Client Profile

Mr. J, a 55-year-old male and retired self-employed carpenter, is readmitted to the hospital after being discharged two weeks ago. He is 5′10″ and weighs 230 pounds. At readmission he complains of pleuritic chest pain and generalized weakness. His vital signs on admission are:

> Blood pressure: 150/90
> Pulse: 100
> Respirations: 30
> Temperature: 101.0° F

Case Study

On physical assessment, Mr. J's chest wall motion is reduced, palpation and percussion reveal flat sounds, and breath sounds are decreased. Medical history reveals history of hypertension, past history of lung abscess and bacterial pneumonia, past history of pulmonary tuberculosis, recurrent left pneumothorax, and frequent upper respiratory infections. Mr. J reports gastric ulcer, which he relates to alcohol intake for several years, and allergies to contrast dye, radiographic dye, and thorazine. His social history involves several years of cigarette smoking. A chest X-ray is ordered and confirms pleural effusion. The health care provider determines the need to remove pleural fluid and explains the purpose and plan to Mr. J. An informed consent for a thoracentesis is signed by the client. The thoracentesis is done, and pleural fluid is sent to the lab for color, red blood cell count, white blood cell count and differential, and glucose and protein levels. The results are:

> Appearance: cloudy
> Red blood cell (RBC) count: >1000/mm^3
> White blood cell (WBC) count: >1000/mm^3
> pH: <7.4
> Glucose: 68 mg/dL
> Protein: >3.0 g/dL

A gram stain and acid fast stain are ordered and yields gram-negative species. Blood is positive for Staphylococcus aureus, and WBC is 15,000/mm^3. A diagnosis of pulmonary empyema is confirmed and a treatment plan is discussed with Mr. J that includes the placement of chest tubes attached to water-seal drainage and wall suction.

The following are prescribed:

- Cefuroxime sodium (Zinacef) 1.5 g IV before the procedure/750 mg IV q8h × 24 hours
- Gentamicin sulfate (Garamycin) 2.5 mg/kg IV q8h
- Morphine sulfate (Duramorph) 2 mg IV q1–2h PRN
- Rabeprazole sodium (Aciphex) 60 mg PO once daily
- Chest tube to 20 cm wall suction via Pleur-evac

Questions

1. Discuss the pathophysiology of pulmonary empyema.

2. Discuss the findings on auscultation if pleural effusion is present with empyema.

3. What are management strategies for clients with pulmonary empyema?

4. Discuss pleural abnormalities as they relate to pulmonary empyema.

5. How would the health care provider determine that the client is experiencing compression of lung tissue due to the effusion?

6. What are the purposes for the prescribed medications?

7. What are the most common adverse reactions, drug-to-drug, drug-to-food/herbal interactions of the prescribed medications?

8. A tube thoracotomy is done, with chest tube for drainage. What are specific nursing interventions for managing chest drainage systems?

9. What are common nursing diagnoses for post–chest tube insertion?

10. Discuss client education for pulmonary empyema.

CASE STUDY 5

Non-Small Cell Adenocarcinoma of the Right Lung

GENDER

F

AGE

60

SETTING

- Hospital

ETHNICITY/CULTURE

- African/Nigerian

PREEXISTING CONDITIONS

- Recurrent pneumonias
- Pulmonary fibrosis

COEXISTING CONDITIONS

- Chronic obstructive pulmonary disease

LIFESTYLE

- Smoked three packs of cigarettes per day for 15 years

COMMUNICATION

DISABILITY

SOCIOECONOMIC STATUS

- Middle

SPIRITUAL/RELIGIOUS

- Attends Sunday Mass
- Spiritual counseling

PHARMACOLOGIC

- Ibuprofen (Motrin)
- Vinorelbine tartrate (Navelbine)
- Ondansetron HcL (Zofran)

PSYCHOSOCIAL

- Anxiety
- Fear
- Denial

LEGAL

ETHICAL

- Is it a nurse's responsibility to educate clients and others on the dangers of "secondhand smoke"?

ALTERNATIVE THERAPY

- Meditation
- Herbalism

PRIORITIZATION

- Reduce anxiety
- Prepare client for diagnostic tests

DELEGATION

- RN certified in oncology management
- Client education

THE RESPIRATORY AND IMMUNE SYSTEMS

Level of difficulty: Moderate

Overview: This case involves a thorough assessment of the client's condition, past medical history, social habits, and current medications including herbal and over-the-counter drugs. The nurse must use critical thinking and prioritization to meet the immediate needs of clients who are diagnosed with different types of cancer at different stages of progression. Nurses must be vigilant with assessment skills when caring for clients receiving chemotherapeutic agents that suppress bone marrow.

Client Profile

Ms. Y is a 60-year-old female who is admitted by her primary health care provider to the hospital after her annual physical examination. Ms. Y has never been married and has been unemployed for the past three years. She was employed as a "private" home health aide, but after the death of that client, she was unable to find employment.

Case Study

During the initial nurse interview, Ms. Y reports seeking her primary health care provider's advice because of a persistent cough for the past month. Ms. Y reports a history of smoking three packs of cigarettes per day for 15 years. Ms. Y admits to being anxious but does not believe she has cancer. She denies weight loss or unusual physical changes except the unusual cough. She reports occasional use of Advil (ibuprofen) for infrequent headaches and use of herbal medicines, especially at breakfast and before retiring to bed. Admission vital signs are:

Blood pressure: 140/84

Pulse: 80

Respirations: 18

Temperature: 98.2° F

Auscultation reveals unilateral wheeze in the right lower lobe of the lung. Respiratory assessment is occasionally interrupted because of her need to cough. After the physical assessment is complete, the following diagnostic studies and labs are prescribed: cytologic examination of sputum; chest X-ray; pulmonary function tests (PFTs); computed tomography (CT) scan of the lung; positron emission test (PET); serum sodium, potassium (K+), and calcium, platelet count, hematocrit, hemoglobin, white blood cell count, and creatinine. The results of the diagnostic tests reveal: sputum for cytology with malignant cells; chest X-ray shows lesion on the right lung; vital capacity (VC) is 75%, FEV_1 80%, FEF 68%; CT scan identifies the lesion and scans and measures it at 10 cm; PET is negative for metastasis. Results of the serum labs are:

Sodium (Na): 133

Potassium (K+): 4.2

Calcium: 8.4

Platelet count (PLT): 2,500,153

Hematocrit (Hct): 32.8%

Hemoglobin (Hgb): 11.5 g/dL

White blood cell (WBC) count: 10,000/mm^3

Creatinine: 0.9 mg/dL

After the diagnostic tests and lab results are reviewed and discussed with the medical, surgical, and oncology teams, a diagnosis of non–small squamous cell adenocarcinoma of the right lung is made. The findings are discussed and explained with Ms. Y, and a decision for plan of care is made. Serum sodium, calcium, complete blood count will be done twice weekly.

The following are prescribed:

- Vinorelbine tartrate (Navelbine) 30 mg/m^2 weekly at oncology clinic
- Ondansetron HcL (Zofran) 8 mg PO 30 minutes before chemotherapy

Questions

1. Discuss the pathophysiology of lung cancer.

2. Compare tobacco smoke, secondhand smoke, and environmental and occupational exposure and their effects on the development of lung cancer.

3. Discuss non-small cell lung cancer.

4. Discuss the clinical manifestations of lung cancer.

5. Discuss the different stages of lung cancer as designated by the tumor-mode-metastasis (TNM) classification system.

6. Discuss diagnostic tests use to confirm lung cancer.

7. What are the purposes for the prescribed orders?

8. What are the most common adverse reactions, drug-to-drug, drug-to-food/herbal interactions of the prescribed medications?

9. What process does the nurse use when administering medications to this client?

10. Discuss client education for lung cancer.

Questions

Pulmonary Emphysema

GENDER

M

AGE

62

SETTING

- Hospital

ETHNICITY/CULTURE

- Italian American

PREEXISTING CONDITIONS

- History of cigarette smoking

COEXISTING CONDITIONS

- Hyperinflated lung

LIFESTYLE

- Supervisor, 20 years in garment industry

COMMUNICATION

DISABILITY

- Easy fatigability
- Dyspnea on slight exertion

SOCIOECONOMIC STATUS

- Middle

SPIRITUAL/RELIGIOUS

- Catholic

PHARMACOLOGIC

- Theophylline ethylenediamine
- Methylprednisolone sodium succinate (Solu-Medrol)
- Cromolyn sodium (Intal)
- Albuterol (Proventil)
- Ampicillin sodium/sulbactam sodium (Unasyn)
- Pneumococcal 0.5 mL and influenza vaccine
- Metered-dose inhaler – Albuterol (Proventil)

PSYCHOSOCIAL

- Depression
- Anxiety

LEGAL

ETHICAL

ALTERNATIVE THERAPY

- Fish oil
- Garlic

PRIORITIZATION

- Airway management
- Prevent respiratory failure

DELEGATION

- RN
- CNA

MODERATE

THE RESPIRATORY AND IMMUNE SYSTEMS

Level of difficulty: Moderate

Overview: This case involves a thorough assessment of the client's condition including recent exposure to risk factors, pattern of symptom development, past medical history, current medications, and available social and family support. It involves prioritization of care. The nurse must be skilled at assessing respiratory status and competent in managing respiratory emergencies. The certified nursing assistant (CNA) can take height and weight, vital signs, and assist with hygiene care as needed.

Client Profile

Mr. X is a 62-year-old thin, underweight male who is accompanied by his wife to the respiratory unit after brief triage in the emergency department (ED). His wife is in the waiting room of the unit while the receiving nurse makes Mr. X comfortable before initiating the history and physical.

Case Study

Report from the triage nurse indicates that on arrival to the ED, Mr. X demonstrates signs of mild anxiety but his chief complaint is "increased difficulty breathing after climbing three flights of stairs today." He reports that his breathing has become progressively worse to the point where it interferes with activities of daily living (ADL). He concludes by saying that the breathing is worse today, which is the reason he came to the ED. His vital signs are:

Blood pressure: 140/78

Pulse: 88

Respirations: 24

Temperature: 99.8° F

On assessment, he has a barrel chest and uses his accessory muscles of respiration to assist with breathing. He frequently does pursed-lip breathing during the interview and coughs and expectorates moderate amount of yellowish sputum. He has auscultatory rales at the base of the lung fields. His social history includes smoking three packs of cigarettes per day for 40 years.

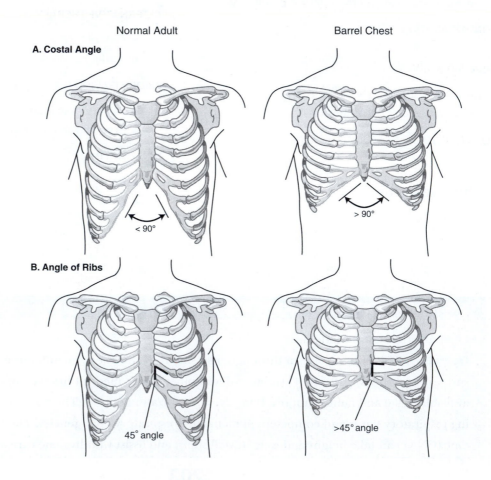

Mr. X reports not having gotten the pneumococcal and influenza vaccines for a long period of time but is not specific about the length of time. A health care provider completes the history and physical and orders a stat arterial blood gas (ABG) and complete blood count (CBC). The results of the ABG tests are:

pH: 7.36

$PaCO_2$: 48 mm Hg

PaO_2: 80%

HCO_3: 25

Complete blood count (CBC):

White blood cell (WBC) count: 7.1

Hematocrit (Hct): 38%

Hemoglobin (Hgb): 15 mg/dl

Two liters of oxygen via nasal cannula are initiated. A chest X-ray shows a flattened diaphragm but no infiltrates. Pulmonary function studies reveal FEV-1/FVC 60% and increased residual volume (RV). Sputum analysis identifies Haemophilus influenza. A diagnosis of chronic obstructive pulmonary disease (pulmonary emphysema) is confirmed. Mr. X is admitted to the hospital for respiratory and oxygen therapy and pharmacological therapy.

The following are prescribed:

- Albuterol (Proventil) aerosol metered-dose inhalant (MDI) two puffs stat and q4h PRN
- Oxygen/nasal cannula to maintain oxygen saturation greater than 89% but not to exceed two liters
- Dextrose 5% and 0.45% sodium chloride intravenous infusion at 100 ml/hr
- Theophylline ethylenediamine (with 20 mg theophylline, 25 mg aminophylline) 0.3 mg/kg/hr continuous intravenously administration
- Ampicillin sodium/sulbactam sodium (Unasyn) 1.5 gm IV q6h
- Cromolyn sodium (Intal) two metered sprays q6h
- Pneumococcal 0.5 mL single dose and influenza vaccine 0.5 mL single dose prior to discharge

Questions

1. Discuss the types of emphysema and the most common risk factor for the development of pulmonary emphysema.

2. Discuss the complications associated with emphysema.

3. Discuss the enzyme inhibitor that predisposes young clients who do not smoke to rapid development of lobular emphysema.

4. Pulmonary function tests (PFTs) are used to confirm pulmonary emphysema. What are the specific findings of the PFTs?

5. Discuss the clinical manifestations of pulmonary emphysema.

6. What are common nursing diagnoses for clients with pulmonary emphysema?

7. What are the purposes for the prescribed medications?

8. What are the most common adverse reactions of the prescribed medications?

9. Discuss the drug-to-drug and drug-to-food/herbal interactions of the prescribed medications.

10. Discuss the surgical approaches that might be used for the client with emphysema.

11. Discuss client education for pulmonary emphysema.

Acute Respiratory Distress Syndrome

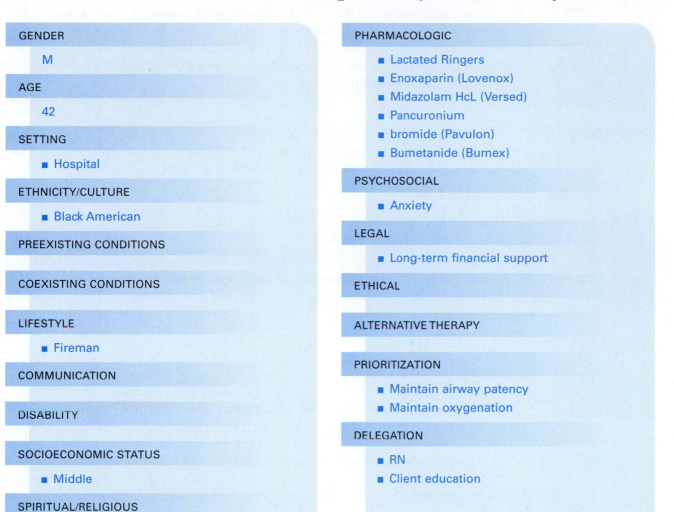

GENDER

M

AGE

42

SETTING

- Hospital

ETHNICITY/CULTURE

- Black American

PREEXISTING CONDITIONS

COEXISTING CONDITIONS

LIFESTYLE

- Fireman

COMMUNICATION

DISABILITY

SOCIOECONOMIC STATUS

- Middle

SPIRITUAL/RELIGIOUS

- Catholic

PHARMACOLOGIC

- Lactated Ringers
- Enoxaparin (Lovenox)
- Midazolam HcL (Versed)
- Pancuronium
- bromide (Pavulon)
- Bumetanide (Bumex)

PSYCHOSOCIAL

- Anxiety

LEGAL

- Long-term financial support

ETHICAL

ALTERNATIVE THERAPY

PRIORITIZATION

- Maintain airway patency
- Maintain oxygenation

DELEGATION

- RN
- Client education

THE RESPIRATORY AND IMMUNE SYSTEMS

Level of difficulty: Difficult

Overview: This case involves a quick assessment of the client and presenting symptoms while maintaining airway patency. It involves prioritization of care to other clients when the burn client arrives on the unit. It involves a complete physical examination that includes the client's general appearance on arrival to the unit.

DIFFICULT

Client Profile

Mr. T is a 42-year-old firefighter assigned to an engine company located in a poor urban neighborhood. Mr. T has been acknowledged by the mayor of the city on three occasions for bravery, which includes going beyond the call of duty to save lives from actively burning buildings. One month ago, Mr. T was brought to the hospital emergency department (ED) for smoke inhalation after combating a fire for several hours. Mr. T was discharged and returned to work after clearance from his primary health care provider.

Case Study

Today, Mr. T is brought to the ED from his place of employment. On arrival at the ED, he is restless, complains of fatigue, headache, and difficulty breathing even when in an upright position. An arterial blood gas (ABG) test reveals:

pH: 7.30

PCO_2: 48

HCO_3^- done with a PaO_2 of 58

The test indicates respiratory acidosis. He is started on a non-rebreather mask and pulse oximeter to monitor oxygen saturation. Physical assessment by the nurse finds the use of accessory muscles with decreased breath sounds. Vital signs are:

Blood pressure: 100/72

Pulse: 114

Respirations: 22

Temperature: 99.4° F

Mr. T is 5′6″ and weighs 205 pounds. Pulmonary function tests (PFTs) show decreased lung compliance with reduced vital capacity, minute volume and functional vital capacity. On auscultation of the lungs, the health care provider auscultates bilateral rales. Results of a chest X-ray done in the ED show diffuse haziness, "whited-out" (ground-glass) appearance of the lung. A repeat ABG reveals PaO_2 of 58 even after the implementation of four liters of oxygen. The client is intubated and placed on mechanical ventilation with positive-end expiratory pressure (PEEP) setting and placed in semi-Fowler's position. A pulmonary artery catheter is inserted. After review of physical findings, response to increase in oxygen, chest X-ray findings, and pulmonary capillary wedge pressure readings, the diagnosis of acute respiratory distress syndrome (ARDS) is made. Plans to initiate enteral feeding or parenteral nutrition (hyperalimentation) will be included in the treatment regimen.

The following are prescribed:

- Lactated Ringers 1,000 mLs at 125 mLs per hour
- Enoxaparin (Lovenox) injection 40 mg/0.4 ML SC daily
- Midazolam HcL (Versed) 0.02 mg/kg/h by continuous infusion
- Pancuronium bromide (Pavulon) 0.1 mg/kg IV initial dose
- Bumetanide (Bumex) 1 mg IV q6h for 24 hours

Questions

1. Discuss your understanding of the client's situation.

2. Discuss the pathophysiology of ARDS and the leading cause of death in clients with ARDS.

3. Discuss the usual cause of refractory hypoxemia in ARDS.

4. Discuss the purpose and benefits for the positive-end expiratory pressure (PEEP) setting on the ventilator.

5. Discuss the significance of pulmonary capillary wedge pressure (PCWP) in diagnosing ARDS.

6. What are common nursing diagnoses for clients with ARDS?

7. What are the purposes for the prescribed orders?

8. What are the most common adverse reactions of the prescribed medications?

9. Discuss the drug-to-drug and drug-to-food/herbal interactions of the prescribed medications.

10. Discuss essential nursing responsibilities when caring for mechanically ventilated clients on neuromuscular blockers.

Acquired Immunodeficiency Syndrome

GENDER

M

AGE

40

SETTING

- Hospital

ETHNICITY/CULTURE

- Hispanic American

PREEXISTING CONDITIONS

- HIV

COEXISTING CONDITIONS

- Peripheral neuropathy
- Hepatitis C
- Recurrent bacterial pneumonia

LIFESTYLE

- Cab driver for eight years

COMMUNICATION

- Spanish and English as a second language

DISABILITY

SOCIOECONOMIC STATUS

- Low

SPIRITUAL/RELIGIOUS

- Nondenominational

PHARMACOLOGIC

- Interferon alfa-2b (Intron A)
- Amikacin sulfate (Amikin)
- Bleomycin sulfate (Blenoxane)
- Nystatin (Mycostatin)
- Trimethoprim/sulfamethoxazole (Bactrim)

PSYCHOSOCIAL

- Fear

LEGAL

- Financial support
- Advance directives
- Counseling

ETHICAL

- Discrimination and denial have decreased national response to the AIDS epidemic. Strong, positive leadership for care and prevention is needed.

ALTERNATIVE THERAPY

- Aloe vera
- Echinacea

PRIORITIZATION

- Body substance isolation
- Confidentiality

DELEGATION

- RN
- LPN
- CNA

THE RESPIRATORY AND IMMUNE SYSTEMS

Level of difficulty: Difficult

Overview: This case involves thorough knowledge of the complexities of acquired immunodeficiency syndrome (AIDS) and is void of values that cloud professional approach to delegation of assignments and optimum care (i.e., immediate and general). The nurse must be familiar with the mix of medications usually prescribed for Persons With AIDS (PWAs). The licensed practical nurse (LPN) can administer medications as prescribed after the registered nurse (RN) has completed the initial assessment. The certified nursing assistant (CNA) can provide routine hygiene care and take vital signs, reporting abnormal readings to the LPN.

DIFFICULT

Client Profile

Mr. C is a 40-year-old male who was diagnosed with human immunodeficiency virus (HIV) five years ago and has been under outpatient medical supervision at a community health center affiliated with a medical center in the community in which he resides. Mr. C lives with his aunt, who is 68 years old and is his primary caregiver. Mr. C was seen in the outpatient clinic two weeks ago with complaints of nausea, vomiting, and diarrhea. Review of laboratory data and diagnostic studies from previous clinic visits indicate progression of the disease as evidenced by axilary adenopathy, decrease in CD+W cells of 300 mm^3, and oral candidiasis.

Case Study

Today Mr. C is seen in the outpatient clinic with complaints of severe diarrhea for two days, fever, and dry, productive cough. He reports being able to walk for approximately four feet without assistance but becomes extremely fatigued afterward. The nurse practitioner completes a history and physical examination and, after reviewing Mr. C's previous clinic records, refers him to the hospital for further evaluation and possible admission. At the hospital, Mr. C's vital signs are:

Blood pressure: 110/86

Pulse: 106

Respirations: 28 and shallow

Temperature: 102.6° F

He is sent from the admission's department to the AIDS unit and is assigned to a private room. Mr. C is placed on three liters of oxygen as per the unit's protocol. An arterial blood gas (ABG) is done and reveals:

pH: 7.35

pCO$_2$: 45

HCO$_3$: 28

pO$_2$: 78

The health care provider is notified, and the nurse initiates a brief history and physical, taking into consideration the physical and emotional state of the client. The nurse briefly discusses the Patient's Bill of Rights and the American Health Insurance Portability and Accountability Act of 1996 (HIPPA) with Mr. C and informs him that the documents will be given to him before the completion of the nurse's work schedule. Mr. C is seen by a health care provider who continues with the history and physical assessment then reviews Mr. C's medical records sent from the clinic, which include a diagnosis of AIDS. Current laboratory data from the clinic indicate values of: CD+4/CD8+ ratio less than 2 and CD4+ count of 200/mm^3, positive ELISA and Western Blot tests. Current blood cultures reveal Escherichia coli, Pseudomonas aeruginosa, and Klebsiella pneumoniae. After the multidisciplinary team reviews current data and physical assessment findings, an admitted with diagnosis is made for AIDS complicated with pneumocystis carinii pneumonia (PCP), cytomegalovirus (CMV) retinitis, Kaposi's sarcoma (KS), and oral candidiasis.

The following are prescribed:

- Interferon alfa-2b (Intron A) 20,000,000 IU/M^2 SC for five consecutive days pr week for four weeks
- Amikacin sulfate (Amikin) 7.5 mg/kg IV q12h

- Trimethoprim/sulfamethoxazole (Bactrim) 5mg/kg IV q6h for seven days and then PO q6h for seven days
- Bleomycin sulfate (Blenoxane) 0.5 U/kg IV × two weekly
- Nystatin suspension (Mycostatin) 500,000 U PO three times per day, swish and swallow
- Ondansetron 32 mg IV 30 minutes before bleomycin therapy
- Dextrose 5% in 0.45% normal saline at 125 mL/hr

Questions

1. Define PCP.

2. Discuss the clinical manifestations of PCP associated with AIDS.

3. Discuss the enteric pathogen that may occur in the stool of the client with AIDS.

4. Discuss the two cytokines that play an important role in AIDS-related wasting syndrome.

5. The Centers for Disease Control and Prevention (CDC) has included Kaposi's sarcoma (KS) in the classification of AIDS-related malignancies. Discuss how KS diagnosis is confirmed.

6. Discuss priority nursing diagnoses associated with AIDS.

7. What are the purposes for the prescribed medications?

8. What are the most common adverse reactions of the prescribed medications?

9. Discuss the drug-to-drug and drug-to-food/herbal interactions of the prescribed medications.

10. Discuss how the nurse can promote home- and community-based care.

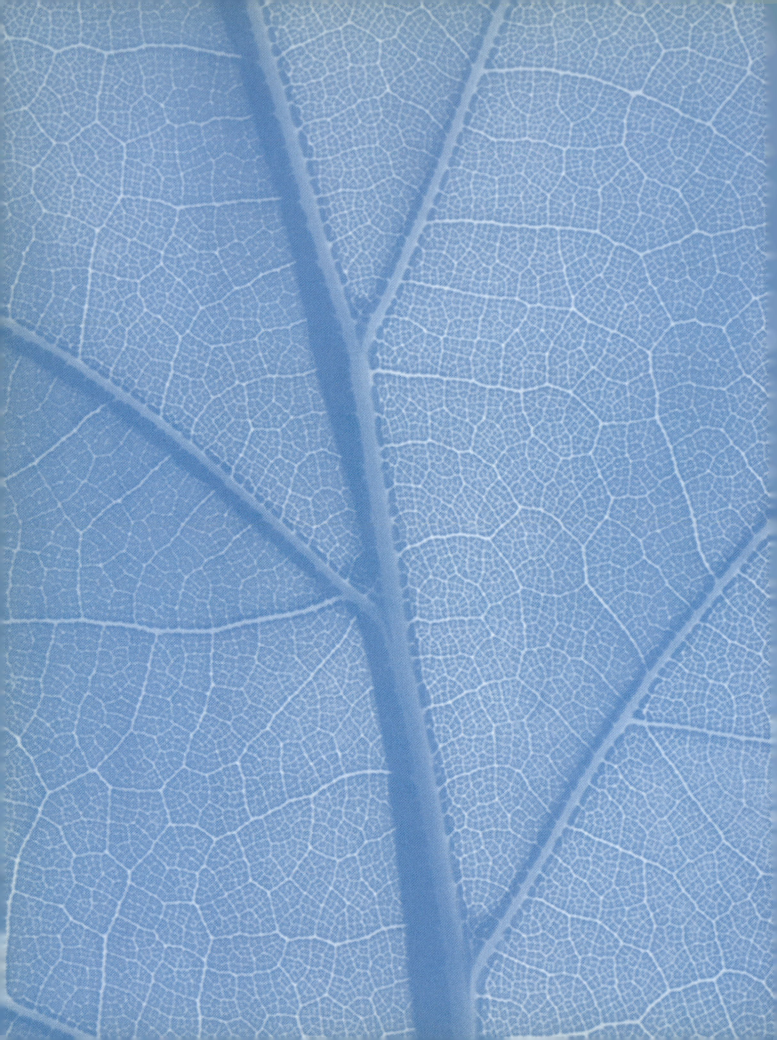

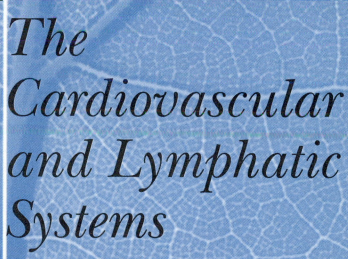

PART THREE

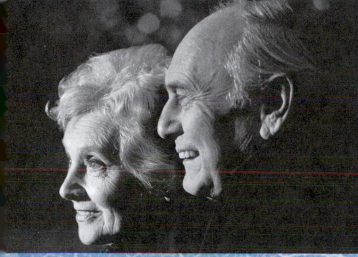

The Cardiovascular and Lymphatic Systems

Primary (Essential) Hypertension

GENDER

M

AGE

65

SETTING

- Hospital emergency department

ETHNICITY/CULTURE

- Black American

PREEXISTING CONDITIONS

- High blood pressure

COEXISTING CONDITIONS

- Family history: mother with history of hypertension died at age 70.

LIFESTYLE

- Part-time school bus driver. Work hours are 11:00–3:00, three days per week.
- Diet includes moderate amount of sodium.

COMMUNICATION

DISABILITY

SOCIOECONOMIC STATUS

- Low

SPIRITUAL/RELIGIOUS

- Baptist

PHARMACOLOGIC

- Furosemide (Lasix)
- Captopril (Capoten)
- Hydrochlorothiazide (HydroDIURIL)
- Spironolactone (Aldactone)
- Ezetimibe (Zetia)

PSYCHOSOCIAL

- Anxiety

LEGAL

ETHICAL

ALTERNATIVE THERAPY

- Listens to different kinds of music

PRIORITIZATION

- Interview
- Physical examination
- Evaluation of information
- Accurate monitoring of blood pressure

DELEGATION

- RN
- Client education

THE CARDIOVASCULAR AND LYMPHATIC SYSTEMS

Level of difficulty: Easy

Overview: This case involves understanding essential hypertension, monitoring blood pressure, administering prescribed medications, and clarifying the client's understanding of the disease. The case also involves client education and discharge planning with emphasis on follow-up care at the clinic or primary health care provider.

Client Profile

Mr. J is a 65-year-old male who has been visiting his primary health care provider yearly for annual examinations specifically related to history of mild congested heart failure (CHF). Over the past year, Mr. J notices that he gets infrequent headaches even though he is not stressed. Mr. J is 5′5″ and weighs 240 pounds.

Case Study

Mr. J reports a family history of hypertension and was diagnosed with primary hypertension at the age of 64. He reveals he likes foods that are high in sodium content. His father is alive and well, but his mother died at age 70 from a cerebral vascular accident related to hypertension. His social history reveals alcohol consumption of beer during the day and a glass of wine at dinner. Mr. J is seen by a nurse practitioner (NP) at the community clinic for complaints of headache and dizziness, which he reports experiencing while shopping at a department store. Upon admission, his vital signs are:

Blood pressure: 190/110

Pulse: 104 and regular

Respirations: 18

Temperature: 98.4° F

He is transferred to the local hospital's emergency department (ED) for further evaluation. On arrival at the ED, he is seen by an NP who initiates a systems assessment and finds his blood pressure reading to be 180/110 × two readings with the use of appropriate blood pressure cuff size. Mr. J reports current medications of captopril and metoprolol tartrate. He is kept in the ED for three hours on continuous telemetry while awaiting a bed on a medical unit. He is later transferred to a medical unit for further evaluations. Lab values are prescribed and include: urine for urinalysis, complete blood count, serum potassium (K+), sodium (Na), glucose, blood urea nitrogen (BUN), creatinine, cholesterol and triglyceride levels, serum aldosterone, and 24-hour urine aldosterone. His body mass index (BMI) is done and is 35, indicating that Mr. J is moderately obese for his height. The following are Mr. J's laboratory results:

Urinalysis: negative

White blood cell (WBC) count: 8,500 cells/mm³

Hematocrit (Hct): 33%

Hemoglobin (Hgb): 15 g/dL

Platelet count: 150,000 cells/mm³

Glucose: 80 mg/dL

Blood urea nitrogen (BUN): 14 mg/dL

Creatinine: 1.2 mg/dL

Potassium (K+): 3.7 mEq/L

Sodium (Na): 158 mEq/L

Albumin: 3.4 gm/dL

Calcium: 9 mg/dL

Cholesterol: 218 mg/dL

Triglyceride: 180 mg/dL

Urine aldosterone: 30 ug/24 hr

Serum aldosterone: 28 ng/dL

A fundoscopic examination of the eyes is done and indicates the retinal structures of the eyes are within normal limits. A 12-lead electrocardiogram (EKG) shows sinus rhythm, and a chest X-ray reveals normal heart size and normal lung structures. The dietitian sees the client and performs a three-day dietary recall, and plans to suggest a two-gram sodium diet to the multidisciplinary team. After the health care provider, pharmacist, NP, RN, and dietitian review the diagnostic tests and the laboratory data, a diagnosis of primary hypertension is confirmed.

The following are prescribed:

- Furosemide (Lasix) 40 mg IV stat
- Captopril (Capoten) 25 mg PO three times per day
- Hydrochlorothiazide (HydroDIURIL) 12.5 mg PO daily
- Spironolactone (Aldactone) 50 mg PO two times per day
- Ezetimibe (Zetia) 10 mg PO daily
- Two-gram sodium diet

Questions

1. What are specific cultural considerations in the United States for hypertension?

2. What are some common nursing diagnoses for clients with hypertension?

3. After the diagnosis of essential hypertension is confirmed with initial studies, what further evaluations are necessary?

4. What is the purpose of the registered dietitian in the multidisciplinary team conference with the client who is diagnosed with essential hypertension?

5. What are the purposes for the prescribed medications?

6. What are the most common adverse reactions of the prescribed medications?

7. Discuss drug-to-drug and drug-to-herbal interactions of the prescribed medications.

8. What is the ultimate goal of antihypertensive therapy?

9. Discuss the effects of angiotensin converting enzyme (ACE) on hypertension and nursing priority of care when caring for clients taking ACE inhibitor agents.

10. What are some complementary modalities clients with hypertension may use to decrease blood pressure?

11. Discuss client education for a captopril (Capoten) prescription upon discharge to home.

CASE STUDY 2

Coronary Artery Disease (Atherosclerosis)

GENDER

F

AGE

68

SETTING

- Hospital's outpatient clinic

ETHNICITY/CULTURE

- White American

PREEXISTING CONDITIONS

- Obesity

COEXISTING CONDITIONS

- Peripheral vascular disease

LIFESTYLE

- Unemployed

COMMUNICATION

DISABILITY

SOCIOECONOMIC STATUS

- Low

SPIRITUAL/RELIGIOUS

- Anglican

PHARMACOLOGIC

- Lipid-lowering agents
- Diuretics
- Cardiotonic
- Vasodilator
- Calcium-channel blocker
- Anticoagulant

PSYCHOSOCIAL

- Anxiety

LEGAL

- Financial resources

ETHICAL

ALTERNATIVE THERAPY

PRIORITIZATION

- Accurate systems assessment
- Continuous telemetry

DELEGATION

- RN
- LPN
- Client education

THE CARDIOVASCULAR AND LYMPHATIC SYSTEMS

Level of difficulty: Easy

Overview: The nurse will elicit appropriate nursing history to more accurately identify appropriate nursing diagnoses. The nurse also will use critical-thinking skills in identifying the client's immediate needs during triage. Client education is important before discharge from the hospital.

Client Profile

Ms. Z is a 68-year-old female who is 5′5″ and weighs 248 pounds. Her cardiologist refers her to the clinic of the community hospital after several complaints of fatigue and decrease in energy over the past month.

Case Study

Ms. Z is seen in the hospital outpatient clinic following the cardiologist's referral. She denies chest pain or palpitations on admission but reports frequent episodes of dizziness and inability to concentrate for "long periods of time." Her past medical history (PMH) includes hypercholesterolemia, chronic atrial fibrillation, episodes of syncope, occasional anginal type pain, and peripheral vascular disease (PVD). Past surgical history (PSH) includes a right femoral popliteal bypass. On initial assessment at the clinic, a complete physical examination is done and reveals bruits on auscultation of the left carotid artery. An electrocardiogram (EKG) shows atrial fibrillation. Her vital signs are:

> Blood pressure: 170/100
>
> Pulse: 78 and irregular
>
> Respirations: 20
>
> Temperature: 98.4° F

Lab reports from the clinic reveal:

> Prothrombin time (PT): 13.4 seconds, Control: 12.9 seconds
>
> Partial thromboplastin time (PTT): 30 seconds, Control: 29.9 seconds
>
> Glucose: 109 mg/dL
>
> Blood urea nitrogen (BUN): 9 mg/dL
>
> Creatinine: 0.8 mg/dL
>
> Sodium (Na): 136 mEq/L
>
> Potassium (K+): 3.9 mEq/L
>
> Calcium: 9 mg/dL
>
> Protein total: 7.8 g/dL
>
> Albumin: 3.2 g/dL
>
> Total bilirubin: 0.6
>
> White blood cell (WBC) count: 10,300/mm^3
>
> Red blood cell (RBC) count: 4.26 million/mm^3
>
> Hemoglobin (Hgb): 11.7 g/dL
>
> Hematocrit (Hct): 34.6%
>
> Platelet count: 258,000/mm^3
>
> Low-density lipoprotein (LDL): 127 mg/dL
>
> High-density lipoprotein (HDL): 46 mg/dL
>
> Total cholesterol: 257 mg/dL
>
> Triglyceride: 220 mg/dL

Medications taken at home are brought to the clinic and include: simvastatin, felodipine, lisinopril, hydrochlorothiazide, and aspirin 325 mg (EC). Carotid duplex ultrasonography is done and reveals marked narrowing of proximal left external carotid artery with area of plaque noted. Her ejection fraction is 30%. Magnetic resonance imaging (MRI) is done and compared with carotid duplex ultrasonography; the results are similar. After a complete history and physical and review of serum labs and diagnostic studies, the diagnosis of atherosclerosis is confirmed. Ms. Z will be discharged to home and will return to the hospital as scheduled for possible carotid endarterectomy after reevaluation of current medication regimen and repeat carotid duplex ultrasonography. Ms. Z is referred to physical therapy for physical strengthening exercises.

The following are prescribed:

- Cholestyramine resin (Questran) 4 g PO four times per day, before meals
- Colestipol HcL (Colestid) 15 g two times per day, before meals and at bedtime
- Digoxin (Lanoxin) 0.125 mg PO daily
- Dipyridamole (Persantine) 75 mg PO four times per day
- Diltiazem HcL (Cardizem) 30 mg PO four times per day
- Warfarin sodium (Coumadin) 5 mg PO today

Questions

1. What are the most common cited coronary artery disease risk equivalents for atherosclerosis?

2. What are the prominent modifiable and non-modifiable risk factors of atheroslcerosis?

3. What are common nursing diagnoses for the client with atherosclerosis?

4. What are the purposes for the prescribed medications?

5. What are the most common adverse reactions of the prescribed medications?

6. Discuss the drug-to-drug and drug-to-food/herbal interactions of the prescribed medications.

7. What are some physical findings in carotid stenosis?

8. What are some psychosocial stressors that can worsen hypertension and affect the client's ability to collaborate with treatment?

9. If Ms. Z is noncompliant with medical regimen after discharge and develops hypertensive crisis and is brought to the emergency department (ED), what are the indicators the nurse should focus on eliciting from the client on initial contact?

10. How should the nurse discuss discharge plans with Ms. Z in regard to her admission weight, at 5′5″, of 248 pounds?

Chronic Vascular Ulcers of the Right Foot

GENDER

M

AGE

78

SETTING

- Hospital

ETHNICITY/CULTURE

- Black American

PREEXISTING CONDITIONS

- Diabetes
- Hypertension

COEXISTING CONDITIONS

- Coronary artery bypass stroke
- Stroke

LIFESTYLE

- Retired

COMMUNICATION

DISABILITY

- Immobility

SOCIOECONOMIC STATUS

- Middle

SPIRITUAL/RELIGIOUS

- Baptist

PHARMACOLOGIC

- Rosiglitazone maleate (Avandia)
- Ticarcillin disodium/clavulanate potassium (Timentin)
- Gentamicin sulfate (Garamycin)
- Gabapentin (Neurontin)
- Enoxaparin (Lovenox)

PSYCHOSOCIAL

- Anxiety

LEGAL

ETHICAL

ALTERNATIVE THERAPY

Prayer

PRIORITIZATION

- Microbiological control
- Metabolic control
- Vascular control
- Wound control

DELEGATION

- RN
- Wound care specialist
- CNA

THE CARDIOVASCULAR AND LYMPHATIC SYSTEMS

Level of difficulty: Moderate

Overview: This case involves accurate identification of weak or absent peripheral pulses; sensation of bilateral extremities; pain on toes, between toes, and on upper aspect of the foot. Critical-thinking skills are used to prioritize effective care.

Client Profile

Mr. M is a 78-year-old retired lieutenant of the U.S. Army. He is 5′10″ and weighs 190 pounds. He is admitted from a nursing home with ulcers on the right great toe and plantar surface of the right foot.

Case Study

On admission to the hospital, Mr. M's vital signs are:

Blood pressure: 170/98

Pulse: 76

Respirations: 20

Temperature: 100.9° F

He is alert and oriented to time, place, and person. He has an indwelling Foley catheter in place to straight drainage, which is draining amber-colored urine. The following lab reports are sent from the nursing home:

White blood cell (WBC) count: 18,000/mm³

Red blood cell (RBC) count: 3,000,000/uL

Hemoglobin (Hgb): 16.4 g/dL

Hematocrit (Hct): 34%

Platelet count (PLT): 298,000/mm³

Glucose: 208 mg/dL

Blood urea nitrogen (BUN): 12 mg/dL

Past medical history (PMH) includes type 2 diabetes mellitus (non-independent diabetes mellitus [NIDDM]), peripheral vascular disease (PVD), hypertension, benign prostatic hyperplasia (BPH), depression, status-post (S/P) cerebrovascular accident (CVA) two years ago. Past surgical history (PSH) includes status-post (S/P) coronary artery bypass graft (CABG) and S/P femoral popliteal bypass and femoral endarterectomy one year ago. Medications sent with certified nursing assistant (CNA) who accompanied him to the hospital include: fluoxetine HcL, aspirin EC, ferrous sulfate, folic acid, gemfibrozil, finasteride, furosemide, metoprolol tartrate, omeprazole, and rosiglitazone maleate. Plans to review the medications brought to the hospital at a later time and renew them as appropriate are discussed by the health care provider and the primary nurse, the wound care specialist, and a pharmacist. Blood and wound culture is done and reveals Pseudomonas aeruginosa. The health care provider does a history and physical including a head-to-toe assessment. During the assessment of the lower extremities, the client reports pain in the lower right extremity during ambulation and at rest. Bilateral lower extremities are thoroughly assessed for color, temperature, pulses, odor, or drainage from the ulcer. An ankle brachial index (ABI) is done on both extremities and reveals an ABI 0.6 of the right lower extremity and a 0.9 of the left lower extremity. A surgical consult is requested and done, and the health care provider orders a duplex ultrasonography with color flow Doppler that shows chronic ischemic areas of the foot. After the multidisciplinary team reviews the labs and diagnostic reports, a medical diagnosis of vascular ulcers of the right foot is made. A discussion with Mr. M is done pertaining to management of the wound. Surgical débridement is discussed, and informed consent witnessed and signed by Mr. M. The débridement is scheduled for the next day. The débridement is successful. The client returns from the surgical procedure with an intact transparent wound barrier dressing to the foot and a vacuum-assisted pump applied with negative pressure to the ulcer area.

The following are prescribed:

- Morphine sulfate (Duramorph) 8 mg IM q4h PRN pain × 3 days
- Ticarcillin disodium/clavulanate potassium (Timentin) 3.1 g q6h
- Rosiglitazone maleate (Avandia) 8 mg PO daily
- Metoprolol tartrate (Lopressor) 75 mg PO daily
- Furosemide (Lasix) 49 mg PO daily
- Gabapentin (Neurontin) 400 mg PO q8h
- Enoxaparin (Lovenox) 30 mg/0.3 ML SC q12h
- Oxycodone/acetaminophen (Endocet) 5/325 MG 2 tablets PO q4h PRN
- Fingerstick glucose every shift and PRN
- Serum labs: glucose, WBC

Questions

1. Discuss risk factors and pathophysiology of vascular ulcers of the lower extremities.

2. Discuss the clinical manifestations for vascular disease of the lower extremities.

3. Discuss diagnostic studies used to confirm the diagnosis of vascular ulcers of the lower extremities.

4. Discuss common nursing diagnoses for vascular ulcers of the lower extremities.

5. What are the purposes for the prescribed orders?

6. What are the most common adverse reactions, drug-to-drug, drug-to-food/herbal interactions for the prescribed medications?

7. Discuss surgical management for peripheral artery disease of the lower extremities.

8. Discuss client education for vascular ulcers of the lower extremities.

CASE STUDY 4

Disseminated Intravascular Coagulation

GENDER

F

AGE

56

SETTING

- Hospital

ETHNICITY/CULTURE

- Black American

PREEXISTING CONDITIONS

- History of intestinal obstruction

COEXISTING CONDITIONS

LIFESTYLE

- Health educator who lectures four days per week at a senior college

COMMUNICATION

DISABILITY

SOCIOECONOMIC STATUS

- Middle

SPIRITUAL/RELIGIOUS

- Evangelical

PHARMACOLOGIC

- Gentamicin sulfate (Garamycin)
- Clindamycin HcL (Cleocin Hydrochloride)
- Cryoprecipitate
- Aminocaproic acid
- Vancomycin HcL (Vancocin)
- Metronidazole (Flagyl)

PSYCHOSOCIAL

- Anxiety
- Pain

LEGAL

ETHICAL

- The right to make decisions related to care

ALTERNATIVE THERAPY

- Prayer

PRIORITIZATION

- Patent airway
- Improve circulatory volume
- Supportive therapy with blood components

DELEGATION

- RN
- Client education

THE CARDIOVASCULAR AND LYMPHATIC SYSTEMS

Level of difficulty: Moderate

Overview: The case involves critical-thinking skills to prioritize and delegate care efficiently and appropriately. It involves clinical expertise in caring for the client with potential for thrombi and bleeding, and acute renal failure (ARF). It requires a multidisciplinary team with a clear understanding of the physiological changes that occur in disseminated intravascular coagulation.

Client Profile

Mrs. L is a 56-year-old female who for the past month has experienced occasional nausea and dizziness. After returning home from her teaching assignment, Mrs. L experienced a moderately sharp pain across her umbilicus. She had a cup of tea then went to rest and fell asleep. Upon awakening, Mrs. L experienced a more severe, intolerable pain of the abdomen. She is accompanied by a neighbor to her family health care provider and, on arrival at the health care provider's office, is immediately transferred to the emergency department (ED) of a nearby hospital.

Case Study

In the ED, a quick systems assessment is done followed by an upper gastrointestinal radiographic series (UGIS), which is ineffective because she vomits contents of the barium sulfate, including fecal content seen in the vomitus. Mrs. L is transferred to a surgical unit, and a systematic approach is used in doing the nursing history. Serum, urine specimens, and blood cultures are collected and sent to the laboratory. A chest X-ray, abdominal X-ray, and electrocardiogram (EKG) are completed, and the informed consent is signed. The abdominal X-ray reveals large amounts of fecal contents resting in the small intestines. Mrs. L's husband is notified of the plans for surgery, and Mrs. L is prepared for emergency laparotomy. A nasogastric tube (NGT) is inserted and attached to low continuous suction, and a Foley catheter is inserted and placed to straight drainage. Mrs. L is transferred to the operating room (OR) with a tentative diagnosis of mechanical obstruction of the small intestines. The initial surgery is successful and Mrs. L is returned to the surgical unit. On arrival, there is gentamicin 80 mg IV, Ringers Lactate at 125 cc/hr, morphine sulfate via PCA at 1 mg continuous, 5 mg PCA dose every eight minutes, and Foley catheter draining amber-colored urine at 50cc/hr. Mrs. L is drowsy but responsive to name and painful stimuli. Vital signs are:

Blood pressure: 130/80

Pulse: 100

Respirations: 16

Temperature: 98.0° F

On post-op day one, a consultation is written for an infectious disease health care provider to approve intravenous clindamycin due to the large strains of gram-positive cocci, including E. coli and C. diffcile, which were cultured from fecal contents of the intestines. Clindamycin 1500 mg is prescribed and is started on post-op day two. Within minutes after clindamycin is started, Mrs. L develops large wheals over her entire body, with pustules over the face and upper and lower extremities, and profuse watery diarrhea. Clindamycin is immediately discontinued and intravenous diphenhydramine HcL is administered. Ceftriaxone sodium IV is initiated. Mrs. L's condition worsens with evidence of high fever of 106.6° F, shaking chills, B/P 90/60, respirations 24, and pulse 120. She is immediately transferred to the surgical intensive care unit and is placed on four liters of oxygen via nasal cannula and 0.9% NaCL initiated at 150 mL/hr. Continuous monitoring of oxygen saturation with pulse oximeter, frequent arterial blood gases (ABGs), and accurate urinary output from indwelling catheter are maintained. On post-op day three, her condition deteriorates and a tentative diagnosis of sepsis-induced distributive shock is made. Laboratory data reveal:

Fibrinogen level: 200 mg/dL

D-dimer: 150 ng/mL

Bleeding time: 20 minutes

Platelet count (PLT): 100,000/mm³

Prothrombin time (PT) with INR: 3.8

Activated partial thromboplastin time (aPTT): 80 seconds

Partial thromboplastin time (PTT): 90 seconds

White blood cell (WBC) count: 20,000/mm³

After the labs are reviewed, a diagnosis of disseminated intravascular coagulation (DIC) secondary to sepsis-induced distributive shock is made.

The following are prescribed:

- Gentamicin sulfate (Garamycin) 2 mg/kg IV stat, followed by 3 mg/kg IV q8h
- Clindamycin HcL (Cleocin Hydrochloride) 1,500 mg q6h IV
- Metronidazole (Flagyl) 7.5 mg/kg q6h IV
- Diphenhydramine HcL (Benadryl) 50 mg IV stat
- Ceftriaxone sodium (Rocephin) 2 g q12h IV
- Fresh frozen plasma 1 unit IV
- Drotrecogin alfa (Activated) (Xigris) 24 mcg/kg/h continuous infusion × 96 h
- Daily serum labs: fibrinogen, D-dimer, bleeding time, PLT, PT, PTT

Questions

1. Discuss some specific factors that cause DIC.

2. Discuss common nursing diagnoses for clients with DIC.

3. What was the main purpose for the NGT to suction while the client was in the ED?

4. What is the reason for withholding opioid analgesic from Mrs. L, even though she is complaining of severe abdominal pain on arrival to the ED?

5. What are the purposes for the prescribed medications post-surgery?

6. If the client has developed anaphylaxis due to adverse reaction to the clindamycin, what reversal agent would most likely be prescribed?

7. What are the most common adverse reactions of the prescribed medications?

8. Why are the specified serum labs ordered for Mrs. L?

9. Discuss the drug-to-drug and drug-to-food/herbal interactions for the prescribed medications.

10. What is an important reminder for Mrs. L prior to her discharge?

11. You are a community-based nurse for a visiting nurse service. You are assigned to supervise home-care management in preparation for Mrs. L to return home upon discharge. A home health aide (HHA) is assigned to Mrs. L's care, with RN visits five days per week for the first week, three days per week for the second week, and one day per week for two additional weeks. Develop a community-based plan of care for the HHA to follow in the absence of the RN.

CASE STUDY 5

Unstable Angina Pectoris (Acute Myocardial Ischemia)

GENDER

F

AGE

60

SETTING

- Hospital

ETHNICITY/CULTURE

- Hispanic American

PREEXISTING CONDITIONS

- Atherosclerosis
- Coronary spasms
- Anemia

COEXISTING CONDITIONS

- Hyperthyroidism
- Stimulant abuse

LIFESTYLE

- Accounting department supervisor

COMMUNICATION

- Spanish and English

DISABILITY

SOCIOECONOMIC STATUS

- Middle

SPIRITUAL/RELIGIOUS

- Nondenominational

PHARMACOLOGIC

- Nitrates
- Beta-adrenergic blockers
- Calcium-channel blockers
- Aspirin

PSYCHOSOCIAL

- Anxiety

LEGAL

ETHICAL

ALTERNATIVE THERAPY

- Acupuncture
- Ginseng

PRIORITIZATION

- Obtain description of client's chest discomfort
- Obtain 12-lead EKG
- Provide measures to enhance tissue perfusion

DELEGATION

- RN
- Client education

THE CARDIOVASCULAR AND LYMPHATIC SYSTEMS

Level of difficulty: Moderate

Overview: This case involves a thorough assessment and critical-thinking skills to identify the classic symptoms of unstable angina so that appropriate medical interventions can be implemented effectively and to prioritize clients, because clients with unstable angina can progress to myocardial infarction or even death.

Client Profile

Ms. T, a 60-year-old female, is brought to the hospital emergency department (ED) due to intolerable chest pain after climbing several flights of stairs at her place of employment. Ms. T is 5'5" and weighs 206 pounds. Ms. T is an accounting department supervisor. She is a good historian and is able to explain quality and intensity of the present symptoms that warranted her access to the hospital ED.

Case Study

Ms. T reports taking nitroglycerin (NTG) for chest pain but says she did not take her NTG tablets to work with her, therefore, the pain was worse than she had experienced with previous attacks. However, on arrival to the ED, she reports that the severity of the pain has subsided. Ms. T's vital signs on arrival to the ED are:

> Blood pressure: 118/84
>
> Pulse: 74 and irregular
>
> Respirations: 22
>
> Temperature: 98.2° F

A 12-lead electrocardiogram (EKG) is done and reveals ST depression, T-wave inversion, atrioventricular conduction delay, and atrial fibrillation. Ms. T presently denies any discomfort and is waiting to be seen by the nurse practitioner (NP). The NP in the ED is given the report of the 12-lead EKG and will collaborate with the health care provider. As the interview with the NP continues, Ms. T reports inability to walk more than two blocks without difficulty breathing. She further reports noticing these occurrences increasing over the past three weeks. Her past medical history (PMH) includes aortic stenosis and hyperlipidemia and a right- and left-heart catheterization seven years ago. She reports being monitored in a cardiology clinic by a team of cardiologists. Reports from her medical records indicate moderate stenosis of the left anterior descending (LAD) artery. She has mild pulmonary hypertension, mild coronary atherosclerosis, and a mildly increased left ventricular hypertrophy. Her right coronary artery (RCA) shows mild calcification, and the LAD and the circumflex artery have moderate lesions. She is admitted to the coronary care unit (CCU), and continuous telemetry is initiated. The health care provider prescribes an echocardiogram and exercise stress test. The findings are positive for myocardial ischemia with decreased ejection fraction noted. Current laboratory values reveal:

> White blood cell (WBC) count: 10,000/mm³
>
> CK-MB: 132 U/L
>
> Hematocrit (Hct): 32%
>
> Hemoglobin (Hgb): 12 g/dL
>
> Potassium (K+): 4 mEq/L
>
> Sodium (Na): 145 mEq/L
>
> Troponin: T_1 0.1 ng/mL
>
> LDH_1: 38%
>
> LDH_2: 40%
>
> Total serum cholesterol: 185 mg/dL
>
> Triglyceride: 165 mg/dL

After review of diagnostic studies, laboratory data, physical assessment, and client's subjective data, a diagnosis of unstable angina pectoris is made. The health care team decides that Ms. T can return home, with follow-up care with her primary health care provider within two weeks from today's date. A repeat 12-lead EKG is done without any changes noted from the initial one. Ms. T is resting and her vital signs are:

Blood pressure: 118/78

Pulse: 74 irregular

Respirations: 18

Temperature: 98.2° F

The cardiologist and the NP discuss the discharge criteria with Ms. T, and she is to be discharged within 24 hours. The social worker and registered dietitian will visit with Ms. T in preparation for discharge.

The following are prescribed at discharge:

- Nitroglycerin (NTG) tab 0.4 mg SL for chest pain PRN
- Propranolol HcL (Inderal) 40 mg PO two times per day
- Nifedipine (Procardia) 20 mg PO three times per day
- Clopidogrel bisulfate (Plavix) 75 mg PO daily

Questions

1. What is your understanding of the above situation?

2. What is the incidence according to the American Heart Association (AHA) in regard to being overweight and obesity?

3. Discuss the relationship between gender and acute coronary syndrome (angina).

4. Explain the two predominant types of angina.

5. Discuss common nursing diagnoses for clients with angina pectoris.

6. If the following diagnostic tests were ordered for Ms. T, what would be the expected results?

- Chest radiography
- Echocardiogram

7. When would surgical intervention be considered for Ms. T?

8. What are the purposes for the prescribed medications?

9. What are the most common adverse reactions of the prescribed medications?

10. Discuss the drug-to-drug and drug-to-food/herbal interactions for the prescribed medications.

11. Discuss client education for unstable angina and aortic stenosis.

Sternal Wound Infection

GENDER

M

AGE

66

SETTING

- Hospital

ETHNICITY/CULTURE

- White American

PREEXISTING CONDITIONS

COEXISTING CONDITIONS

- Coronary artery bypass graft

LIFESTYLE

- Self-employed construction worker

COMMUNICATION

DISABILITY

SOCIOECONOMIC STATUS

- Middle

SPIRITUAL/RELIGIOUS

- Catholic

PHARMACOLOGIC

- Morphine sulfate (Duramorph)
- Piperacillin sodium/Tazobactam sodium (Zosyn)
- Ciprofloxacin HcL (Cipro)

PSYCHOSOCIAL

- Anxiety

LEGAL

ETHICAL

- Quality care
- Decrease in income
- Health care benefits

ALTERNATIVE THERAPY

- St. John's Wort

PRIORITIZATION

- Room assignment
- Antimicrobial management

DELEGATION

- RN
- Wound care specialist
- CNA

MODERATE

THE CARDIOVASCULAR AND LYMPHATIC SYSTEMS

Level of difficulty: Moderate

Overview: This case focuses on the use of critical thinking to provide effective prioritization in a triage situation in a busy urban medical center emergency department. It also involves management of sternal wound infection secondary to post-coronary artery bypass graft. A wound care specialist is important to management of an infected wound. The certified nursing assistant (CNA) can help with assembling necessary equipment in preparation for wound care and can position the client for the performance of the wound care.

Client Profile

Mr. Y is a 66-year-old male who was discharged from the hospital six weeks ago after an emergency quadruple coronary artery bypass graft (CABG) surgery. His post-op recovery was uneventful, and he was discharged ten days after the surgery. He returns to the chief surgeon's private office on the tenth day post-discharge prior to readmission because the sternal incisional site is red and inflamed with an unusual odor from the site of the wound. He reports pain at the site during hygiene care and a temperature of 101.2° F during the five days prior to seeing the health care provider. Mr. Y believes the redness at the incisional site is normal after surgery. However, because of the unusual odor, he goes to the health care provider's office to have the wound evaluated. Mr. Y is 5′8″ and weighs 206 pounds.

Case Study

Mr. Y is referred to the hospital for further evaluation. On initial interview his vital signs are:

> Blood pressure: 130/84
>
> Pulse: 78 and regular
>
> Respirations: 20
>
> Temperature: 102.4° F

The sternal incision is red, raised, and moderately warm to touch. There are no signs of dehiscence although the wound edges are not completely approximated. Mr. Y reports a 30-year history of cigarette smoking, three packs per week. His past medical history (PMH) includes hyperlipidemia, stable angina, and past surgical history of left cardiac catheterization and percutaneous transluminal coronary angioplasty (PTCA) with stent two years ago. Lab test results sent from the health care provider's office reveal:

> White blood cell (WBC) count: 12,000/mm^3
>
> Red blood cell (RBC) count: 4.6/mm^3
>
> Calcium: 9 mg/dL
>
> Sodium (Na): 142 mEq/L
>
> Potassium (K+): 4.9 mEq/L
>
> Chloride: 100 mEq/L
>
> Blood urea nitrogen (BUN): 15 mg/dL
>
> Creatinine: 1.4 mg/dL
>
> Glucose: 130 mg/dL
>
> Platelet count (PLT): 300, 000/cm
>
> Prothrombin time (PT): 14 seconds, Control: 15.1 seconds
>
> Hematocrit (Hct): 42%
>
> Hemoglobin (Hgb): 16 g/dL
>
> Low-density lipoprotein (LDL): 130 mg/dL
>
> Total cholesterol: 200 mg/dL

Medications brought to the hospital include: lovastatin (Mevacor), nitroglycerin (NTG) sublingual, isosorbide dinitrate (Isordil), warfarin sodium (Coumadin) 7.5 mg, and rabeprazole sodium (Aciphex). Mr. Y is transferred to a cardio-thoracic unit. A computed tomography (CT) scan of the chest is done in the ED and there is no evidence of infection in the deeper structures of the thoracic cavity.

On continued interview, Mr. Y reports self-medication with St. John's Wort whenever he feels anxious. His sternal wound is inspected by the receiving nurse who documents and reports the finding. Wound specimen for culture and sensitivity, and blood for gram stain are done and sent to the lab. An electrocardiogram (EKG) and a chest X-ray are done upon arrival to the unit, nursing assessment is completed, Mr. Y is placed on telemetry, and the nurse documents assessment findings. A nurse practitioner (NP) reviews the medications with the client and will discuss with the cardiologist before including them in current orders. The lab sends the report of the cultures, and the results are positive for Staphylococcus aureus and Enterococcus species. Mr. Y is informed that he will be admitted for further evaluation and antibiotic therapy. A diagnosis of sternal wound infection is made.

The following are prescribed:
- Piperacillin sodium/tazobactam sodium (Zosyn) 3 g IV q8h
- Morphine sulfate (Duramorph) PRN 2 mg IV prior to each dressing change
- Oxycodone (Roxicodone) 5–10 mg q4h PRN for mild to moderate pain
- Lovastatin (Mevacor) 40 mg PO two times per day
- Isosorbide dinitrate (Isordil) 10 mg four times per day PO, before meals and at bedtime
- Rabeprazole sodium (Aciphex) 20 mg PO daily
- Warfarin sodium (Coumadin) 7.5 mg PO daily after checking PT level
- Wound irrigation with 0.9% normal saline solution two times per day, followed by a wet-to-moist packing with 0.9% normal saline solution

Questions

1. What is a local factor that has affected Mr. Y's wound healing?

2. How do age, chronic disease, and vascular problems delay Mr. Y's wound healing?

3. Discuss common nursing diagnoses related to wound management.

4. What are the purposes for the prescribed medications?

5. What are the most common adverse reactions of the prescribed medications?

6. Discuss the drug-to-drug and drug-to-food/herbal interactions of the prescribed medications.

7. How do drugs such as corticosteroids, anti-inflammatory agents, and chemotherapy delay wound healing?

8. How do years of cigarette smoking delay wound healing?

9. What are the benefits of wound irrigation?

10. Discuss the phases of wound healing.

11. Discuss client education at time of discharge for an unhealed wound.

CASE STUDY 7

Valvular Heart Disease – Aortic Stenosis

GENDER

M

AGE

56

SETTING

- Hospital

ETHNICITY/CULTURE

- Hispanic/American

PREEXISTING CONDITIONS

- Angina

COEXISTING CONDITIONS

LIFESTYLE

- Supervisor for a community department store

COMMUNICATION

- Spanish and English

DISABILITY

SOCIOECONOMIC STATUS

- Middle

SPIRITUAL/RELIGIOUS

- Catholic

PHARMACOLOGIC

- Calcium-channel blocker
- ACE inhibitor
- Cardiotonic
- Oxygen

PSYCHOSOCIAL

- Anxiety

LEGAL

ETHICAL

ALTERNATIVE THERAPY

- Holy Communion

PRIORITIZATION

- Maintain cardiac output
- Monitor vital signs
- Administer oxygen

DELEGATION

- RN
- Client education

THE CARDIOVASCULAR AND LYMPHATIC SYSTEMS

Level of difficulty: Moderate

Overview: This case involves the use of the nursing process and critical thinking to appropriately assess the client and delegate effectively so that care can be implemented. The case requires health care personnel who are competent in cardiac assessment, identifying heart sounds and dysrhythmias, and intervening effectively.

Client Profile

Mr. W is a 56-year-old male who is 5′6″ and weighs 190 pounds. His past medical history includes childhood rheumatic heart disease with one occurrence of strep throat at the age of 30. Mr. W is married, and there is one young adult living at home with him and his wife. They live in a private home with four flights of steps going up to the bedrooms.

Case Study

Mr. W is referred to the hospital by his primary health care provider after frequent complaints of difficulty breathing when climbing stairs and a report of feeling tired after walking only two blocks. Mr. W also reports anginal-type chest pain and infrequent syncope. He reports loss of appetite and loss of 12 pounds over one month. On admission to the hospital, his vitals signs are:

> Blood pressure: 150/68
>
> Pulse: 64 and irregular
>
> Respirations: 16
>
> Temperature: 98.6° F

On auscultation, there is a harsh systolic murmur in the second intercostal space at the right sternal border. An arterial blood gas (ABG) is done and reveals hypoxemia. Oxygen, three liters via nasal cannula, is initiated. Mr. W denies surgical history but reports having a cardiac catheterization that was done two months ago at another hospital and chronic atrial fibrillation. The result of the catheterization is sent from Mr. W's primary health care provider's office. The report of the catheterization is:

> Routine blood pressure in brachial artery: 120/50 mm Hg
>   (normal = 90–140/60–90 mm Hg)
>
> End-diastolic volume (EDV): 80 ml/m^2 (normal = 50–90 ml/m^2)
>
> Ejection fraction: 0.58 (normal = 0.67 ± 0.07)
>
> Cardiac output: (CO) 4 liters/min (normal = 3–6 liters/min)

A thorough history and physical is completed by a health care provider and a registered nurse (RN). A multidisciplinary team reviews the current data gathered from the history, physical, and reports of the previous diagnostic tests. A chest X-ray reveals mid-left ventricular enlargement, and echocardiography provides data of the cardiac structure, movement of the valve leaflets, and the size and function of the cardiac chambers, which aids in diagnosis. An EKG confirms chronic atrial fibrillation. Admission lab tests reveal:

> White blood cell (WBC) count: 9,000/mm^3
>
> Red blood cell (RBC): 3.4 million/mm^3
>
> Hemoglobin (Hgb): 10 g/dL
>
> Hematocrit (Hct): 28%
>
> Platelet: 150,000/mm^3
>
> Glucose: 116 mg/dL
>
> Blood urea nitrogen (BUN): 15 mg/dL
>
> Creatinine: 0.9 mg/dL
>
> Sodium (Na): 135 mEq/L
>
> Potassium (K+): 4.6 mEq/L

Albumin: 3.3 mg/dL

Calcium: 8.6 mg/dL

Digoxin level: 1.3 ng/dL

After review of collected data and collaborative discussion with the multidisciplinary team, a diagnosis of aortic stenosis is confirmed. The findings are discussed with Mr. W and his wife, and a surgical consultation is done. Elective surgery for aortic valve repair is planned and will be scheduled within three days. A prosthetic valve will be used. In preparation for the aortic valve repair, Mr. W is to be transfused as prescribed with two units of packed red blood cells (PRBCs) because of the low Hgb and Hct.

The following new medications are prescribed:

- Digoxin (Lanoxin) 0.125 mg PO
- Diltiazem (Cardizem) 40 mg PO two times per day
- Amiodarone HcL (Cardarone) 200 mg PO daily
- Warfarin sodium (Coumadin) 5 mg PO today

Questions

1. Discuss common nursing diagnoses for clients with valvular heart disease.

2. Why is cardiac catheterization usually done when clients are diagnosed with aortic stenosis?

3. Why is atrial fibrillation a common finding in aortic stenosis?

4. What is a long-term complication of aortic stenosis?

5. What are the purposes for the prescribed orders?

6. What are the most common adverse reactions of the prescribed medications?

7. Discuss the drug-to-drug and drug-to-food/herbal interactions of the prescribed medications.

8. Which modality is the definitive treatment of aortic stenosis for clients with complaints of dyspnea, fatigue, and chest pain?

9. Identify the different types of valves used in valvular replacement procedures.

10. What are the two post-surgery complications the nurse should monitor for when a client has a valvular replacement?

11. Discuss client education for post-valvular surgery?

CASE STUDY 8

Hodgkin's Disease

GENDER

M

AGE

54

SETTING

- Outpatient clinic of a medical center

ETHNICITY/CULTURE

- White Englishman

PREEXISTING CONDITIONS

- Enlarged, painless, freely movable mass in the neck

COEXISTING CONDITIONS

- History of viral infection

LIFESTYLE

- Worked as a subway worker before immigrating to the U.S.

COMMUNICATION

DISABILITY

SOCIOECONOMIC STATUS

- Middle

SPIRITUAL/RELIGIOUS

- Anglican

PHARMACOLOGIC

- Mechlorethamine HcL (Mustargen)
- Vincristine sulfate (Oncovin)
- Procarbazine HcL (Matulane)
- Prednisone (Deltasone)
- Ondansetron HcL (Zofran)

PSYCHOSOCIAL

- Anxiety

LEGAL

- Assistance with financial resource

ETHICAL

- Do recent immigrants to the U.S. have a right to optimum health care benefits in lieu of unemployment related to work status?

ALTERNATIVE THERAPY

PRIORITIZATION

- Physical assessment
- Prepare for staging of lymph node

DELEGATION

- RN
- Client education

THE CARDIOVASCULAR AND LYMPHATIC SYSTEMS

Level of difficulty: Moderate

Overview: This case study involves a thorough assessment of the client's condition with careful palpation for lymphadenopathic lesions. It also involves critical questioning pertaining to night sweats and weight loss of more than 10%, unusual headaches, dry cough, and neck or back pain.

Client Profile

Mr. O is a 54-year-old male who has been a resident of the United States for the past three years after relocating from London, England, where he worked as an underground railroad employee. He is 5′8″ and weighs 165 pounds.

Case Study

Mr. O is seen in the outpatient clinic of a major medical center with complaints of gradual fatigue and weight loss over the past two months. He also reports fever of unknown cause, unusual pruritus on the trunk and chest of his body, headaches, and vertigo. After initial interview by the nurse, Mr. O is seen by a health care provider, who continues with the history and physical examination. Large, painless lymph nodes are found in the neck and axilla areas. Mr. O denies the use of medications or herbal supplements and denies past medical or surgical history. Vital signs on admission reveal:

> Blood pressure: 120/80
>
> Pulse: 78
>
> Respirations: 16
>
> Temperature: 98.4° F

Lab results reveal:

> White blood cell (WBC) differential:
>> Lymphocytes: 22%
>>
>> Segmented neutrophils: 60%
>>
>> Monocytes: 6.2%
>>
>> Eosinophils: 0.9%
>>
>> Basophils: 1.1%
>>
>> Bands: 5%
>
> Red blood cell (RBC) count: 4 million/mm^3
>
> Hematocrit (Hct): 42%
>
> Hemoglobin (Hgb): 13 g/dL
>
> Platelet count: 267,000/mm^3
>
> Granulocyte: 20.4%
>
> Sodium (Na): 138 mEq/L
>
> Potassium (K+): 3.9 mEq/L
>
> Calcium: 8.4 mg/dL
>
> Blood urea nitrogen (BUN): 15 mg/dL
>
> Creatinine: 0.7 mg/dL
>
> Magnesium: 2 mg/dL

After the labs and physical assessment findings are reviewed by the health care provider and a hematologist, Mr. O is admitted to a medical unit for further evaluation. A positron emission test (PET) shows cancer cells in the peripheral lymph node and peripheral lymph node enlargement. A chest X-ray and an abdominal computed tomography (CT) scan are done, but the findings for lymphadenopathy in the thoracic and abdominal areas are negative. Mr. O is advised of the need for lymph node biopsy, and he signs an informed witnessed consent. The biopsy is positive for Reed-Sternberg cells. Staging procedures reveal stage IIa lymphoma. After the health care provider and hematologist review the results of the labs and diagnostic reports, a diagnosis of stage IIa Hodgkin's disease is confirmed and discussed with the client, who agrees with the treatment plan.

The following are prescribed:

- MOPP combination therapy q4 weeks for six cycles:
- Mechlorethamine HcL (Mustargen) IV 6 mg/m^2 on day one and eight of a 28-day cycle
- Vincristine sulfate (Oncovin) IV 1.4 mg/m^2 weekly
- Procarbazine HcL (Matulane) PO 2 mg/kg/d for one week, then 6 mg/kg/d
- Prednisone (Deltasone) 30 mg PO daily
- Ondansetron HcL (Zofran) 32 mg IV 30 minutes before chemotherapy

Questions

1. Discuss the prevalence, incidence, risk factors, and pathophysiology of Hodgkin's disease.

2. Discuss clinical manifestations of Hodgkin's disease.

3. Discuss diagnostic studies used to confirm Hodgkin's disease.

4. Discuss medical management for Hodgkin's disease.

5. Discuss complications of Hodgkin's disease.

6. What are the purposes for the prescribed medications?

7. What are the most common adverse reactions, drug-to-drug, drug-to-food/herbal interactions of the prescribed mediations?

8. Discuss staging classification for Hodgkin's disease.

9. Discuss management for vincristine infusion therapy.

10. Discuss client education for Hodgkin's disease.

Multiple Myeloma (Plasma Cell Myeloma)

GENDER

F

AGE

64

SETTING

- Hospital

ETHNICITY/CULTURE

- Black American

PREEXISTING CONDITIONS

COEXISTING CONDITIONS

- Renal failure

LIFESTYLE

- Worked 15 years for a company that sells wood and soil for agricultural and building purposes

COMMUNICATION

DISABILITY

- Difficulty ambulating independently

SOCIOECONOMIC STATUS

- Middle

SPIRITUAL/RELIGIOUS

- Baptist

PHARMACOLOGIC

- Acetaminophen (Tylenol)
- Melphalan (Alkeran)
- Prednisone (Deltasone)
- Pamidronate disodium (Aredia)
- Cyclophosphamide (Cytoxan)
- Furosemide (Lasix)
- Palonosetron HcL (Aloxi)

PSYCHOSOCIAL

- Anxiety

LEGAL

- Supplemental resource to defray hospital expenses

ETHICAL

- The right to receive disability benefits if illness is job related

ALTERNATIVE THERAPY

- Fish oil

PRIORITIZATION

- Assess bone or joint pain
- Promote comfort
- Provide safety

DELEGATION

- RN
- CNA
- Client education

MODERATE

THE CARDIOVASCULAR AND LYMPHATIC SYSTEMS

Level of difficulty: Moderate

Overview: This case involves a thorough assessment of the client's condition with focus on bone and joint pain, easy bruising, and signs of renal insufficiency. It involves nursing measures to avoid exposure to infections. The certified nursing assistant (CNA) can be delegated the duty of observing for discoloration while assisting with hygiene care.

Client Profile

Mrs. R, a 64-year-old widow for the past ten years, is accompanied by her home health aide (HHA) via ambulance to the hospital's emergency department (ED) after falling at home. Mrs. R is 4′5″ and weighs 120 pounds.

Case Study

On arrival in the triage area, she reports pain of the right upper extremity, which she said began after she fell at home. The nurse attempts to assess the upper extremity but is unable to do so because of the pain and the guarding of the extremity by Mrs. R. On initial interview, she reports being fatigued, weak, anorexic, and constipated for the past four days. She describes back and joint pain that is not related to her recent fall and explains that the pain is worse in the supine position and is not relieved by ibuprofen or acetaminophen. Mrs. R points to bluish discoloration on areas of her body, which she believes occur whenever she bumps on an object in her apartment. The HHA confirms the report of easy bruising, telling the nurse that Mrs. R bruises even with the slightest contact on soft furniture, and informs the nurse that Mrs. R has been showing signs of confusion and occasional disorientation for the past two weeks. Mrs. R denies significant past medical history but reports fracture of the left ankle that occurred six months ago due to a fall while ambulating in her apartment. Mrs. R is seen by the health care provider and a history and physical are done. She is then admitted to a medical unit for further evaluation and diagnosis. Serum lab reports reveal:

Calcium: 16.5 mg/dL

Phosphorous: 2.5 mg/dL

Neutrophils: 2,500%

Lymphocytes: 2,000/mm^3

Monocytes: 150/mm^3

Eosinophils: 200/mm^3

Basophils: 80/mm^3

Red blood cell (RBC) count: 4.2 mm^3

Platelet count: 140,000 cells/mm^3

Creatinine: 1.5 mg/dL

Blood urea nitrogen (BUN): 9 mg/dL

A bone marrow biopsy is done, after an informed consent is signed, and shows significant presence of sheets of malignant plasma cells. A 24-hour urinalysis by protein electrophoresis is positive for Bence Jones protein, and X-ray studies of bones find thinning and signs of osteoporosis and osteopenia. A diagnosis of multiple myeloma is confirmed.

The following are prescribed:
- Cyclophosphamide (Cytoxen) 10 mg/kg IV once daily × five days
- M combined with elphalan (Alkeran) 9 mg/PO daily × four days; alternate with 6 mg PO daily × seven days
- Prednisone (Deltasone) 50 mg PO two times per day × four days; alternate with 100 mg PO daily × seven days
- Pamidronate disodium (Aredia) 30 mg once daily IV × three days
- Palonosetron HcL (Aloxi) 0.25 mg IV 30 minutes before administration of antineoplastic

- Monitor serum labs daily: WBC count, Hct, Hgb, leukocytes, PLT, calcium, creatinine, BUN, and phosphorous
- Monitor urine for blood each void
- Maintain fluid hydration 3,000 mL daily and monitor intake and output and urine specific gravity

Questions

1. Discuss the pathophysiology of multiple myeloma.

2. Discuss clinical manifestations of multiple myeloma.

3. Discuss assessment and diagnostic findings.

4. Discuss different steps of diagnostic staging used to guide and manage treatment of multiple myeloma.

5. Discuss nursing diagnoses for multiple myeloma.

6. Discuss common complications of multiple myeloma.

7. What are the purposes for the prescribed orders?

8. What are the most common adverse reactions to the prescribed medications?

9. Discuss the drug-to-drug and drug-to-food/herbal interactions for the prescribed medications.

10. Discuss client educational for the client with multiple myeloma.

CASE STUDY 10

Chronic Myelogenous Leukemia

GENDER

M

AGE

60

SETTING

- Hospital health clinic

ETHNICITY/CULTURE

- White/Portuguese

PREEXISTING CONDITIONS

COEXISTING CONDITIONS

LIFESTYLE

- Retired plastic factory employee

COMMUNICATION

DISABILITY

- Yes

SOCIOECONOMIC STATUS

- Middle

SPIRITUAL/RELIGIOUS

- Anglican

PHARMACOLOGIC

- Imatinib mesylate (Gleevec)
- Leucovorin calcium (Folinic acid)
- Hydroxyurea (Hydrea)
- Interferon alfa-2b (Intron-A)

PSYCHOSOCIAL

- Depression

LEGAL

- If work-related factors are the cause of CML, employers should help with treatment costs, and the client should receive lifelong compensation.

ETHICAL

- Clients should be informed of risk factors in the workplace and educated on how to prevent direct exposure to those risks.

ALTERNATIVE THERAPY

- Naturopathy
- Ginseng
- Soy foods

PRIORITIZATION

- Private room
- Monitor platelet function

DELEGATION

- RN
- Client education

THE CARDIOVASCULAR AND LYMPHATIC SYSTEMS

Level of difficulty: Moderate

Overview: This case involves a thorough history that should include questions pertaining to risk factors and causative factors, occupation, and hobbies to detect causative environmental factors that may have aggravated leukemic process. The case involves questioning the client about frequency and severity of infectious process during the preceding six months, because the risk for infection is increased in clients with leukemia. It requires asking about overt or hidden excessive bleeding episodes, because platelet function is usually diminished with leukemia. Aggressive treatment is needed with chronic myelogenous leukemia (CML), because it can and often does progress to acute leukemia.

Client Profile

Mr. K is a 60-year-old client who came to the hospital outpatient clinic complaining of increased sensitivity at his right side, unusual loss of appetite, and weight loss, which he believes is due to lack of appetite. He reports discomfort in the right and left upper quadrants and informs the nurse that he is concerned about his health because of a family history of leukemia. Mr. K is 5′6″ and weighs 285 pounds. On initial discussion with a nurse, he remarks that he is wondering if his symptoms are early signs of recurring leukemia because he was diagnosed with "childhood leukemia" at the age of 12. However, "he had complete remission" after several treatments at a children's hospital in Portugal. Mr. K reports that he was employed for ten years in a factory that manufactures plastic covers for furniture and household items.

Case Study

Mr. K is known to the clinic and is a reliable historian. Mr. K informs the nurse he has been seeing a naturopathic practitioner, he is currently taking ginseng, and he has recently included soy foods in his diet. The nurse assesses Mr. K and, on physical exam, finds an enlarged spleen and liver and a palpable mass on palpation. Upon completion of the nursing history and assessment, the nurse informs the nurse practitioner (NP) of the findings. The NP continues with further physical assessment on Mr. K and elicits that he has been experiencing weakness, early satiety, and sweating more frequently over the past week. He also reports easy fatigability with minimal activities of daily living (ADLs) and occasional "gouty attacks." After the NP reviews the assessment findings with a medical doctor and a hematologist, the following serum labs are ordered: complete blood count (CBC) with peripheral blood smear, serum acid levels, and alkaline phosphatase. The CBC reveals:

High numbers of mature white blood cells (WBCs): 30,000/mm³

Decreased hematocrit (Hct): 33.2%

Hemoglobin (Hgb): 12.9%

Platelet counts: elevated at 480,000/mm³

The peripheral smear reflects the presence of granulocytes at all levels of maturation, serum uric acid level is elevated (9.2 mg/dl), and alkaline phosphatase (LAP score) is reduced (28 U/L). The multidisciplinary team reviews the recent serum lab data and determines that a bone marrow aspiration and biopsy would enhance the diagnosis. Mr. K is informed of the need for the procedures, agrees, and signs an informed witnessed consent. Mr. K is given two oxycodone/acetaminophen 5/325 mg tablets prior to the bone marrow aspiration and biopsy procedure. The bone marrow aspiration and biopsy reveal hypercellularity, megakaryocytosis, and B-cell proliferation. After reviewing the results and report from the hematologist, the oncologist assigns the diagnosis of CML. The health care provider discusses the diagnosis and chemotherapy treatment plan with Mr. K, and refers him to the dietitian, who, in collaboration with the health care team, plans a balanced diet with supplemental vitamins and iron.

The following are prescribed:

- Imatinib mesylate (Gleevec) 400 mg PO four times per day
- Leucovorin calcium (Folinic acid) 10 mg/M² IV q6h until serum methotrexate level is less than 0.05 micromolar
- Hydroxyurea (Hydrea) 30 mg/kg PO daily
- Interferon alfa-2b (Intron-A) 2 million U/m² three times per week

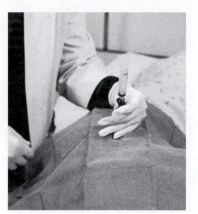

Bone marrow biopsy/aspiration.

Questions

1. Discuss the incidence and prevalence of CML.

2. Discuss the pathophysiology of CML.

3. Discuss diagnostic studies for CML.

4. Discuss main prognostic indicators of CML.

5. Discuss common nursing diagnoses and expected outcome criteria for adult clients with CML.

6. What are the purposes for the prescribed medications?

7. What are the most common adverse reactions of the prescribed medications?

8. Discuss the drug-to-drug and drug-to-food/herbal interactions for the prescribed medications.

9. Discuss health care resources that are usually needed by clients with CML.

10. Discuss client education for CML.

CASE STUDY 11

Femoral-Popliteal Bypass for Peripheral Vascular Disease

GENDER

M

AGE

72

SETTING

ETHNICITY/CULTURE

- White/American

PREEXISTING CONDITIONS

COEXISTING CONDITIONS

LIFESTYLE

- Retired computer sales manager

COMMUNICATION

DISABILITY

SOCIOECONOMIC STATUS

- Middle

SPIRITUAL/RELIGIOUS

- Catholic

PHARMACOLOGIC

- Morphine sulfate (Duramorph)
- Dipyridamole (Persantine)
- Piperacillin sodium/tazobactam sodium (Zosyn)

PSYCHOSOCIAL

- Anxiety

LEGAL

ETHICAL

ALTERNATIVE THERAPY

PRIORITIZATION

- Assess and manage pain
- Peripheral vascular assessment
- Increase tissue perfusion

DELEGATION

- RN
- Client education

THE CARDIOVASCULAR AND LYMPHATIC SYSTEMS

Level of difficulty: Moderate

Overview: This case requires critical post-operative care for the client with peripheral vascular disease. The nurse must use critical decision making in pain management and be able to critically assess for signs or symptoms of reocclusion of the graft.

Client Profile

Mr. T is a 72-year-old male admitted to the surgical intensive care unit (SICU) following a femoral-popliteal bypass graft of the right lower extremity for peripheral vascular disease. Mr. T is initially admitted to the emergency department (ED) of the hospital with complaints of severe pain of the extremity even at rest (ischemic rest pain). He reports a long history of cigarette smoking and history of hypertension and coronary artery disease (atheroclesrosis) and denies surgical history in the past. A Doppler study is done; peripheral pulses of the right extremity are faint and are absent on palpation, peripheral pulses of the left lower extremity are weak, and bilateral extremities are cool to touch.

Case Study

During the history and physical in the ED by a health care provider, Mr. T's pain becomes so unbearable even at rest that he is transported to the operating room for emergency surgery. The surgery is completed, and Mr. T is transferred to the SICU. On arrival, Mr. T is alert but drowsy. However, he moves his head and responds to his name when called, and is responsive to tactile stimuli. He has an arterial line in place, intravenous catheter with Ringer's lactate infusing at 125 mL per hour via electronic pump. He is attached to telemetry, with normal sinus rhythm and occasional unifocal premature ventricular contractions (PVCs) noted. He has a face mask with 40% oxygen in place and a Foley catheter in situ with clear, amber-colored urine draining in a urometer. He has an arterial line in situ, and on arrival to the unit, his vital signs are:

Blood pressure: 140/82

Pulse: 98

Respirations: 18

Temperature: 99.4° F

His leg is wrapped with a light dressing and orders are written to keep the leg flat in bed. His chart reveals post-embolectomy. The receiving nurse completes the assessment, provides initial care to the client, and proceeds to document the data.

The following are prescribed:
- Morphine sulfate (Duramorph) 2 mg IV q1–2h PRN
- Dipyridamole (Persantine) 100 mg PO four times per day
- Piperacillin sodium/tazobactam sodium (Zosyn) 3 g IV q6h
- Serum PTT, aPTT, CBC, and INR daily
- Bed rest with extremity straight

Questions

1. Discuss the factors from Mr. T's past medical history that predispose him to the need for femoral popliteal bypass.

2. Discuss the femoral-popliteal bypass procedure.

3. Discuss a specific diagnostic test to determine that the bypass procedure is needed and how the test is performed

4. Discuss important post-operative assessment findings to which a nurse should give critical attention.

5. Discuss common nursing diagnoses, expected outcomes, and nursing interventions for the client with post-femoral-popliteal bypass.

6. Discuss the potential complications post femoral-popliteal bypass graft.

7. What are the purposes for the prescribed orders?

8. What are the common adverse reactions, drug-to-drug, drug-to-food/herbal interactions of the prescribed drugs?

9. Discuss client education for post-femoral-popliteal bypass.

CASE STUDY 12

Premature Ventricular Contractions

GENDER

M

AGE

72

SETTING

- Adult home and hospital

ETHNICITY/CULTURE

- Black American/West Indian

PREEXISTING CONDITIONS

- Premature ventricular contractions and atrial fibrillation

COEXISTING CONDITIONS

- Left-sided heart failure

LIFESTYLE

- Retired farmer

COMMUNICATION

DISABILITY

- Reduced ability to perform ADL

SOCIOECONOMIC STATUS

- Low

SPIRITUAL/RELIGIOUS

- Anglican

PHARMACOLOGIC

- Atropine sulfate (Atropine)
- Amiodarone HcL (Cardarone)
- Lidocaine HcL (Xylocaine)
- Carvedilol (Coreg)

PSYCHOSOCIAL

- Anxiety

LEGAL

ETHICAL

- Availability of place of residence upon discharge

ALTERNATIVE THERAPY

PRIORITIZATION

- Stabilize heart rate and rhythm

DELEGATION

- RN
- Client education

THE CARDIOVASCULAR AND LYMPHATIC SYSTEMS

Level of difficulty: Difficult

Overview: This case involves a thorough assessment of the client's condition with focus on his cardiac status, including the drugs he is presently on and those brought to the hospital. The case involves prioritization in a triage situation and critical thinking to appropriately delegate and transfer the client to the appropriate unit for continued observation.

Client Profile

Mr. J is a 72-year-old male admitted to the emergency department (ED) from an adult home where he has been living for the past two years. Vital signs on admission are:

Blood pressure: 110/74

Pulse: 54

Respirations: 18

Temperature: 98.4° F

Case Study

On admission, Mr. J is alert and oriented to person, date, and current year. He complains of occasional pressure in his chest, and reports feeling tired and dizzy when he keeps his head down for short periods of time. Past medical history (PMH) reveals myocardial infarction five years ago and current left-sided heart failure. The certified nurse's assistant (CNA) who accompanies him to the ED informs the triage nurse that he self medicates with digoxin (Lanoxin), docusate sodium (Colace), and furosemide (Lasix) daily, but the CNA does not know the dosages of the mentioned medications. A chest X-ray is done and reveals pulmonary congestion and a 12-lead EKG shows decrease tissue perfusion, but no signs of new injury to the myocardium. An IV line is inserted and atropine sulfate 0.5 mg IV administered × one, with a noted increase of heart rate of 68. Mr. J is placed on continuous telemetry that reveals unifocal premature ventricular contractions (PVCs) that developed into coupling then trigeminy. Mr. J complains of chest discomfort, the health care provider is informed and reviews the current serum levels:

Serum digoxin: 2.6 ng/dL

Sodium (Na): 135 mEq/L

Potassium (K+): 3 mEq/L

Blood urea nitrogen (BUN): 15 mg/dL

Calcium: 8.5 mg/dL

Magnesium: 2 mg/dL

The drugs brought to the hospital with the client are reviewed and digoxin and furosemide are held. Mr. J is transferred to the coronary care unit (CCU) with a diagnosis of PVCs.

The following are prescribed:

- Dextrose 5% and 0.45% sodium chloride with 20 mEq KcL IV infusion at 100 ml/hr
- Atropine sulfate (Atropine) 0.5 mg IV q1h PRN for a maximum of 2 mg
- Lidocaine HcL (Xylocaine) 50 mg IV bolus at 20 mg/min, repeat in 5 min, then start infusion of 20 mcg/kg/min immediately after first bolus
- Amiodarone HcL (Cardarone) 150 mg IV over 10 mg followed by 360 mg slow infusion over 6 hours followed by 540 mg at 0.5 mg/min over 18 hours
- Place client on continuous telemetry
- Monitor continuous oxygen saturation/pulse oximetry
- Oxygen to maintain oxygen saturation greater than 94%
- Serial arterial blood gas (ABG)
- Carvedilol (Coreg) 3.125 mg two times per day for two weeks
- Serum digoxin levels two times per day until stable
- Monitor serum sodium, potassium, and magnesium levels

Questions

1. Discuss PVCs or complexes.

2. Discuss some risk factors for the development of PVCs.

3. Discuss the effects of atropine sulfate in treating bradycardia and the development of PVCs.

4. Discuss clinical manifestations of PVCs.

5. Discuss the complications that can result from PVCs, especially in Mr. J's case.

6. Discuss common nursing diagnoses for clients with dysrhythmias.

7. Discuss the reasons why Mr. J's digoxin and furosemide are being held.

8. Discuss the reason digoxin immune fab (Ovine) was not prescribed for Mr. J.

9. What are the purposes of the prescribed orders?

10. What are the most common adverse reactions, drug-to-drug, drug-to-food/herbal interactions of the prescribed medications?

11. Discuss the psychosocial impact of being in an intensive care unit (ICU).

12. Discuss client education for a multiple diagnosis of left-sided heart failure and current episodes of PVCs.

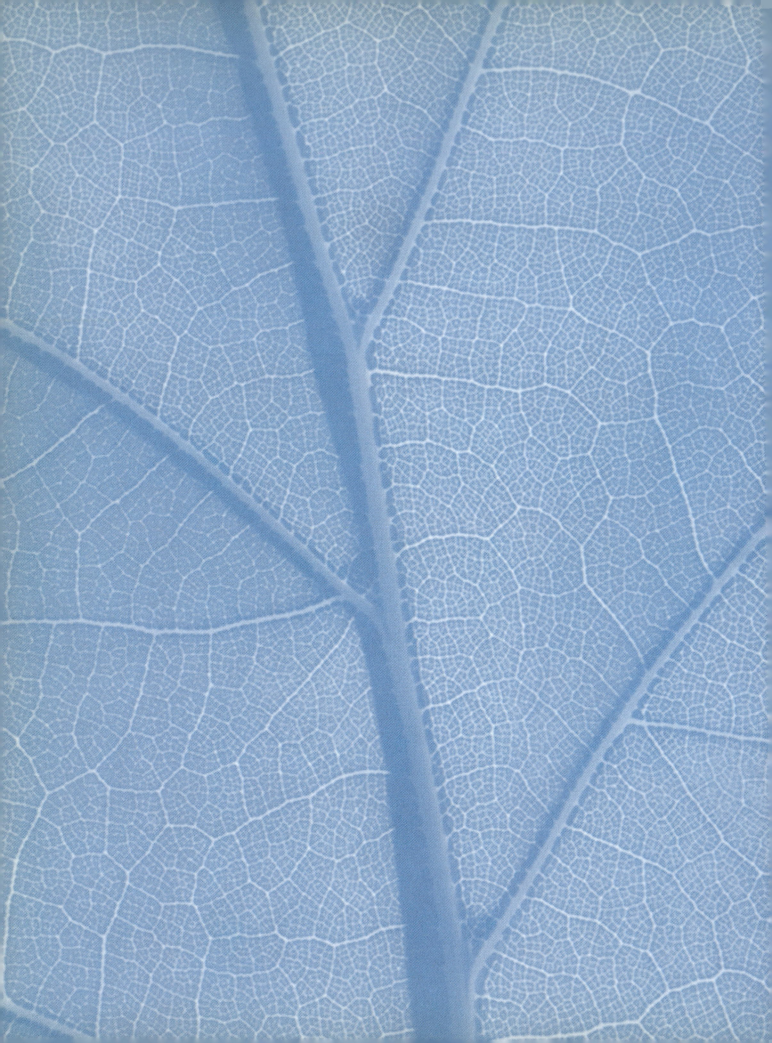

PART FOUR

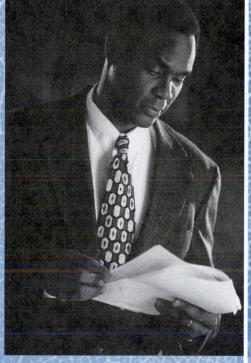

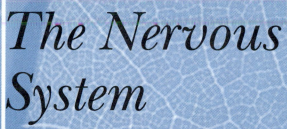

The Nervous System

Unilateral Ménière's Disease

GENDER

M

AGE

30

SETTING

- Clinic

ETHNICITY/CULTURE

- Hispanic American

PREEXISTING CONDITIONS

COEXISTING CONDITIONS

- Allergic reactions to sulfur, feathers

LIFESTYLE

- Licensed mechanic

COMMUNICATION

Spanish and English

DISABILITY

SOCIOECONOMIC STATUS

- Middle

SPIRITUAL/RELIGIOUS

- Evangelical

PHARMACOLOGIC

- Meclizine HcL (Antivert)
- Diazepam (Valium)
- Hydrochlorothiazide (HydroDIURIL)
- Nicotinic acid (Nicobid)
- Dimenhydrinate (Dramamine)

PSYCHOSOCIAL

- Anxiety
- Fear

LEGAL

ETHICAL

- Drugs that cause drowsiness will prohibit the client from working.

ALTERNATIVE THERAPY

PRIORITIZATION

- Maintain safety

DELEGATION

- RN
- Client education

THE NERVOUS SYSTEM

Level of difficulty: Easy

Overview: This case involves a thorough assessment of the client's condition including all drugs he may be currently taking. The case also involves a careful history for vertigo, the extent of disability, and implementing of measures to stabilize balance.

Client Profile

Mr. S is a 30-year-old single client who is employed by a major motor vehicle department as a licensed mechanic. Mr. S is seen in the clinic with complaints of imbalance, which he relates to a roaring sound and a feeling of fullness in his left ear for the past two weeks. On further history gathering by the nurse, Mr. S reports that periods of whirling infrequently last for a few minutes, but during the past two days, vertigo has lasted for 30 minutes.

Case Study

On further assessment, Mr. S complains of nausea, vomiting, diaphoresis, and a persistent feeling of imbalance, which occurred while he was on the job the previous day, causing him to request time off to seek medical assistance. History and physical are continued by a nurse practitioner (NP), who documents a normal physical examination, with the exception of evaluation of cranial nerve VIII, indicating impairment of the left ear. An audiogram is done, and reveals a sensorineural hearing loss in the left ear. An electronystagmogram is done and shows reduced vestibular response in the left ear. Physical examination findings and diagnostic results are discussed and a diagnosis of Ménière's disease is made in collaboration with a health care provider. Mr. S will be given prescriptions and instructions to return to the clinic in two weeks for follow-up evaluation. The registered dietitian discusses the need for a low sodium diet with Mr. S, and the RN provides him with a list of foods that are both high and low in sodium.

The following are prescribed:

- Meclizine HcL (Antivert) 50 mg PO daily
- Diazepam (Valium) 5 mg PO two times per day
- Hydrochlorothiazide (HydroDIURIL) 50 mg PO daily
- Nicotinic acid (Nicobid) 10 mg PO daily
- Dimenhydrinate (Dramamine) 50 mg PO q6h

Questions

1. Discuss the pathophysiology of Ménière's disease.

2. Discuss the incidence and prevalence of Ménière's disease.

3. Discuss clinical manifestations of Ménière's disease.

4. Discuss diagnostic studies for Ménière's disease.

5. Discuss common nursing diagnoses and goals for vertigo.

6. What are the purposes for the prescribed medications?

7. What are common adverse reactions of the prescribed medications?

8. Discuss drug-to-drug and drug-to-food/herbal interactions of the prescribed medications.

9. Surgical treatment of Ménière's disease is a last resort. When medical therapy is ineffective, discuss surgical procedures that may be performed.

10. Discuss client education for Ménière's disease.

CASE STUDY 2

Multiple Sclerosis

GENDER

F

AGE

38

SETTING

- Hospital

ETHNICITY/CULTURE

- White American

PREEXISTING CONDITIONS

COEXISTING CONDITIONS

LIFESTYLE

- Accountant

COMMUNICATION

DISABILITY

- Impaired mobility

SOCIOECONOMIC STATUS

- Middle

SPIRITUAL/RELIGIOUS

- Baptist

PHARMACOLOGIC

- Interferon beta-1a (Avonex)
- Mitoxantrone HcL (Novantrone)
- Baclofen (Lioresal)
- Carbamazepine (Tegretol)
- Methylprednisolone (Medrol)
- Amantadine HcL (Symmetrel)

PSYCHOSOCIAL

- Anxiety
- Emotional instability
- Depression

LEGAL

ETHICAL

- Confidentiality
- Client and family involvement in decision making
- Disability issues
- Quality of life

ALTERNATIVE THERAPY

- Meditation

PRIORITIZATION

- Systems assessment
- Monitor temperature and serum calcium levels

DELEGATION

- RN
- Client education

THE NERVOUS SYSTEM

Level of difficulty: Moderate

Overview: This case uses systems assessment to detect features of multiple sclerosis (MS). It involves a thorough assessment of the client's condition including prescribed drugs and alternative therapy used to help relieve distressing symptoms. The nurse must use critical-thinking skills to prioritize and implement quality care, with the use of therapeutic management aimed at treating the disease process and providing symptomatic relief.

Client Profile

Mrs. N is a 38-year-old married woman with three children, ages 9, 11, and 13. She has been active with her family and community activities. She has worked as a certified accountant in a law firm for more than ten years. Her husband has been employed at a major bank in the city for 15 years. Mrs. N's husband accompanies her to the hospital's emergency department (ED) because of complaints of increased fatigue and stiffness in the lower extremities and double vision. She is 5′8″ and weighs 195 pounds. She is a good historian who responds to questions in a detailed manner. Mrs. N denies family history of neurological diseases and reports that her parents are alive and well.

Case Study

Ms. N's complaints on arrival to the ED include increased fatigue and stiffness of the lower extremities with unsteady gait and sudden fuzziness of the eyes followed by double vision (diplopia). She reports that similar symptoms were noticed two years ago, with brief periods of decreased visual acuity that disappeared after a while. Therefore, medical attention was not sought. Mrs. N is transferred to a medical unit of the hospital for continued assessment and evaluation. Her vital signs are:

Blood pressure: 130/78

Pulse: 78

Respirations: 16

Temperature: 98.6° F

The health care provider completes a thorough history and physical with focus on basic motor skills and sensory assessments which elicited positive indications for MS. A magnetic resonance imaging (MRI) is scheduled and the health care provider discusses ongoing plans with the primary nurse who continues with the nursing history and assessment. Further neurological assessment finds increased deep tendon reflexes, and the client's report of numbness, paresthesia, tingling, and burning in the lower extremities. Babinski reflex is positive, and abdominal reflexes are slow. Serum calcium level is drawn and sent to the lab, revealing a result of 9 mg/dL. The health care provider returns soon after the completion of the nursing assessment with a multidisciplinary team of a neurologist, medical doctor, pharmacist, a nurse practitioner, dietitian, and social worker. After further discussion with Mrs. N pertaining to the physical assessments, the following diagnostic studies are prescribed: Cerebrospinal fluid (CSF) analysis, CSF electrophoresis, MRI of the spine. The neurologist explains the need for a lumbar puncture to Mrs. N and how the procedure would be done. Mrs. N then signs an informed witnessed consent for the lumbar puncture. The social worker remains in the client's room after the rest of the team leaves to discuss the possible need for help at home while she remains in the hospital for continued evaluation. The diagnostic studies are completed and reviewed by the team, then discussed with Mrs. N and her husband as per her request. A diagnosis of MS is confirmed.

The following are prescribed:
- Inteferon beta-1a (Avonex) 30 mcg IM every week
- Mitoxantrone HcL (Novantrone) IV 12 mg/M² over 5–15 minutes
- Baclofen (Lioresal) 5 mg PO three times per day
- Methylprednisolone (Medrol) 40 mg PO daily
- Amantadine HcL (Symmetrel) 100 mg PO q12h5

Questions

1. Why is a lumbar puncture used as a diagnostic test for MS?

2. Discuss the guideline for lumbar puncture.

3. What are the expected findings of the diagnostic tests that aided in the confirmation of the diagnosis of MS?

4. What are some common nursing diagnoses for clients with MS?

5. What are the purposes for the prescribed medications?

6. What are the most common adverse reactions of the prescribed medications?

7. Discuss the drug-to-drug and drug-to-food/herbal interactions of the prescribed medications.

8. What are some complementary and alternative therapies that may be included in the comprehensive treatment plan for the client with MS after the client has discussed his or her plan to include these therapies?

9. Why is it important to discharge the client with MS to a rehabilitation center for a brief period of time after discharge from the hospital?

10. Explain a significant psychosocial problem for Mrs. N as it relates to discharge to a rehabilitation center briefly instead of to home.

11. What should the client with MS do to help maintain a sense of well-being upon discharge to home?

CASE STUDY 3

Generalized Tonic-Clonic Seizure

GENDER

F

AGE

24

SETTING

- Emergency department

ETHNICITY/CULTURE

- Black American/West Indian

PREEXISTING CONDITIONS

- Head injury two years ago

COEXISTING CONDITIONS

LIFESTYLE

- Nursing student

COMMUNICATION

DISABILITY

SOCIOECONOMIC STATUS

- Middle

SPIRITUAL/RELIGIOUS

- Baptist

PHARMACOLOGIC

- Phenytoin (Dilantin)
- Carbamazepine (Tegretol)
- Diazepam (Valium)

PSYCHOSOCIAL

- Anxiety

LEGAL

- If client injures a person while operating a moving vehicle due to a seizure attack, should the client be liable?

ETHICAL

- Does the client with history of seizure have the right to operate a moving vehicle?

ALTERNATIVE THERAPY

PRIORITIZATION

- Maintain safety
- Control seizure

DELEGATION

- RN
- Client education

THE NERVOUS SYSTEM

Level of difficulty: Difficult

Overview: This case involves a through assessment of the client's presenting symptoms and maintaining a patent airway. The case involves prioritization in a triage situation at a busy urban hospital emergency department (ED).

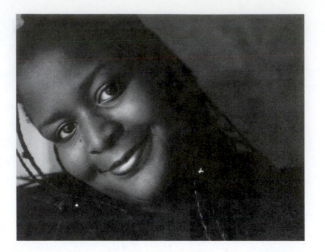

Client Profile

Ms. D is a 24-year-old nursing student who, after leaving the clinic for home via public transportation, complains to her classmates of an unusual feeling that she is not able to describe. A few minutes after her remarks, Ms. D starts to fall but is assisted to the ground by one of her classmates. Emergency medical service (EMS) is contacted, and Ms D's airway is maintained with the help of a passerby while waiting for EMS arrival. The EMS arrives in five minutes and, after a "quick assessment," applies a high-flow oxygen via a non-rebreather mask.

Case Study

Ms. D is taken to the emergency department (ED) of a hospital in a busy section of a large city. On arrival to the hospital triage area, the client is responsive to tactile and verbal stimuli, but not capable of giving an appropriate report of the occurrence. The report is given by a classmate, who describes a tonic phase seizure, with the client uttering a cry then slumping to the ground. The classmate describes Ms. D saying that she felt uneasy and saw unusually bright light, and a smell as though rubber was burning. There was an abrupt increase in muscle tone, loss of consciousness, and loss of postural control, and Ms. D began to fall to the ground but was assisted by her classmate and a passerby. The passerby dialed "911" as the classmate remained with Ms. D. Ongoing observation of Ms. D finds an opisthotonic posture (evidence of acute arching of the back, the head bent back on the neck, the heels bent back on the legs, and the arms and hands flexed rigidly at the joints due to prolonged and severe spasm of the muscles). Ms. D became unconscious, with urinary incontinence; pupils were fixed and dilated, lasting for approximately 45 seconds. Continued observation by the classmate describes alternating contraction and relaxation of the muscles in all the extremities along with hyperventilation. Ms. D is now in the ED, alert, and oriented to her name and place, but not to time of day. A triage nurse continues collection of additional data from the client and her classmate, while an ED clerk notifies the health care provider of Ms. D's arrival. She is placed in a single room, in a side-lying position, and a suction machine and apparatus are at the bedside. Vital signs are:

Blood pressure: 130/80

Pulse: 82

Respirations: 20

Temperature: 98.6° F

Serum labs are drawn: glucose, sodium, total calcium. The bed is placed in low position and side-rails are padded. A stat dose of diazepam (Valium) 10 mg IV is administered by the triage nurse while awaiting the arrival of the health care provider. Thirty minutes after the valium is administered, Ms. D responds appropriately to verbal and tactile stimuli. The health care provider arrives and orders a loading dose of phenytoin which is initiated by the triage nurse. The health care provider continues with a history and physical, history of seizures, psychosocial assessment and mental status examination, and a detailed neurologic examination. Ms. D denies history of seizure or prior episode before today. Upon completion of a neurological assessment, the health care provider orders an electroencephalogram (EEG), and a computed tomography (CT) scan. Result of an ECG shows brain wave abnormalities and the CT scan negative for congenital abnormalities or masses. Based on the documentation of the presenting symptoms on arrival to the ED, and the ECG brain wave abnormalities, a diagnosis of tonic-clonic seizure is confirmed.

The following are prescribed:

- Phenytoin (Dilantin) 100 mg three times per day × seven days then return to health care provider for evaluation
- Carbamazepine (Tegretol) 200 mg PO two times per day
- Complete blood count and serum electrolyte levels
- Carbamazepine and phenytoin levels in the morning

Questions

1. What is the incidence and prevalence of seizure (epilepsy) in the United States?

2. Discuss the pathophysiology of seizures.

3. What is a tonic-clonic seizure?

4. What are common nursing diagnoses for the client with seizure?

5. What is the focus of documentation for a client having a seizure?

6. What is included in the diagnostic assessment of seizures?

7. What are the purposes for the prescribed orders, including diazepam administered in the ED?

8. What are the most common adverse reactions of the prescribed medications, including diazepam?

9. Discuss the drug-to-drug and drug-to-food/herbal interactions for the prescribed medications, including diazepam.

10. What is a major complication of seizure activity?

11. Discuss client education for seizures.

Subarachnoid Hemorrhage – Grade II

GENDER

F

AGE

42

SETTING

- Hospital

ETHNICITY/CULTURE

- Mixed race

PREEXISTING CONDITIONS

- Hypertension

COEXISTING CONDITIONS

LIFESTYLE

- Bank supervisor

COMMUNICATION

DISABILITY

SOCIOECONOMIC STATUS

- Middle

SPIRITUAL/RELIGIOUS

- Baptist

PHARMACOLOGIC

- Mannitol (Osmitrol)
- Nimodipine (Nimotop)
- Phenobarbital sodium (Luminal Sodium)
- Phenytoin (Dilantin)
- Valsartan (Diovan)
- Ducosate sodium (Colace)

PSYCHOSOCIAL

- Anxiety
- Denial

LEGAL

ETHICAL

ALTERNATIVE THERAPY

PRIORITIZATION

- Brief mental status exam
- Prevent increase in intracranial pressure

DELEGATION

- RN
- Client education

THE NERVOUS SYSTEM

Level of difficulty: Difficult

Overview: This case involves emergency management. The nurse must use critical-thinking skills to prioritize care in a busy triage area to prevent increase in intracranial pressure. The nurse must be skilled and competent at implementing care to maintain cerebral perfusion pressure, controlling intracranial pressure (ICP), managing cardiac dysrhythmias, and preventing rebleeding with ongoing neurologic assessment.

DIFFICULT

Client Profile

Mrs. M-W is a 43-year-old client who has been experiencing bouts of headache for the past two months. The headaches have become worse, increasing in severity and frequency over the past two weeks. Today, Mrs. M-W experienced a sudden onset of severe headache while preparing a meal for her family. She yells to her husband saying, "I just had a sudden headache that is so severe, I feel weak. It is the worst one I have had." The husband enters the kitchen to find Mrs. M-W projectile vomiting. Mr. W calls his brother-in-law (his neighbor) and they accompany Mrs. M-W to the emergency department (ED) in their community.

Case Study

On arrival at the ED, Mrs. M-W describes the pain as "awful" and sudden. She complains of nausea, and tells the nurse her eyes are blurred. The nurse examines the client, while the certified nursing technician requests that the ED health care provider be paged, then notifies the intensive care unit of the pending transfer. Mrs. M-W is awake, alert, and oriented to person, place, and time. Her conversation and response to questions are comprehensible and easily understood. Mrs. M-W reports a history of hypertension for ten years, and social drinking at dinner time. She is currently taking Valsartan 80 mg PO daily. She follows complex commands, her facial structure is normal, and she is able to move all extremities with equal strength. Her pupils are equal and reactive to light and accommodation. However, her neck is stiff and painful with positive Kernig's and Brudzinski's sign. Her vital signs are:

> Blood pressure: 170/96
>
> Pulse: 90
>
> Respirations: 18
>
> Temperature: 98.6° F

The health care provider orders a noncontrast computed tomography (CT) scan of the brain, which reveals blood in the subarachnoid space, intracerebral clots, and large clots surrounding an aneurysm. A transcranial doppler ultrasonography (TCD) is done with evidence of minimal vasospasms. The client is transferred to the medical intensive care unit (MICU) and is placed on complete bed rest, with the head of the bed elevated at 45 degrees, while the nursing team prepares her for possible surgery. An arterial line is inserted, and neurological assessment is ongoing, including blood pressure readings and monitoring of arterial pressure. An intravenous line of D 5.45% NS at 100 mL per hour is initiated. The client is instructed to avoid coughing, sneezing, or straining and is given reasons for these instructions. Bilateral pneumatic compression devices to lower extremities are applied as per protocol for subarachnoid hemorrhage (SAH). Seizure precautions are initiated as per protocol for SAH. After the interdisciplinary team reviews the history and physical and diagnostic studies, the neurologist decides that the diagnosis is grade II SAH secondary to cerebral aneurysm rupture. The treatment plan for a craniotomy is discussed with Mrs. M-W and her husband. An informed consent is signed by Mrs. M-W.

The following are prescribed:

- Neurologic assessment and blood pressure q1h and PRN
- Mannitol (Osmitrol) IV 0.5–1 g/kg over five to ten minutes, may repeat 0.25–1 g/kg q4h per critical-care protocol
- Furosemide (Lasix) 40 mg IV prior to administration of mannitol

- Phenobarbital sodium (Luminal Sodium) 100 mg IV two times per day
- Phenytoin (Dilantin) 1 g loading dose IV, 100 mg q8h
- Nimodipine (Nimotop) 60 mg PO q4h for 21 days. Start in morning
- Ducosate sodium (Colace) 100 mg PO three times per day
- Serum labs: sodium, platelet count
- Insert indwelling urinary catheter
- Hourly urine outputs

Questions

1. Which factors in the case study indicate that Mrs. M-W has suffered an SAH?

2. Discuss precautions to avoid SAH.

3. Discuss the incidence and socioeconomic impact of intracranial aneurysm and SAH.

4. Discuss common nursing diagnoses and expected outcomes for the client with SAH

5. Discuss the conditions that occur after an aneurysm ruptures.

6. Discuss specific factors related to the treatment of SAH that may cause hyponatremia and complications in clients with SAH.

7. Discuss the advantages and disadvantages of early or delayed surgery for SAH.

8. Discuss the types of surgeries that can be done for the client with SAH secondary to ruptured aneurysm.

9. What are the purposes for the prescribed medications?

10. Discuss the most common adverse reactions of the prescribed medications.

11. Discuss drug-to-drug and drug-to-food/herbal interactions for the prescribed medications.

12. Discuss discharge instructions for the client with post-craniotomy related to SAH secondary to cerebral aneurysm.

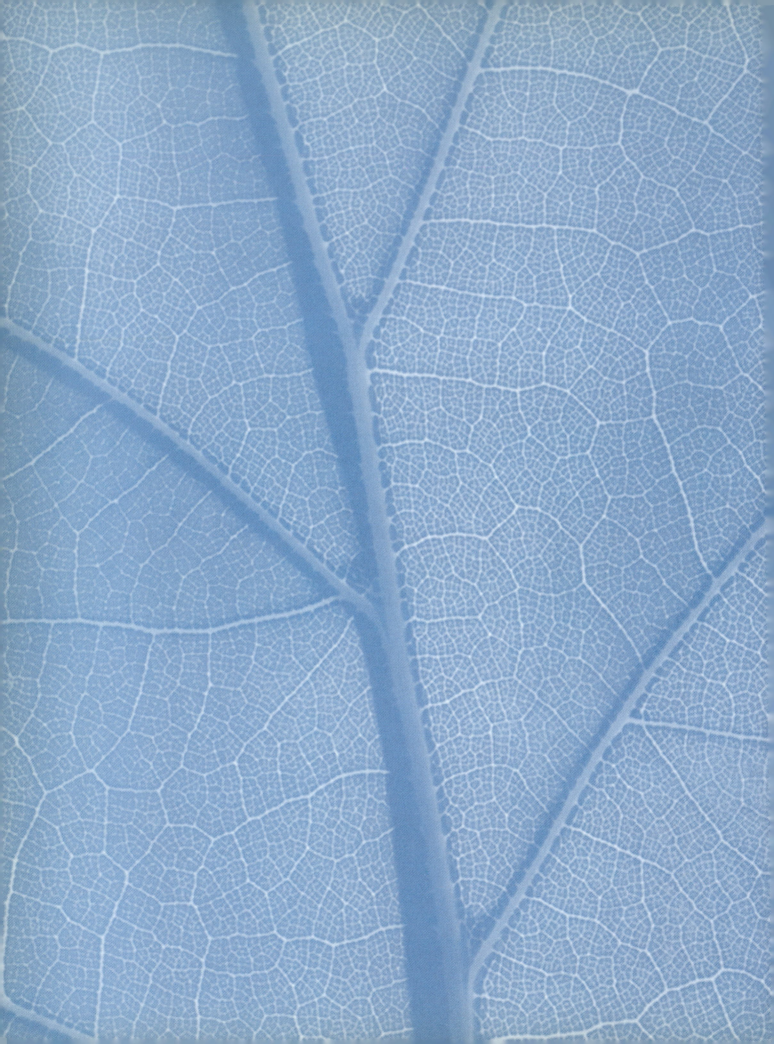

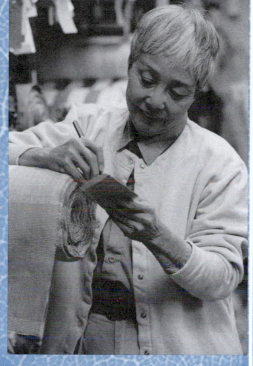

## PART FIVE

The Endocrine System

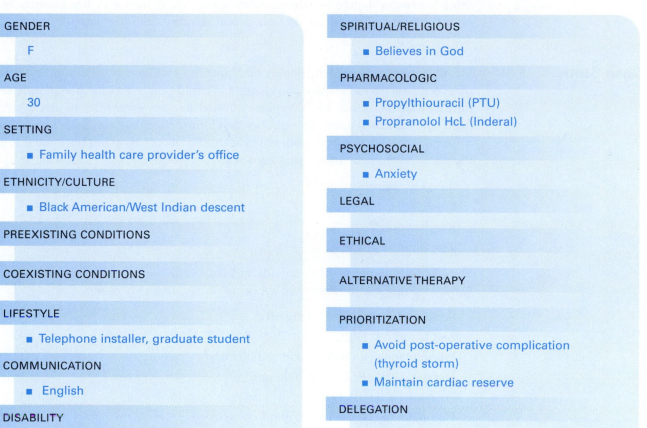

GENDER

F

AGE

30

SETTING

- Family health care provider's office

ETHNICITY/CULTURE

- Black American/West Indian descent

PREEXISTING CONDITIONS

COEXISTING CONDITIONS

LIFESTYLE

- Telephone installer, graduate student

COMMUNICATION

- English

DISABILITY

SOCIOECONOMIC STATUS

- Middle

SPIRITUAL/RELIGIOUS

- Believes in God

PHARMACOLOGIC

- Propylthiouracil (PTU)
- Propranolol HcL (Inderal)

PSYCHOSOCIAL

- Anxiety

LEGAL

ETHICAL

ALTERNATIVE THERAPY

PRIORITIZATION

- Avoid post-operative complication (thyroid storm)
- Maintain cardiac reserve

DELEGATION

- RN
- Client education

THE ENDOCRINE SYSTEM

Level of difficulty: Easy

Overview: This case involves thorough assessment of the client's condition including health history. Physical assessment should focus on testing muscle strength, vital signs, size of thyroid, and presence of bruits over the thyroid gland. The nurse must use critical thinking to prioritize care in a busy triage area in the event the client goes into thyroid crisis.

Client Profile

Ms. C is a 30-year-old female who is employed as a telephone installer for a major cable company. She is 5′7″ with previous weight of 200 pounds. She is presently pursuing a masters degree in telecommunication. Ms. C lives with her parents, but reports that she pays rent for a one-bedroom apartment in her parent's home.

Case Study

Ms. C is seen at her family health care provider's office for follow-up review of observed patterns of behavior and changes in health status over the past month. On interview by the nurse, Ms. C reports unusual hunger, even after having a large meal. She has noted unusual weight loss that is not related to exercise or stress, diarrhea, and inability to tolerate normal heat that she would have not responded to in the past. On assessment, her vital signs are:

Blood pressure: 150/92

Pulse: 120

Respirations: 22

Temperature 101.6° F

She has visible tremors of the hands and her eyeballs are beginning to protrude. Current diagnostic studies reveal abnormal T_3, T_4, and TSH results.

Serum calcium level: 11.2 mg/dL

Red blood cell (RBC) count: 7/mm^3

White blood cell (WBC) count: 4,000/mm^3

Platelet count (PLT): 250,000 /mm^3

Hematocrit (Hct): 34%

Hemoglobin (Hgb): 14 g/100 mL

A thyroid scan with the use of radioactive tracers reveals an enlarged thyroid goiter with increased iodine uptake. Ms. C denies difficulty swallowing or pain upon swallowing. A diagnosis of hyperthyroidism is made by the health care provider, and is discussed with Ms. C, and the possibility for surgery is explained.

The following are prescribed:

- Weekly monitoring of WBC after initiation of PTU
- Propylthiouracil (PTU) 450 mg PO daily
- Strong iodine solution 4 drops three times per day × ten days
- Propranolol HcL (Inderal) 80 mg PO q6h

Questions

1. Discuss the risk factors and pathophysiology of hyperthyroidism.

2. Discuss clinical manifestations of hyperthyroidism.

3. Discuss diagnostic findings of hyperthyroidism.

4. Discuss gerontologic considerations of hyperthyroidism.

5. What are the purposes for the prescribed orders?

6. What are the most common adverse reactions, drug-to-drug, drug-to-food/herbal interactions for the prescribed medications?

7. Discuss complications of hyperthyroidism.

8. Discuss surgical management for hyperthyroidism.

9. Discuss relapse rate and risk for hyperthyroidism after treatment for thyroid storm.

10. Discuss client education for hyperthyroidism.

CASE STUDY 2

Hypercortisolism (Cushing's Syndrome)

GENDER

F

AGE

42

SETTING

■ Hospital

ETHNICITY/CULTURE

■ Native American/Argentina

PREEXISTING CONDITIONS

■ Hypertension

COEXISTING CONDITIONS

■ History of alcohol abuse

LIFESTYLE

■ Self employed, Indian art antique shop

COMMUNICATION

■ Spanish and English

DISABILITY

SOCIOECONOMIC STATUS

■ Middle

SPIRITUAL/RELIGIOUS

■ Roman Catholic

PHARMACOLOGIC

■ Mitotane (Lysodren)

PSYCHOSOCIAL

■ Emotional instability
■ Irritability
■ Depression

LEGAL

■ Does the client have the right to bring charges against health care providers if necessary treatment is withheld?

ETHICAL

■ Will the client have equitable access to essential health care benefits compared to clients with major medical health coverage?

ALTERNATIVE THERAPY

■ Prayer

PRIORITIZATION

■ Decrease cortisol levels
■ Decrease blood glucose levels
■ Provide safety

DELEGATION

■ RN
■ Client education

MODERATE

THE ENDOCRINE SYSTEM

Level of difficulty: Moderate

Overview: This case involves a thorough assessment of the client's condition, including questions related to recent onset of weakness, increase in weight or abdominal girth, bone pain or history of fractures, and history of frequent infections and easy bruising. It involves questioning the client about gastrointestinal (GI) discomfort and the use of steroid drugs and herbals. The nurse must use critical-thinking skills to prioritize care in the event of signs and symptoms indicating the development of adrenal crisis.

Client Profile

Mrs. V is a 42-year-old widow whose husband and only child, who was three years old, died in a motor vehicle accident three years ago, the day before Christmas. Prior to their deaths, Mrs. V and her husband of 12 years had wine as a social appetizer during meal times. Mrs. V is 5'4" and weighs 208 pounds.

Case Study

Mrs. V reports that since her husband's death, she has continued with the practice of having wine with her evening meals. However, she reports that as the years went by, she became lonely, missing her husband and child, especially at holidays, which led to an increase in the amount of wine consumed at meal times. The client reports social drinking with her friends who frequently visit her at the "shop" at which she worked as manager. The client's husband was a real estate broker for a progressive brokerage firm. Mrs. V finds out she had no health insurance when she goes to a community health center for elevated blood pressure and ongoing headaches. Her blood pressure at the time of arrival was 194/98 and she complained of nausea. A history is taken by a nurse practitioner (NP) at the clinic and Mrs. V is referred to the community hospital emergency department (ED), and transported from the clinic to the community hospital. On arrival at the ED, she informs the triage nurse that the headache is less severe in comparison to when she was at the clinic. Mrs. V believes the headache is directly related to her history of hypertension. The NP does the history and physical in the ED, during which time Mrs. V reports periods of emotional instability, with mood swings and depression. She informs the nurse that at times she is unusually irritable for no specific reasons, and experiences frequent urination, muscle weakness, and easy bruising. Physical assessment findings reveal hirsutism and a male pattern type balding of the head, abdominal striae, and dependent edema of the lower extremities. Mrs. V is admitted to a medical unit and will be seen by an endocrinologist for further evaluation. The primary nurse assigned to Mrs. V completes additional nursing history and assessment, after which Mrs. V is seen by an endocrinologist. The following tests are ordered: 24-hour urine for free cortisol and 17-hydroxycorticosteroids and 17-ketosteroids, plasma cortisol, ACTH level, erythro-sedimentation rate (ESR), white blood cell (WBC) count, lymphocyte count, sodium, potassium, and calcium, urine calcium, potassium, and glucose. A computed tomography (CT) of the adrenal gland is ordered, and a high-dose (8 mg) dexamethasone suppression test is ordered for the next day. The nurse instructs Mrs. V on how to collect the 24-hour urine and received verbal feedback that was positive. The results of the diagnostic studies reveal 24-hour urine for 17-hydroxycorticosteroids and 17-ketosteroids elevated (12 mg/24 h), and:

> Plasma cortisol: 30 ug/dL
>
> ACTH in AM: 100 pg/mL; in PM: 75 pg/mL
>
> Erythro-sedimentation rate (ESR): elevated
>
> White blood cell (WBC) count: 12,000/mm^3
>
> Lymphocyte count: 700/mm^3
>
> Sodium (Na): 150 mEq/L
>
> Decrease potassium (K+): 2.8 mEq/L
>
> Calcium: 7 mg/dL
>
> Increase glucose: 140 mg/dL
>
> Urine calcium: 310 mg/24 h, elevated

Urine potassium: 150 mEq/24 h

Urine glucose: 300 mg/24 h

The high dose dexamethasone suppression test reveals reduction in plasma cortisol level less than 50% of the baseline, indicating positive finding for Cushing's syndrome. The CT scan reveals an inoperable adrenal tumor. An endocrinologist reviews the labs and diagnostic reports with the multidisciplinary team; a diagnosis of Cushing's syndrome is confirmed. The multidisciplinary team discusses the plan of care with Mrs. V, and she agrees with the plan.

The following is prescribed:

- Mitotane (Lysodren) 3 g PO three times per day

Questions

1. Discuss the prevalence and pathophysiology of Cushing's syndrome.

2. Discuss clinical manifestations of Cushing's syndrome.

3. Discuss assessment and diagnostic findings of Cushing's syndrome.

4. Discuss common nursing diagnoses for Cushing's syndrome.

5. Discuss a potential complication of Cushing's syndrome.

6. What is the purpose for the prescribed medication?

7. What are the most common adverse reactions, drug-to-drug, drug-to-food/herbal interactions of the prescribed medications?

8. Discuss adrenalectomy for primary adrenal hypertrophy in Cushing's syndrome.

9. Discuss management of adrenal insufficiency post adrenalectomy.

10. Discuss client education after bilateral adrenalectomy.

Diabetes Mellitus Type 1

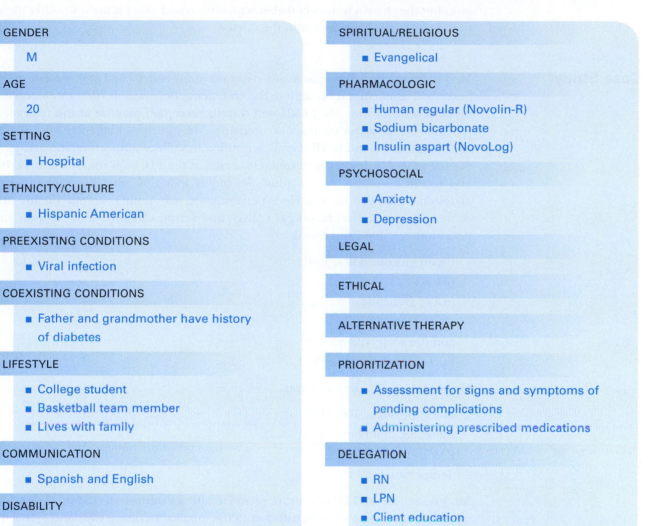

GENDER

M

AGE

20

SETTING

- Hospital

ETHNICITY/CULTURE

- Hispanic American

PREEXISTING CONDITIONS

- Viral infection

COEXISTING CONDITIONS

- Father and grandmother have history of diabetes

LIFESTYLE

- College student
- Basketball team member
- Lives with family

COMMUNICATION

- Spanish and English

DISABILITY

SOCIOECONOMIC STATUS

- Middle

SPIRITUAL/RELIGIOUS

- Evangelical

PHARMACOLOGIC

- Human regular (Novolin-R)
- Sodium bicarbonate
- Insulin aspart (NovoLog)

PSYCHOSOCIAL

- Anxiety
- Depression

LEGAL

ETHICAL

ALTERNATIVE THERAPY

PRIORITIZATION

- Assessment for signs and symptoms of pending complications
- Administering prescribed medications

DELEGATION

- RN
- LPN
- Client education

MODERATE

THE ENDOCRINE SYSTEM

Level of difficulty: Moderate

Overview: This case involves a thorough assessment of the presenting symptoms on arrival to triage, including all medications the client is currently taking. It involves critical thinking to appropriately delegate assignment to nurses highly competent in applying decision-making skills to clients requiring immediate medical and nursing interventions. The nurse must be capable of identifying pending signs of diabetic complications and able to collaborate with the team to prevent occurrences.

Client Profile

Mr. J is a 20-year-old college student with a history of diabetes mellitus type 1 for the past six years. Mr. J lives at home with his extended family. Mr. J's father and grandmother have a history of diabetes mellitus type 1. Mr. J is the only other member of the family diagnosed with the disease.

Case Study

Mr. J is a respiratory therapist major at a community college and is a member of the basketball team. Mr. J is brought to the emergency department (ED) by emergency medical services after Mr. J collapsed during basketball practice at the college. A member of the basketball team accompanies Mr. J in the ambulance. Mr. J is 6′3″ and weighs 220 pounds. His family is notified by college authorities and arrives at the ED while Mr. J is being triaged. On arrival at the ED, he is responsive to verbal and tactile stimuli, is very diaphoretic, mildly lethargic, and is complaining of abdominal pain and nausea. He hyperventilates, manifesting acetone breath. Stat serum glucose, arterial blood gas (ABG), and serum electrolytes for sodium and potassium are done and reveal:

Blood glucose: 450 mg/dL

pH: 6.9

pCO_2: 20 mm Hg

HCO_3: 12 mEq/L

Sodium (Na): 128 mEq/L

Potassium (K+): 3.0 mEq/L

His vital signs on admission are:

Blood pressure: 100/70

Pulse: 88, rapid but regular

Respirations: 22

Temperature: 98.1° F

Mr. J is seen by the ED health care provider, and a diagnosis of diabetic ketoacidosis (DKA) is made. Mr. J is transferred to the medical intensive care unit (MICU).

The following are prescribed:

- 0.9% NaCL at 1 liter per hour × two hours
- Human regular (Novolin-R) initial bolus 0.4 units/kg, followed by 2.4 u/hr continuous infusion
- Sodium bicarbonate ($NaHCO_3$) 5 mEq/kg infusion over four hours and low dose insulin at a continuous rate (five units per hour) at 25 mL per hour.
- Monitor serum glucose and potassium level; if stable, change infusion to 0.45% sodium chloride at 125 mL/hr
- Insulin aspart (NovoLog) insulin 100 U/mL inj four units and NPH ten units in combination SC three times per day, before meals

Questions

1. What are specific cultural considerations of diabetes mellitus?

2. What is an extremely critical indicator of diabetes mellitus?

3. What are common nursing diagnoses for clients with diabetes?

4. What is a primary collaborative problem for Mr. J because of the elevated blood glucose level on arrival to the ED?

5. What are the defining characteristics of DKA?

6. What are the priorities of management for a client experiencing DKA?

7. What are the purposes for the prescribed orders?

8. What are the most common adverse reactions of the prescribed medications?

9. Discuss the drug-to-drug and drug-to-food/herbal interactions for the prescribed medications.

10. Explain the difference between Dawn phenomenon and Somogyi phenomenon.

11. What are the critical areas that should be included in client education for type 1 diabetes mellitus?

12. What are the nursing implications as they relate to diabetes mellitus?

Addison's Disease
(Acute-Primary Hypocortisolism)

GENDER

F

AGE

50

SETTING

- Hospital

ETHNICITY/CULTURE

- White American

PREEXISTING CONDITIONS

- History of pulmonary TB

COEXISTING CONDITIONS

- Pernicious anemia

LIFESTYLE

- Clothing designer

COMMUNICATION

DISABILITY

SOCIOECONOMIC STATUS

- Middle

SPIRITUAL/RELIGIOUS

- Methodist

PHARMACOLOGIC

- Hydrocortisone (Hydrocortone)
- Fludrocortisone acetate (Florinef)

PSYCHOSOCIAL

- Depression

LEGAL

ETHICAL

ALTERNATIVE THERAPY

- Vegetarian

PRIORITIZATION

- Prevent Addisonian Crisis
- Maintain safety

DELEGATION

- RN
- Client education

MODERATE

THE ENDOCRINE SYSTEM

Level of difficulty: Moderate

Overview: This case involves a thorough assessment of the client's condition, including current medications and dietary regimen. It involves prioritization in a triage situation at a busy hospital emergency department (ED) to avoid Ms. X developing Addisonian Crisis.

Client Profile

Ms. X is a 50-year-old client who is seen in a hospital's outpatient clinic as follow-up to her primary health care provider's referral for diagnostic tests to rule out diagnosis of Addison's disease. During an interview by a registered nurse (RN), she reveals past history of pulmonary tuberculosis and fungal lesions of the skin. She reports currently taking oral vitamin B_{12} for history of pernicious anemia. On further collection of data, Ms. X reports weakness, fatigue, anorexia, nausea, vomiting, and weight loss during the past month. Ms. X visited her primary health care provider a month ago because of dizziness and weakness, when rising from bed in the mornings or when standing from a sitting position for an extended period of time. Initial vital signs on arrival to the clinic are:

Blood pressure: 90/64

Pulse: 126

Respirations: 14

Temperature: 98.9° F

Case Study

Physical assessment of Ms. X reveals hyperpigmentation of the hands and lower extremities. Ms. X is later seen by a physician assistant (PA) who completes the history and physical, and informs Ms. X she will be admitted to the hospital for short-term stay. Serum cortisol, fasting blood glucose, sodium, potassium, blood urea nitrogen (BUN), adrenocortical thyroid hormone (ACTH), and eosinophil count are sent to the lab. The results are:

Serum cortisol: 12 ug/dL

Fasting blood glucose: 50 mg/100 mL

Sodium (Na): 128 mEq/L

Potassium (K+): 6 mEq/dL

Blood urea nitrogen (BUN): 26 mg/100 mL

The ACTH stimulation test reveals 100 pg/mL at 6 to 8 AM (after the patient followed a low-carbohydrate diet for 48 hours and fasted from foods for 12 hours before the test). A computed tomography (CT) with contrast reveals beginning atrophy of the adrenal gland, and magnetic resonance imaging (MRI) is negative for tumors or infections. Urinary 17-hydroxycorticosteroids and 17-ketosteroid levels urinary free cortisol are explained to Ms. X and the procedures are appropriately completed. The result reveals low normal levels. After laboratory data and diagnostic tests are reviewed by an endocrinologist and a medical and nursing staff, the diagnosis of Addison's disease is confirmed. The findings, confirmation of the disease, and treatment plan are discussed with Ms. X.

The following are prescribed:

- Hydrocortisone (Hydrocortone) 30 mg IV three times per day
- Fludrocortisone acetate (Florinef) 0.1 mg PO daily

Questions

1. Discuss the incidence, prevalence, and pathophysiology of Addison's disease.

2. Discuss risk factors of Addison's disease.

3. Discuss clinical manifestations of Addison's disease.

4. Discuss nursing diagnoses for Addison's disease.

5. Discuss diagnostic findings of Addison's disease.

6. Discuss urinary 17-hydroxycorticosteroids.

7. What are the purposes for the prescribed medications?

8. What are the most common adverse reactions, drug-to-drug, drug-to-food/herbal interactions for the prescribed medications?

9. Discuss management of hyponatremia and hyperkalemia found in Addison's disease.

10. Discuss client education for Addison's disease.

Pheochromocytoma

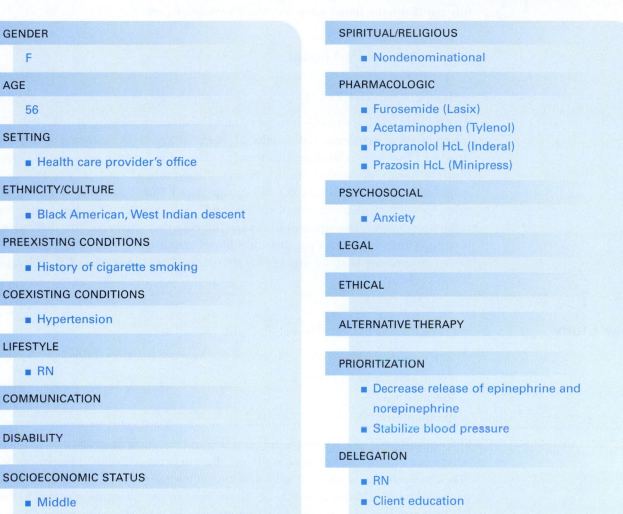

GENDER

F

AGE

56

SETTING

- Health care provider's office

ETHNICITY/CULTURE

- Black American, West Indian descent

PREEXISTING CONDITIONS

- History of cigarette smoking

COEXISTING CONDITIONS

- Hypertension

LIFESTYLE

- RN

COMMUNICATION

DISABILITY

SOCIOECONOMIC STATUS

- Middle

SPIRITUAL/RELIGIOUS

- Nondenominational

PHARMACOLOGIC

- Furosemide (Lasix)
- Acetaminophen (Tylenol)
- Propranolol HcL (Inderal)
- Prazosin HcL (Minipress)

PSYCHOSOCIAL

- Anxiety

LEGAL

ETHICAL

ALTERNATIVE THERAPY

PRIORITIZATION

- Decrease release of epinephrine and norepinephrine
- Stabilize blood pressure

DELEGATION

- RN
- Client education

MODERATE

THE ENDOCRINE SYSTEM

Level of difficulty: Moderate

Overview: This case involves a thorough assessment of the client's condition, including all current medications she is taking. It involves history and physical examination to gather appropriate data to aid in confirming a diagnosis. The nurse must use critical-thinking skills to prioritize care in the event hypertensive crisis develops.

Client Profile

Ms. P is a 56-year-old female who is seen at her primary health care provider's office after experiencing severe headaches. The nurse at the health care provider's office initiates the initial interview. Ms. P's vital signs are:

Blood pressure: 250/110

Pulse: 114, rapid and regular

Respirations: 20

Temperature: 98.4° F

An electrocardiogram (EKG) is ordered and reveals sinus tachycardia. Ms. P denies other medical problems but admits to years of cigarette smoking, which she stopped 15 years ago. Ms. P reports wearing glasses for distance reading but denies blurred vision. Medication history reveals furosemide (Lasix) 50 mg PO daily, amlodipine (Norvasc) 10 mg PO daily, propranolol HcL (Inderal) 40 mg PO two times per day, and acetaminophen (Tylenol) 650 mg PO PRN headache. She reports occasional constipation and uses increased roughage in the diet, which helps ease defecation. Her parents and siblings are alive and well. Ms. P is referred to the community hospital emergency department (ED) because of the elevated blood pressure.

Case Study

On arrival at the ED, Ms. P's vital signs are:

Blood pressure: 250/100

Pulse: 120, rapid and regular

Respirations: 18

Temperature: 98.4° F

She is transferred to a telemetry unit and is seen by a physician assistant (PA), who completes a history and physical while avoiding vigorous abdominal palpation. Ms. P is transferred to a medical unit and the following order is prescribed: nitroprusside sodium (Nitropress) 0.5 mg/kg per minute stat via infusion pump. Serum lab tests ordered are: sodium (Na), potassium (K+), glucose and urine glucose, 24-hour urine collections for vanillylmandelic acid (VMA), computed tomography (CT) scan of the adrenal gland, and abdominal imaging techniques. The results of the serum labs reveal:

Sodium (Na): 145 mEq/L

Potassium (K+): 4 mEq/L

Glucose: 130 mg/dL

Positive glucosuria

The 24-hour urine collections result reveal slight elevation in metanephrine and catecholamines, the CT scan identifies an adrenomedullary tumor on the left adrenal gland, measuring 0.5 cm, but abdominal imaging techniques are negative for metastasis of the tumor. An endocrinology consult is ordered for a team conference to determine surgical interventions. After the health care provider reviews the current labs and diagnostic findings, a diagnosis of pheochromocytoma is made. The health care team decides to begin treatment of the presenting symptoms while waiting for the endocrinology consult. The treatment plans are discussed with Ms. P Her blood pressure is currently 130/80, and her pulse is 102 and regular. She denies headache at this time. The registered dietitian discusses the dietary plan of care with Ms. P. The endocrinologist reviews the collected data, and determines that Ms. P can be monitored on an outpatient basis, and orders repeat CT scan and abdominal X-rays for three months from today's date. Ms. P will be discharged to home within 24 hours and will have follow-up visits with her primary health care provider.

The following are prescribed:

- Prazosin HcL (Minipress) 1 mg PO daily with gradual increase to 6 mg PO daily
- Propranolol HcL (Inderal) 40 mg PO two times per day
- Furosemide (Lasix) 50 mg PO daily
- Acetaminophen (Tylenol) 650 mg PO PRN headache

Questions

1. Discuss the incidence, prevalence, risk factors, and pathophysiology of pheochromocytoma.

2. Discuss clinical manifestations of pheochromocytoma.

3. Discuss assessment and diagnostic findings of pheochromocytoma.

4. Discuss nursing diagnoses to pheochromocytoma.

5. What are the purposes for the prescribed medications?

6. What are most common adverse reactions, drug-to-drug, drug-to-food/herbal interactions of the prescribed medications?

7. Discuss pre-operative intervention for surgical intervention for pheochromocytoma.

8. Discuss surgical management of pheochromocytoma.

9. Discuss client education for pheochromocytoma.

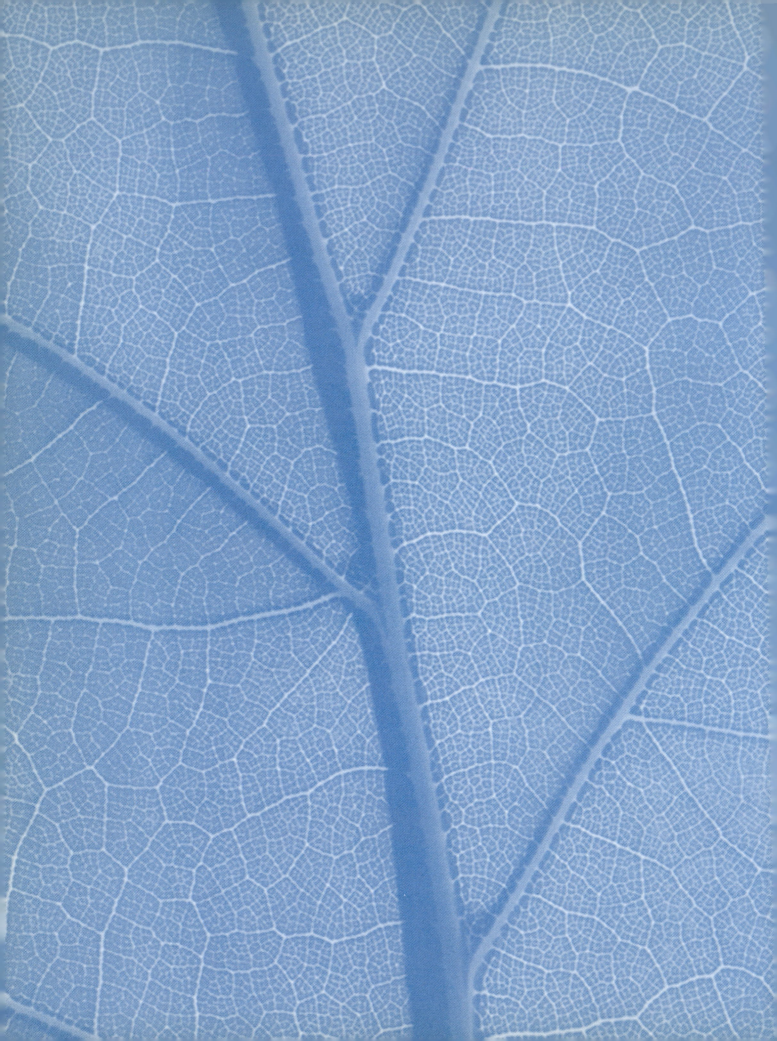

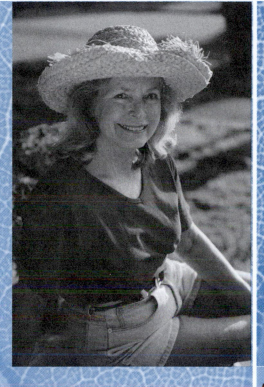

## PART SIX

The Musculoskeletal and Reproductive Systems

Cervical Cancer Stage IA

EASY

GENDER

F

AGE

25

SETTING

- Women's well clinic of a medical center

ETHNICITY/CULTURE

- Native American

PREEXISTING CONDITIONS

- HPV infection

COEXISTING CONDITIONS

- Squamous intraepithelial lesion

LIFESTYLE

- Unemployed college student
- Lives with sister

COMMUNICATION

DISABILITY

SOCIOECONOMIC STATUS

- Low

SPIRITUAL/RELIGIOUS

- Nondenominational

PHARMACOLOGIC

- Codeine sulfate

PSYCHOSOCIAL

- Anxiety
- Fear

LEGAL

ETHICAL

ALTERNATIVE THERAPY

- Meditation

PRIORITIZATION

- Encourage verbalization of feelings
- Prepare for cryosurgery

DELEGATION

- RN
- Client education

THE MUSCULOSKELETAL AND REPRODUCTIVE SYSTEMS

Level of difficulty: Easy

Overview: The case involves a thorough and sensitive assessment of the client's condition, taking into account the client's cultural views on health, wellness, and treatment. The nurse must use communication skills that will enhance trust and optimize the nurse–client relationship.

Client Profile

Ms. R is a 25-year-old female college student who is seen in the women's health clinic of a medical center due to complaints of spotting between menstruation. Ms. R is 5′5″ and weighs 120 pounds.

Case Study

Ms. R reports to the nurse practitioner (NP) on initial interview that her most recent Papanicolaou test (Pap) test is positive and that she had an appointment to see her family health care provider but missed the scheduled date, and the health care provider is away on personal business with an indefinite time of return. She admits to be being sexually active with the same partner for the past five years. Her reason for coming to the women's clinic is due to "spotting between menstruation" at the time of her last menstrual cycle. However, she is not "spotting" at the time of this visit. Her vital signs on admission are:

Blood pressure: 124/78

Pulse: 78 and regular

Respirations: 18

Temperature: 98.6° F

After continuing the history and physical, the NP discusses the need for further diagnostic evaluation, and when it is ascertained that Ms. R understands the need for the presented evaluation, the NP does a pelvic examination, a colposcopy, and an endocervical curettage. After the procedures, specimens are sent to the lab for analysis. Ms. R's vital signs are repeated and reveal:

Blood pressure: 128/80

Pulse: 80

Respirations: 18

Temperature: 98.6° F

The NP gives Ms. R an appointment for follow-up visit and informs her that at the time of that visit, the results of the colposcopy and endocervical curettage will be discussed with her.

The following are prescribed:

- Contact the clinic if you are experiencing excessive bleeding, discharge, or abdominal pain.

- Return to the clinic in one month for discussion on the results of the specimens sent to the lab.

- Codeine sulfate 15 mg PO q6h PRN

Questions

1. Discuss the etiology and pathophysiology of cervical cancer.

2. Discuss cultural and ethnic considerations of cervical cancer.

3. Discuss clinical manifestations of cervical cancer.

4. Discuss diagnostic studies used to confirm cervical cancer.

5. What is the purpose for the prescribed medication?

6. What are the most common adverse reactions, drug-to-drug, and drug-to-food/herbal interactions of the prescribed medication?

7. Discuss surgical management for cervical cancer.

8. Discuss the clinical stages of cervical cancer.

9. Discuss client education for cervical cancer.

GENDER

M

AGE

32

SETTING

- Hospital

ETHNICITY/CULTURE

- Black American/West Indian

PREEXISTING CONDITIONS

COEXISTING CONDITIONS

LIFESTYLE

- Professional painter

COMMUNICATION

DISABILITY

SOCIOECONOMIC STATUS

- Middle

SPIRITUAL/RELIGIOUS

- Methodist

PHARMACOLOGIC

- Morphine sulfate (Duramorph)
- Enoxaparin sodium (Lovenox)
- Docusate sodium (Colace)

PSYCHOSOCIAL

- Anxiety
- Pain

LEGAL

- Worker's compensation should be available until client returns to work.

ETHICAL

ALTERNATIVE THERAPY

PRIORITIZATION

- Stabilize extremity
- Assess and manage pain
- Assess neurological status of lower extremities

DELEGATION

- RN
- CNA
- Client education

THE MUSCULOSKELETAL AND REPRODUCTIVE SYSTEMS

Level of difficulty: Easy

Overview: This case first involves assessment of all major body systems for life-threatening complications, including head, thoracic, and abdominal injuries. The case involves assessment of pain and assessment of the skin for intactness, color, temperature, movement, sensation, pulses, and capillary refill. The triage nurse uses critical thinking to appropriately prioritize care of clients with hip dislocation in a busy emergency department (ED). The certified nursing attendant (CNA) can take vital signs and monitor the client for signs of bleeding, such as restlessness, or unusual findings on the skin (e.g., bruising) and inform the nurse.

Client Profile

Mr. P is a 32-year-old painter who is brought to the ED via emergency medical services (EMS) after falling from a ladder while painting a building under contract by his employer. He is 5′9″ and weighs 150 pounds.

Case Study

On arrival to the ED, Mr. P is alert, oriented to time, person and place, but is voicing intolerable pain in the right thigh with slight movement and moderate pain over his entire back. He denies known allergies to foods or drugs or the use of herbals. Vital signs reveal:

Blood pressure: 130/80

Pulse: 90

Respirations: 20

Temperature: 98.6° F

He is medicated with morphine 10 mg IM for pain as prescribed. Serum labs done in the ED reveal:

Hematocrit (Hct): 36%

Hemoglobin (Hgb): 14%

Serum calcium: 9 mg/dL

Serum phosphorous: 4 mg/dL

Mr. P is transferred from the stretcher that he is brought in on to a ED bed. His right leg remains immobilized by a long backboard. An EMS personnel provides the triage nurse with a detailed report of physical findings and neurovascular status of the injured extremity on arrival to the injury site. The ED health care provider arrives and after gathering additional pertinent history, the health care provider examines Mr. P for other bony injuries and a careful knee examination is also done. Mr. P is transferred to the orthopedic unit, weighed on a bedscale, then placed on bed rest. A complete assessment is done, including assessment of abrasions and other injuries. An EKG shows normal sinus rhythm, and a chest X-ray is negative for rib fracture or diaphragmatic damage. A venography is negative for pulmonary embolism. A pulse oximeter is initiated with a noted oxygen saturation of 98%. At a later time during the shift, a computed tomography (CT) of the spine, pelvis, hip, and leg is done and reveals an intact spine and pelvis, dislocation of the femoral head, and soft tissue damage of the leg and thigh, but no pre-existing disorders. After the multidisciplinary team reviews the data of diagnostic studies and physical findings, a diagnosis of closed femoral head dislocation is made, and plans for surgery are discussed with Mr. P. He is informed that no food or fluids should be taken (NPO) after a scheduled time in preparation for the surgical procedure. A closed reduction/internal fixation of the femoral head is scheduled. An intravenous (IV) line is initiated with IV solution of 0.9% sodium chloride at 125 mL/hr, and a trapeze is placed over the bed with instructions given to Mr. P on its purpose and use.

The following are prescribed:

- Complete bed rest
- Morphine sulfate (Duramorph) 1–2 mg IV PRN for pain
- Enoxaparin sodium (Lovenox) 100 mg/1mL SC daily
- Docusate sodium (Colace) 100 mg PO three times per day

Questions

1. Discuss the different types of fractures, including the closed fracture.

2. Discuss clinical manifestations of clients with closed femoral head fracture.

3. Discuss the potential complications of a closed femoral head fracture.

4. Discuss the use of crutches instead of a walker for this client.

5. Discuss the teaching guidelines for crutch walking.

6. What are common nursing diagnoses for clients with closed femoral head fracture?

7. What are expected outcomes for clients with closed femoral head fracture?

8. What are the purposes for the prescribed orders?

9. What are the most common adverse reactions, drug-to-drug, drug-to-food/herbal interactions for the prescribed medications?

10. Discuss discharge plans for the client following immobilization of the femoral head fracture.

GENDER

M

AGE

64

SETTING

- Hospital

ETHNICITY/CULTURE

- White American

PREEXISTING CONDITIONS

- Status-post femoral-popliteal bypass

COEXISTING CONDITIONS

- Peripheral vascular disease

LIFESTYLE

- CPA

COMMUNICATION

- English

DISABILITY

- Decreased mobility

SOCIOECONOMIC STATUS

- Middle

SPIRITUAL/RELIGIOUS

- Lutheran

PHARMACOLOGIC

- Ticarcillin disodium/clavulanate potassium (Timentin)

PSYCHOSOCIAL

- Anxiety
- Depression

LEGAL

ETHICAL

ALTERNATIVE THERAPY

PRIORITIZATION

- Antibiotic therapy
- Promote wound healing

DELEGATION

- RN
- Client education

THE MUSCULOSKELETAL AND REPRODUCTIVE SYSTEMS

Level of difficulty: Easy

Overview: This case involves assessment of the client's present problems. The nurse must be knowledgeable about osteomyelitis and the need for immediate medical and nursing interventions to prevent systemic complications and chronic osteomyelitis. The case involves pain management and antibiotic administration with knowledge of unintended effects of analgesic and antibiotic medications, and interventions for these effects.

Client Profile

Mr. Y is a 64-year-old certified public accountant who was discharged from the hospital three weeks ago after amputation of the left great toe related to complete loss of circulation in his extremity. Mr. Y is married and has a 28-year-old daughter in college. His wife is an elementary school teacher. He and his family own a three-bedroom co-op in a newly developed neighborhood.

Case Study

Mr. Y's past medical history includes hypertension and arterial insufficiency. He is status-post (S/P) femoral-popliteal bypass three weeks ago. His family history includes diabetes mellitus (mother) and hypertension and peripheral vascular disease (father). Mr. Y reports that both he and his wife have good health insurance and that he receives a salary while recuperating from surgery. However, he says he is concerned about the continuation of his salary, which is dependent on the length of time the infection will take to heal. Vital signs are:

Blood pressure: 140/94

Pulse: 94

Respirations: 20

Temperature: 101.4° F

The entire foot is tender and warm to touch. There is a moderate amount of mildly odorous drainage coming from the wound. The nursing history and physical examination is completed by the nurse, after which the health care provider reviews the data, asks the client about history of allergies, which the client denies. The health care provider continues the history and physical examination, and a specimen from the infected site is sent to the lab for analysis. The following diagnostic studies are ordered: radionuclide bone scan of the left foot, and a magnetic resonance imaging (MRI), blood culture and gram stain, culture and sensitivity of the wound, white blood cell (WBC) count with differential, and erythrocyte sedimentation rate (ESR). The bone scan reveals infection of the bone marrow, and the MRI identifies calcification of the bones of the foot and provides definitive diagnosis for osteomyelitis. The blood culture and gram stain are positive for P. aeruginosa and Staphylococcus aeruginosa. WBC with differential reveals:

White blood cell (WBC) count: 13,000/mm³

Neutrophils: 82%

Eosinophils: 4%

Basophils: 2%

Lymphocytes: 43%

Monocytes: 8%

Erythrocyte sedimentation rate (ESR): elevated, 90%

After the multidisciplinary team reviews the diagnostic studies, a diagnosis of osteomyelitis of the left foot is confirmed; the findings are discussed with the client; and plans for surgical debridement are decided upon by the team and Mr. Y. The debridement is done and the surgical plan is to implement high doses of parenteral antibiotics initially followed by oral antibiotics and serial bone scans. Specific orders are written for the surgical team to change the wound dressing during daily rounds.

The following are prescribed:

- Ticarcillin disodium/clavulanate potassium (Timentin) 3.1 g IV q4h
- 0.9% NaCL at 100 mL per hour
- Vitamin A (Aquasol A) 15,000 IU daily
- Vitamin C (ascorbic acid) 500 mg PO two times per day
- ESR, hemoglobin, WBC, albumin levels

Questions

1. Discuss the pathophysiology of osteomyelitis.

2. Discuss groups of persons in whom osteomyelitis is most difficult to manage.

3. Discuss indirect and direct osteomyelitis.

4. Discuss the organism that is the most common cause of osteomyelitis.

5. Discuss the psychosocial impact of the client's amputation on his well-being and the risk that further surgery may be necessary.

6. Discuss common nursing diagnoses for clients with osteomyelitis.

7. What are the purposes for the prescribed orders?

8. What are the most common adverse reactions, drug-to-drug, drug-to-food/herbal interactions for the prescribed medications?

9. Discuss discharge instructions for the client with osteomyelitis.

GENDER

F

AGE

58

SETTING

- Community health clinic

ETHNICITY/CULTURE

- Black American

PREEXISTING CONDITIONS

- Post menopause
- Lack of exercise

COEXISTING CONDITIONS

- Father has severe OA of the hands

LIFESTYLE

- Laundromat manager

COMMUNICATION

DISABILITY

SOCIOECONOMIC STATUS

- Low

SPIRITUAL/RELIGIOUS

- Baptist

PHARMACOLOGIC

- Aspirin (acetylsalicylic acid)
- Antacid (TUMS)
- Celecoxib (Celebrex)
- Calcium carbonate (Os-Cal)
- Capsaicin (Zostrix)

PSYCHOSOCIAL

- Mood changes
- Difficulty adjusting to limitation of use of hands

LEGAL

ETHICAL

- Client should have the right to use alternative therapy with prescribed medications.

ALTERNATIVE THERAPY

- Vegan diet
- Ginseng
- Cayenne pepper

PRIORITIZATION

- Pain management

DELEGATION

- RN
- LPN
- Client education

MODERATE

THE MUSCULOSKELETAL AND REPRODUCTIVE SYSTEMS

Level of difficulty: Moderate

Overview: This case involves a thorough assessment of the client's condition and current over-the-counter and herbal medications. It involves careful inspection and palpation of joints for symmetry, size, shape, color, appearance, and pain, and the use of arthritis disability and discomfort scales to assess the client's functional level for the past week to help determine assistance needed for activities of daily living (ADL). The licensed practical nurse (LPN) can reinforce teaching, after the registered nurse (RN) has initiated it, and continue with assessment procedures.

Client Profile

Ms. C is a 58-year-old female who is seen at the community health clinic for routine annual evaluation. Ms. C is 5'5" and weighs 150 pounds. The LPN is assigned to take her vital signs, which are:

Blood pressure: 140/84

Pulse: 84

Respirations: 18

Temperature: 98.6° F

Case Study

On initial interview by an RN, Ms. C reports increase in dull, aching pain around the joints of the digits of both hands. Observation of the hands finds evidence of early manifestations of Heberden's and Bouchard's nodes. On further assessment, she reports the use of aspirin to help relieve pain, and antacids (TUMS), to decrease the discomfort in her stomach, which she believes is due to the constant use of aspirin. Continued gathering of data reveals lack of exercise and years of "vegan" diet, but the use of herbs and nuts as supplements. After the RN completes the history and physical, Ms. C is seen by a nurse practitioner (NP) who corroborates data gathered by the nurse, discusses the findings with Ms. C, then orders serum labs to help confirm the presenting symptoms and subjective data. Serum labs are ordered and reveal:

White blood cell (WBC) count: 10,0000 mm^3

Red blood cell (RBC) count: 4.5 million/mm^3

Hemoglobin (Hgb): 13 g/dL

Hematocrit (Hct): 38%

Platelet count (PLT): 250,000 cells/mm^3

Calcium: 8.4 mg/dL

Sodium (Na): 135 mEq/L

Potassium (K+): 4.4 mEq/L

Rheumatoid factor, antinuclear antibody, and erythrocyte sedimentation rate (ESR) are elevated. The labs are reviewed and the client is referred to the community hospital for a magnetic resonance imaging (MRI) of the hands and spine. Ms. C is to return home and have the diagnostic test completed as scheduled, and to continue with follow-up care at the clinic. Ms. C undergoes MRI of the hands and spine, which reveals degenerative changes, especially in the spine. The health care provider discusses the laboratory findings and the result of the MRI with Ms. C, and a diagnosis of osteoarthritis (OA) is confirmed. The health care provider discusses the plan of care for OA, and the following medications are prescribed for her: aspirin (acetylsalicylic acid), topical capsaicin (Zostrix), celecoxib (Celebrex), and calcium (Os-Cal). Ms. C is seen by an RN in the clinic who reviews the prescribed medications with her and allows her to ask questions pertaining to the plan of care as discussed by the health care provider. After dialogue between the client and nurse, Ms. C informs the nurse that she will fill the prescriptions at a pharmacy in her community. A follow-up clinic appointment is scheduled for her, and she leaves the clinic.

The following are prescribed:

- Aspirin (acetylsalicylic acid) 1 g PO three times per day
- Capsaicin (Zostrix) apply to affected areas three to four times per day only
- Celecoxib (Celebrex) 200 mg PO two times per day
- Calcium carbonate (Os-Cal) 1 g PO in the morning and at bedtime

Questions

1. What is your understanding of the above situation?

2. What are some women's health considerations for OA?

3. What is the significance of Heberden's and Bouchard's nodes and their relationship with OA?

4. What are common nursing diagnoses for the client with OA?

5. Discuss nonpharmacologic measures that can be used for clients with OA.

6. What is the role of the physical therapist for clients with OA?

7. What are the purposes for the prescribed medications?

8. What are the most common adverse reactions of the prescribed medications?

9. Discuss the drug-to-drug and drug-to-food/herbal interactions for the prescribed medications.

10. Design a specific pain management plan for the client with OA.

11. What specific information should a nurse provide the client who is discharged to home about topical capsaicin?

CASE STUDY 5

Breast Cancer

GENDER

F

AGE

40

SETTING

- Hospital

ETHNICITY/CULTURE

- Black American

PREEXISTING CONDITIONS

COEXISTING CONDITIONS

- Abscess of the left breast at age 16
- Mother and brother died of breast cancer

LIFESTYLE

- Elementary school teacher
- Uses oral contraceptives

COMMUNICATION

DISABILITY

SOCIOECONOMIC STATUS

- Middle income, but may need supplemental financial support

SPIRITUAL/RELIGIOUS

- Baptist

PHARMACOLOGIC

- Doxorubicin HcL (Adriamycin)
- Cyclophosphamide (Cytoxan)
- Docetaxel (Taxotere)
- Tamoxifen citrate (Nolvadex)
- Ondansetron HcL (Zofran)

PSYCHOSOCIAL

- Anxiety
- Denial
- Fear

LEGAL

ETHICAL

- The client has the right to choose treatment. Is the family able to cope with the present stressors?

ALTERNATIVE THERAPY

- Prayer
- Herbal medications

PRIORITIZATION

- Careful and accurate breast history interview
- Active listening

DELEGATION

- Advanced practice nurse for clinical breast examination
- Client education

THE MUSCULOSKELETAL AND REPRODUCTIVE SYSTEMS

Level of difficulty: Difficult

Overview: This case involves a thorough assessment of the client's condition, including past medical history, family history of cancer including breast cancer, past surgical history, prescribed medications, and herbal supplements the client is currently taking. It requires empathy and the ability to identify with the client's feelings.

Client Profile

Mrs. W is a 40-year-old married client who is seen in the doctor's office for routine examination because she felt a lump in the upper outer quadrant of her left breast during breast self-examination (BSE). Mrs. W is 5′9″ and weighs 194 pounds. During a thorough breast examination, a painless mass that is hard, irregular in shape, and nonmobile in the upper outer quadrant is detected by the health care provider. Her reproductive history reveals one child, age seven years. She reports that her menstrual cycle began at the age of 12. She had used oral contraceptives for several years before her child was conceived. Mrs. W also reports a breast biopsy at the age of 16 for an abscess of the left breast. Her family history includes her mother and a brother who died of breast cancer. Her father, who is 90 years old, and her older sister, who is 42 years old, are both well.

Case Study

Mrs. W is referred for mammography at the community hospital. The mammography is done and reviewed by a radiologist. Mrs. W is later seen by her primary health care provider at his office. The results are discussed, and she is scheduled for diagnostic studies (ultrasound of the left breast and Tru-Cut Core breast biopsy) at a hospital that specializes in oncology. Mrs. W leaves the health care provider's office concerned because of her family history of breast cancer. The diagnostic studies are done and confirm the diagnosis of early stage II cancer of the left breast. Mrs. W is seen by her primary health care provider and an oncologist who discuss her plan of treatment, which will include administration of medication at the hospital and also at home. Mrs. W is admitted to the hospital for treatment for breast cancer and is informed that she will be discharged to home on Tamoxifen citrate (Nolvadex). Her vitals are:

Blood pressure: 134/84

Pulse: 86

Respirations: 18

Temperature: 98.4° F

The following are prescribed:

- Doxorubicin HcL (Adriamycin) 30 mg/m^2 IV for four cycles
- After the four cycles of doxorubicin, start cyclophosphamide (Cytoxan) 4 mg/kg IV over seven days
- Ondansetron HcL (Zofran) 24 mg PO 30 minutes before cyclophosphamide therapy
- Premedicate client with dexamethasone (Decadron) 8 mg two times per day × five days, starting one day prior to docetaxel (Taxotere)

Questions

1. Discuss the various histopathologic types of breast cancer.

2. Discuss etiologies for breast cancer.

3. Discuss cultural and ethnic considerations for breast cancer.

4. Discuss clinical manifestations for breast cancer.

5. Discuss diagnostic studies used to confirm breast cancer.

6. Discuss common nursing diagnoses for breast cancer.

7. What are the purposes for the prescribed medications?

8. What are the most common adverse reactions, drug-to-drug, drug-to-food/herbal interactions of the prescribed medications?

9. Discuss common sites of breast cancer recurrence and metastasis.

10. Discuss client education for breast cancer.

CASE STUDY 6

Myasthenia Gravis

GENDER

M

AGE

30

SETTING

- Hospital

ETHNICITY/CULTURE

- Black American

PREEXISTING CONDITIONS

COEXISTING CONDITIONS

- Respiratory tract infection
- Emotional stress

LIFESTYLE

- Law school student
- Lives with parents

COMMUNICATION

DISABILITY

- Activity intolerance related to muscle weakness and fatigue

SOCIOECONOMIC STATUS

- Low

SPIRITUAL/RELIGIOUS

- Baptist

PHARMACOLOGIC

- Pyridostigmine (Mestinon)
- Prednisone (Deltasone)
- Azathioprine (Imuran)

PSYCHOSOCIAL

- Anxiety
- Depression

LEGAL

- Financial support, depending on extent of medical interventions

ETHICAL

ALTERNATIVE THERAPY

PRIORITIZATION

- Airway patency
- Aspiration precaution

DELEGATION

- RN
- Client education

THE MUSCULOSKELETAL AND REPRODUCTIVE SYSTEMS

Level of difficulty: Difficult

Overview: This case involves a thorough assessment of the client's condition with specific focus on complaints of fatigability. It involves current exposure to infectious agents or current infectious problems. The nurse must use critical-thinking skills to prioritize care for the client in a busy emergency department (ED). Questions pertaining to medications and herbal supplements should be a significant part of the history that is taken.

Client Profile

Mr. T is a 30-year-old law student living at home with his parents. He is expected to graduate at the end of the current semester. Prior to entry into the ED, Mr. T reports having been on amoxicillin as prescribed by his primary health care provider for respiratory infections three weeks ago. Mr. T returned to college after completing the course of amoxicillin but reports feeling unusually tired and was easily fatigued after a two-hour lecture class.

Case Study

In the ED, Mr. T complains of muscle weakness of the eyes and eyelids, has difficulty speaking, and reports noticing that chewing and swallowing were difficult but nonspecific during break period at 10:00 AM. The ED health care provider is notified and immediately responds to the triage nurse's report. Vital signs are:

> Blood pressure: 120/80
>
> Pulse: 78
>
> Respirations: 16
>
> Temperature 98.4° F

History and physical are done and find ptosis (drooping of the eyelids) and weakness of facial muscles. Normal pupillary responses to light and accommodation are present. The following diagnostic tests are ordered: serum T_3, T_4, serum protein electrophoresis, and acetylcholine receptor antibodies (AChR) level. The results of the tests reveal: T_3: 205 ng/dL, T_4: 15 ug/dL, serum protein electrophoresis is negative for rheumatoid arthritis, systemic lupus erythematosus and polymyositis, and the AChR level is elevated (1.2 mmol/L). The findings are discussed with Mr. T and his parents as per his approval, and myasthenia gravis (MG) is diagnosed. Mr. T will be discharged to home in 48 hours. He and his parents are involved in an interdisciplinary team discussion before discharge: speech-language pathologist in collaboration with the primary RN, a registered dietitian, and an occupational therapist. The client will return to the clinic in two weeks for reevaluation of medication regimen.

The following are prescribed:

- Pyridostigmine (Mestinon) 60 mg PO daily
- Prednisone (Deltasone) 2 mg/kg/day × one week
- Azathioprine (Imuran) 1 mg/kg/day as maintenance dose

Questions

1. Discuss the incidence and pathophysiology of MG.

2. Discuss clinical manifestations of MG.

3. Discuss assessment and diagnostic findings of MG.

4. Discuss complications of MG.

5. Discuss the differences in care of the client with myasthenic crisis and cholinergic crisis.

6. Discuss plasmapheresis and its relationship to MG.

7. Discuss surgical management of MG.

8. What are the purposes for the prescribed medications?

9. What are the most common adverse reactions, drug-to-drug, drug-to-food/herbal interactions of the prescribed medications?

10. Discuss client education for MG.

CLINICAL DECISION MAKING

Case Studies in Psychiatric Nursing

Betty K. Richardson

PhD, RN, CNS-MHP, BC, LPC, LMFT

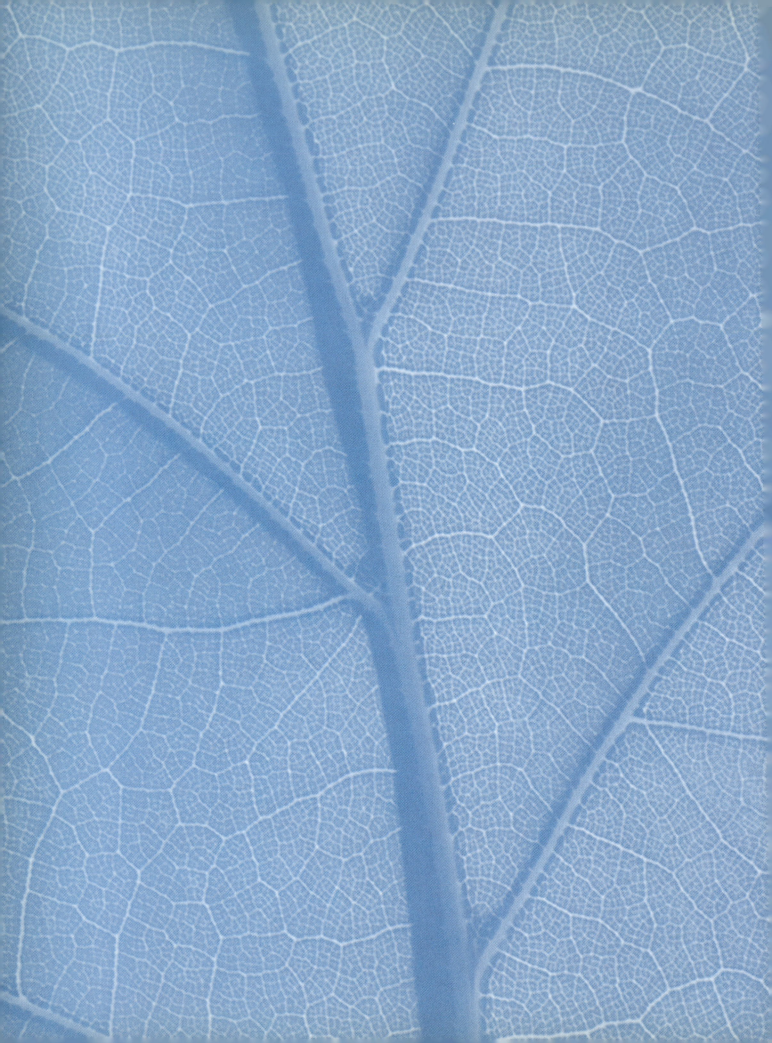

PART ONE

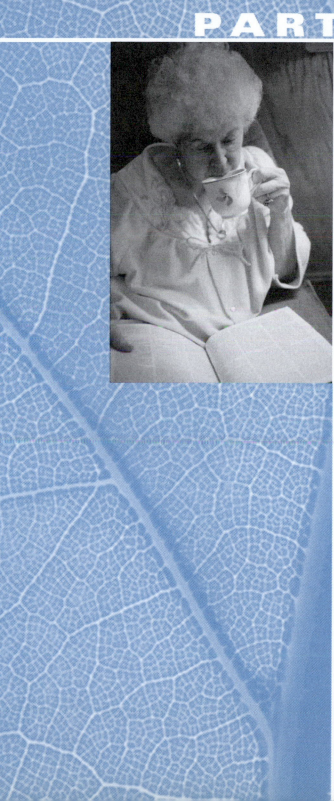

The Client Experiencing Schizophrenia and Other Psychotic Disorders

Sarah

GENDER

Female

AGE

34

SETTING

- Psychiatric hospital

ETHNICITY

- Hungarian American

CULTURAL CONSIDERATIONS

- Hungarian customs

PREEXISTING CONDITION

COEXISTING CONDITION

COMMUNICATION

DISABILITY

SOCIOECONOMIC

SPIRITUAL/RELIGIOUS

PHARMACOLOGIC

- Valproic acid (Depakote)
- Risperodone (Risperdal) liquid
- Venlafaxine hydrochloride (Effexor XR)

PSYCHOSOCIAL

LEGAL

- Confidentiality
- Consent
- Client's rights
- Release of information

ETHICAL

ALTERNATIVE THERAPY

PRIORITIZATION

DELEGATION

MODERATE

SCHIZOAFFECTIVE DISORDER, BIPOLAR TYPE

Level of difficulty: Moderate

Overview: Requires familiarity with the current diagnostic requirements for Schizoaffective Disorder and approaches to the psychotic client, including checking the client's mouth to prevent cheeking of medications. Requires critical thinking about accepting gifts from clients.

Client Profile

Sarah is a 34-year-old female. Born in Hungary, she married an American and came to this country when she was 25 years old. About a year later, Sarah began a series of admissions to psychiatric facilities. She was diagnosed with major depression and later with Schizoaffective Disorder. About a month ago, Sarah stopped keeping outpatient appointments, stopped taking her medication, stopped bathing, and stopped eating, but was sleeping all the time. Sarah's mood symptoms suddenly became less noticeable, and she began wandering her yard after dark, saying the neighbors were in the trees. Sarah began to carry a gun to protect herself against the neighbors, who she thought were out to kill her. When she started to fire the gun into the trees, her brother got a court order to have Sarah committed for treatment.

Case Study

Two deputies, one male and one female, and her brother have brought Sarah to the psychiatric hospital to be admitted. The nurse does an assessment on Sarah and discovers Sarah has been on risperodone (Risperdal) liquid, valproic acid (Depakote), and venlafaxine (Effexor XR). The psychiatrist orders these medications to be continued. At first the nurse is unable to get Sarah to sign consent forms to take the medication, but after a few days, she does sign the forms. By this time, her pregnancy test has come back negative, and she is started back on her usual medication.

The nurse finds Sarah to be somewhat tangential with loose associations. When the nurse assigns Sarah to attend a medication class, she refuses. When asked to interpret a proverb, she refuses.

Sarah begins to talk about her food being poisoned and being "king" of the hospital. She claims to have subjects to take care of the food and those who try to poison it.

Sarah tells the nurse that she has been hospitalized eight times previously at another psychiatric facility. The nurse sends a signed release of information form to the designated psychiatric facility requesting copies of Sarah's latest psychosocial assessment, treatment plan, and discharge summary. The requested information reveals that Sarah's discharge diagnosis at that facility was Schizoaffective Disorder, Bipolar Type.

After three weeks on medication, Sarah no longer seems to have hallucinations and delusions. The psychiatrist is ready to discharge Sarah, but her Depakote level comes back low. A nurse discovers Sarah has been cheeking her morning dose and sometimes her evening dose of Depakote and has been putting the medicine in a pair of shoes.

Sarah hands the nurse an envelope with two hundred dollars and the words "Thank-you nurse" written on the outside. About this time the nurse notices that Sarah has suddenly become hyperverbal, hyperactive, intrusive, and sexually suggestive to peers and staff.

Questions

1. What is Schizoaffective Disorder?

2. Do Sarah's symptoms match those of Schizoaffective Disorder, and if so, how?

3. On what basis do you think Sarah was court committed?

4. Why was Sarah's medication delayed? Why did the nurse not start it on admission?

5. Why does the nurse ask Sarah to interpret a proverb?

6. Does Sarah have hallucinations and/or delusions? What makes you think so?

7. What is the age of onset, the male to female ratio, and the prevalence of Schizoaffective Disorder?

8. Discuss the current theories of etiology, treatment, and prognosis of Schizoaffective Disorder.

9. What nursing diagnoses would you most likely write for Sarah?

10. What goals and interventions do you suggest for Sarah for one of these nursing diagnoses?

11. What are the possible explanations for the client giving the nurse an envelope with money in it? How would you respond to this gift offer if you were the nurse?

Dean

GENDER

Male

AGE

48

SETTING

- Community clinic for low-income clients

ETHNICITY

- American Indian and White American

CULTURAL CONSIDERATIONS

- Pima Indian culture

PREEXISTING CONDITION

- Diabetes

COEXISTING CONDITION

- Cough, fever

COMMUNICATION

DISABILITY

SOCIOECONOMIC

- Homeless

SPIRITUAL/RELIGIOUS

PHARMACOLOGIC

- Metformin (Glucophage)
- Risperodone (Risperdal)
- Trihexyphenidyl (Artane)
- Benztropine (Cogentin)

PSYCHOSOCIAL

- Isolating

LEGAL

- Confidentiality
- Consent for release of information

ETHICAL

- Respect for client's lifestyle choices (paternalism vs. autonomy)

ALTERNATIVE THERAPY

- Medicine man to overcome sources of evil influence on his life

PRIORITIZATION

DELEGATION

MODERATE

SCHIZOPHRENIA

Level of difficulty: Moderate

Overview: Requires the nurse to self-assess feelings about working with a homeless mentally ill client with diabetes and symptoms of Tardive Dyskinesia. The nurse must consider the client's Native American culture.

Client Profile

Dean, a 48 year-old male, grew up on a Pima Indian reservation in Arizona. He left the reservation after high school to serve in the army but was diagnosed and treated for Schizophrenia at age 21 and was discharged early. He has been in and out of psychiatric facilities for several years. He periodically takes a bus back to the reservation to see a medicine man, but he does not stay as he has no work and only distant, poor family there.

Case Study

Dean has come to the community health center. While he is sitting in the lobby, the nurse observes Dean without him being aware of this. The nurse notices that at times he seems to be talking to the air around him. She also notices that Dean is smacking his lips, his tongue protrudes at times, and he periodically coughs without covering his mouth.

When it is time for the nurse to do an assessment on Dean, the receptionist notifies the nurse that Dean has not filled out the intake form. The nurse tries to help him by asking him for his address. Although his speech is somewhat disorganized at times, the nurse finds out from Dean that he is homeless and currently living on the streets. His chief complaint is "not feeling well." The nurse takes Dean's vital signs, which are: T. 100.4, R. 22, P. 100, BP 152/98. He is 5 foot 8 inches tall and weighs 235 pounds. When weighed he says he has recently lost thirty pounds.

When the nurse asks Dean what medications he is on, he shows her some empty medicine bottles, saying he has run out of his medication and does not have the money to buy more. The labels on the bottles indicate he is on metformin (Glucophage), an oral antidiabetic medication, and risperodone (Risperdal). The nurse asks him why he takes Risperdal and also inquires about other medication he has taken in the past. He replies that he was diagnosed with Schizophrenia at age 21 and that he was on Thorazine for several years, then Haldol, then Prolixin injections, and maybe some he forgot before the current Risperdal. He explains that he has gone to the community mental health center twice to get more Risperdal samples

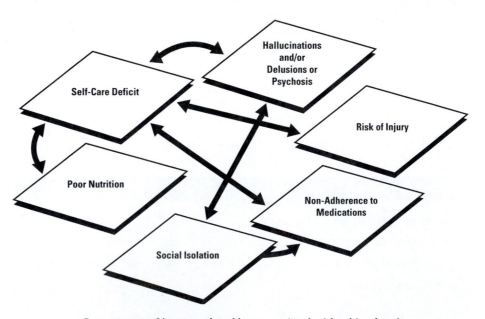

Concept map of issues and problems associated with schizophrenia

and waited most of the day each time without being seen by the psychiatrist. Dean says he either lost, or someone stole, his last supply of Risperdal, so he has not been taking it for about a month. The nurse suspects Dean is hearing voices.

When asked about any health problems, he says he has diabetes, which he is supposed to "keep under control with diet and pills." He also complains of a cough, something the nurse noticed earlier. After the nurse develops some rapport with Dean, he tells her about seeing and hearing an owl that frightens him. He talks about needing to see a medicine man.

Questions

1. What are some feelings that nurses could have about working with people who are homeless and mentally ill, and why would it be important for a nurse to think about his or her feelings toward this population?

2. Discuss the possible significance of Dean's appearance and observed behaviors.

3. What screening tests and/or lab procedures seem to be indicated?

4. What is Tardive Dyskinesia, how common is it, and what is the treatment for it? What did the nurse observe about Dean that would suggest Tardive Dyskinesia?

5. Is diabetes common among persons with a diagnosis of Schizophrenia? Is diabetes more common among Native American Indians? Discuss the possibility of persons with Schizophrenia having medical problems.

6. What precautions should the nurse take with the homeless population?

7. What additional information about Dean would be helpful, and how could this be obtained? What reason can you think of for Dean wanting to see a medicine man?

8. What findings by the health team would be sufficient to get Dean hospitalized in a psychiatric facility, and what opportunities might hospitalization present?

9. What findings might get this client hospitalized in a general hospital, and what opportunities might that present?

10. If you were the nurse in this case, would you want to get Dean off the street and into some other type of living situation? Why or why not? What reasons could he have for wanting to continue living on the streets?

11. Discuss resources likely to be available in the community for the homeless mentally ill, such as food, clothing, shelter, and medical care.

12. What nursing diagnoses and interventions would you write for this client?

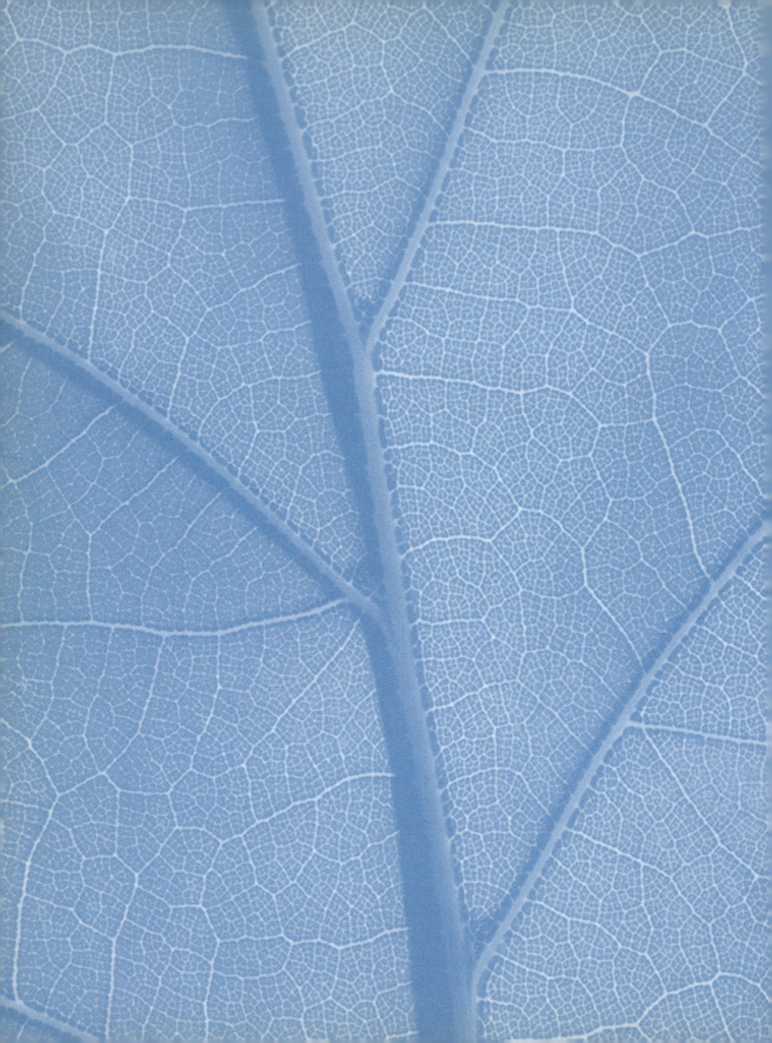

PART TWO

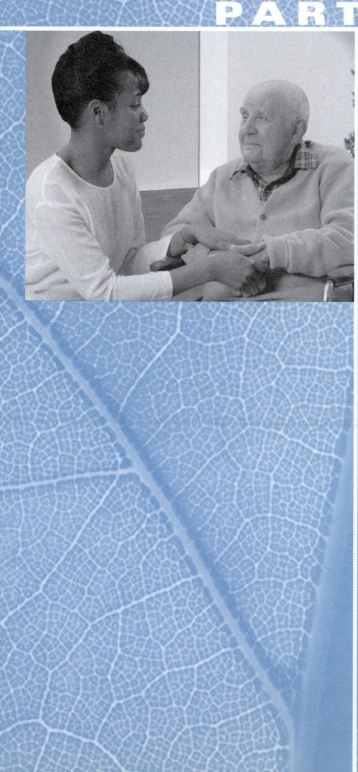

*The Client
Experiencing
Anxiety*

GENDER

Male

AGE

26

SETTING

- Evening outpatient treatment program

ETHNICITY

- White American

CULTURAL CONSIDERATIONS

PREEXISTING CONDITION

COEXISTING CONDITION

- Alcoholism

COMMUNICATION

DISABILITY

SOCIOECONOMIC

SPIRITUAL/RELIGIOUS

PHARMACOLOGIC

- Refusal to eat with or in front of others limits socialization
- Socialization revolves around alcohol

PSYCHOSOCIAL

LEGAL

- Confidentiality
- Informed consent
- DWI

ETHICAL

ALTERNATIVE THERAPY

PRIORITIZATION

DELEGATION

SOCIAL PHOBIA (SOCIAL ANXIETY DISORDER)

Level of difficulty: Moderate

Overview: Requires nurse to use therapeutic communication techniques. The nurse must also use critical thinking to identify her own thinking errors, teach the client and peers to recognize and correct thinking errors, and develop a care plan for a client with dual diagnosis: Social Phobia and Alcohol Abuse.

Client Profile

Jim is a 26-year-old husband and father of a preschool child. He lives and works in a small town in the finance department of an automobile dealership. The main places to gather socially in this small town are churches and bars. Jim prefers the bars where he can watch sports on T.V., talk to people, and drink "a couple of beers" with coworkers and friends. Jim's plan to drink a couple of beers usually turns into a dozen or more beers.

Jim never eats with anyone from work and usually turns down all social engagements that he and his wife are invited to. If he has to attend a work-related social event, he has a feeling that others are looking at him and judging him and he experiences tremors, palpitations, and sweating. Jim never accepts anything to eat at these events. Friends have stopped inviting Jim and his wife to dinner as the invitations are always declined. Jim tells his best friend: "I just don't feel comfortable eating in front of other people. I am afraid I will do something embarrassing and humiliate myself. This sounds unreasonable, even to me; but that is just the way that I am." Jim has been offered a job that pays more money and has better hours, but he would have to take clients to lunch and dinner. He has turned this job down due to his extreme discomfort with eating in public or with anyone other than his immediate family.

Case Study

Jim is attending a nightly outpatient chemical abuse treatment program as part of his follow-up after an inpatient program for substance abuse, a deal his lawyer worked out after he was found guilty of driving while intoxicated. The nurse at the treatment program notices that Jim does not go to the cafeteria with the rest of his group for the evening meal but sits alone in the lobby watching sports on television. The nurse wonders if Jim has enough money to buy dinner and begins to worry that he will be hungry when she does the medication education group later. She thinks about offering him half of her sandwich she brought from home, but stops herself from doing this as she recognizes she has committed a thinking error. The nurse has begun to wonder about Jim and why he seems so reticent, so hesitant to answer questions or share in group sessions or the community meetings. Last time

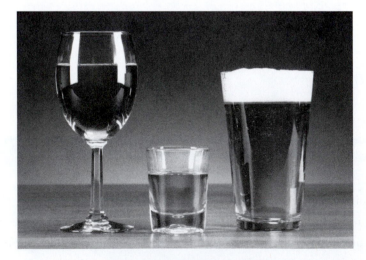

About 20% of clients with social anxiety disorder also have an alcohol use disorder.

she asked him a question in the community meeting, his face flushed and peers teased him, saying he was blushing like a girl and accusing him of having a crush on the nurse.

The nurse approaches Jim and says: "I notice you did not go to eat with your group."

Questions

1. Was the nurse's decision not to offer Jim half of her sandwich a good idea or not? Give a rationale for your answer. What else could the nurse do?

2. What do you think is the rationale for the nurse's opening remark: "I notice you did not go to eat with your group"? What therapeutic communication techniques are you familiar with that could be used in communication with Jim?

3. How do you think the nurse could best deal with the peers' comments about Jim blushing?

4. What is Social Phobia? Do you think this client has signs and symptoms that match those of Social Phobia (Social Anxiety Disorder)? Give a rationale for your answer.

5. Are there any differences in the signs and symptoms of children with Social Phobia compared to those of adults?

6. What are some theories of causation of Social Phobia?

7. What is the incidence of Social Phobia?

8. What other disorders or problems are common in the population experiencing Social Phobia? Could there be a connection between this client's drinking and Social Phobia (Social Anxiety Disorder)? If so, how would you assess for a connection?

9. What is the current thinking about heredity and alcohol abuse? What are some current treatments for those with early onset alcoholism?

10. What are some of the current treatments being used to treat Social Phobia?

11. What nursing diagnoses would you likely write for this client?

12. Discuss possible goals and interventions for this client. Is it possible to treat the alcoholism and the Social Phobia concurrently?

GENDER

Female

AGE

50

SETTING

- Community mental health center

ETHNICITY

- Mexican American

CULTURAL CONSIDERATIONS

- Hispanic

PREEXISTING CONDITION

COEXISTING CONDITION

COMMUNICATION

DISABILITY

SOCIOECONOMIC

- Daughter of migrant farmers; currently middle class

SPIRITUAL/RELIGIOUS

PHARMACOLOGIC

- Calcium
- Vitamins
- Hormone replacement
- Buspirone (BuSpar)

PSYCHOSOCIAL

- Impaired social isolation

LEGAL

ETHICAL

ALTERNATIVE THERAPY

- Herbal treatments containing Kava and Passaflora obtained from a curandara

PRIORITIZATION

DELEGATION

GENERALIZED ANXIETY DISORDER

Level of difficulty: Moderate

Overview: Requires critical thinking to understand and manage the common Hispanic practice of extended family being with a client for health care visits. The nurse must also identify behaviors common in clients with a diagnosis of Generalized Anxiety Disorder (GAD) and become knowledgeable about treatment modalities, including the antidepressant BuSpar.

Client Profile

Betty, a 50-year-old woman, came to this country with her parents when she was 7 years old. The family members worked as migrant farm workers until they had enough money to open a restaurant. Betty married young. She and her husband worked in the family restaurant and eventually bought it from the parents. They raised seven children, all grown and living on their own. Betty and her husband live in a mobile home close to the restaurant. She does not work in the family restaurant anymore because she worries excessively about doing a poor job. Betty no longer goes out if she can help it. She stays at home worrying about how she looks, what people think or say, the weather or road conditions, and many other things. Betty is not sleeping at night and keeps her husband awake when she roams the house. She keeps her clothing and belongings in perfect order while claiming she is doing a poor job of it. She does not prepare large family dinners anymore, though she still cooks the daily meals; one daughter has taken over the family dinners. This daughter has become concerned about Betty being isolated at home and worrying excessively and calls the community mental health center for an appointment for Betty.

Case Study

Betty presents at the community mental health center accompanied by her husband, her children and their spouses, several grandchildren, and a few cousins. When Betty's name is called and she is told that the nurse is ready to see her, she frowns and says: "What will I say? I don't know what to say. I think my slip is showing. My hem isn't straight."

Betty says she wants her whole family to go in to see the nurse with her. The nurse notices that Betty is extremely well groomed and dressed in spite of concerns she has been voicing about her appearance. Before the psychiatric nurse interviews Betty alone, she hears from the daughter that Betty "worries all the time" and although she has always been known to be a worrier, the worrying has become worse over the past six or eight months. The husband shares that his wife is keeping him awake at night with her inability to get to sleep or stay asleep.

The nurse interviews Betty alone. The nurse notices that Betty casts her eyes downward, speaks in a soft voice, does not smile, and seems restless as she taps her foot on the floor, drums her fingers on the table, and seems on the verge of getting out of her chair. Themes in the interview include: being tired, getting tired easily, not being able to concentrate, not getting work done, trouble sleeping, worrying about whether her husband loves her anymore and whether she and her husband have enough money, and not having the energy to attend to the housework or her clothing.

The nurse has the impression that Betty's anxiety floats from one worry to another. There is no convincing Betty that she looks all right. Any attempt to convince her that she need not worry about something in particular leads to a different worry before coming back to the earlier worry.

The community mental health psychiatrist examines Betty and, after a thorough physical examination and lab studies, finds nothing to explain her fatigue and difficulty sleeping other than anxiety. Betty produces her medicine bottles and says she is currently taking only vitamins, hormone replacement, and calcium. The psychiatrist asks the nurse to contact Betty's family health care provider to get information on any medical or psychiatric conditions he is treating her for; the report comes back that she has no medical diagnoses and the family health care provider thinks she suffers from anxiety. The psychiatrist prescribes buspirone (BuSpar) for Betty.

Two weeks later, during a home visit to Betty, the nurse learns, with some probing, that Betty is upset with her husband for loaning all their savings to the daughter and her husband to build a new home, while they continue to live in an older mobile home. At the end of the nurse's home visit, Betty's daughter arrives and tells the nurse that she wonders if Betty is making any progress. Betty also worries she is not getting better and asks the nurse about taking some herbal medicines containing Kava and Passaflora that her sister got from a curandara (folk healer); her sister wants to take her to see the curandara and have her do a ritual to cure the evil eye that was placed on Betty and made her sick.

Questions

1. What behaviors does this client have that match the criteria for a diagnosis of Generalized Anxiety Disorder?

2. How common is the diagnosis of Generalized Anxiety Disorder? Is it common for clients with GAD to have comorbidity, and should this client be assessed for any particular condition?

3. What explanation do you have for the number of family members coming to the community mental health center with this client? If you were the nurse, how would you deal with Betty's request for her whole family to accompany her to see you?

4. Before the nurse, or any other staff at the community mental health center, can talk with Betty's family health care provider, what do they need to do?

5. What does the nurse need to know about buspirone? What teaching needs to be done with the client in regard to buspirone? What medications other than buspirone are being used in the treatment of GAD, and how effective are they?

6. What are some of the interventions, in addition to antianxiety drugs, that are being used with clients who have GAD?

7. At one point the daughter says that she thinks Betty is not showing progress. What progress, if any, do you think has been made? What can you tell the daughter?

8. What do you think about Betty's sister using herbal remedies and rituals for driving out evil spirits in trying to cure Betty? Do herbal remedies work?

9. What nursing diagnoses would you write for Betty related to her Generalized Anxiety Disorder?

GENDER

Female

AGE

19

SETTING

- Day treatment program in psychiatric hospital

ETHNICITY

- White American

CULTURAL CONSIDERATIONS

- Cajun, voodoo beliefs

PREEXISTING CONDITION

COEXISTING CONDITION

- Agoraphobia

COMMUNICATION

DISABILITY

SOCIOECONOMIC

SPIRITUAL/RELIGIOUS

- Voodoo

PHARMACOLOGIC

- Paroxetine (Paxil)

PSYCHOSOCIAL

LEGAL

ETHICAL

ALTERNATIVE THERAPY

PRIORITIZATION

DELEGATION

PANIC DISORDER WITH AGORAPHOBIA

Level of difficulty: High

Overview: Requires the nurse to develop an understanding of Agoraphobia and Panic Disorder and to use critical thinking to teach the client ways to minimize symptoms of a panic attack and overcome a fear of leaving her house. The nurse must also help a client's peers understand that voodoo beliefs can be cultural practices, not psychosis.

DIFFICULT

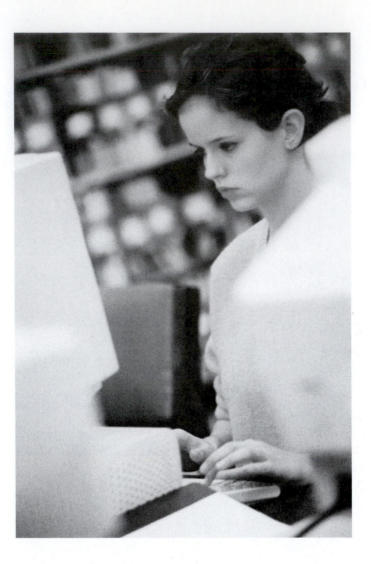

Client Profile

Caroline, a 19-year-old college student from rural Louisiana, is attending a large university in a nearby state. Caroline was doing well at the university until she experienced several unexpected panic attacks. She had a panic attack in the undergraduate library and another one when she went to the gym to work out. The most recent attack occurred about a month ago when she was driving her car. Suddenly and for no reason she could think of, she began feeling short of breath. It "felt like someone was smothering" her, but she was alone in the car. She was afraid she was going to die. Her heart was going very fast; she became dizzy and was feeling numbness and tingling in her hands. She felt a sense of impending danger and wanting to escape. She was so panicked that she had to pull over into a convenience store parking lot and wait until she felt better to call her boyfriend and ask him to come and take her home.

Caroline rode the bus to campus to classes for a while after this panic attack. She parked her car and refused to drive anywhere. She began fearing another panic attack and started skipping classes. A big school football game and party is coming up, and the boyfriend threatens to break up with Caroline if she does not "get a grip."

Case Study

Caroline's mother receives a call from Caroline's roommate telling her of the situation. Her mother takes Caroline to see a psychiatrist who prescribes paroxetine (Paxil) 10 mg/day and suggests an outpatient evening treatment program. Treatment in the evening allows Caroline to go to classes in the daytime. Caroline attends the first two nights of group and individual therapy. Her mother drives Caroline to the evening program on these nights. During group therapy Caroline reveals a fear that she has some life-threatening illness that the doctor has not found on a recent annual physical. Later in group she says she thinks someone has put a voodoo spell on her.

On the third night, Caroline is to take a cab or bus to the evening sessions because her mother has gone back home. It is two hours before the evening program is to begin. Caroline calls the nurse in the outpatient evening treatment program, saying: "I am too afraid to leave the house. I'm sorry. I just can't come tonight. Perhaps I will be able to come tomorrow." The nurse responds, "I want you to take several deep breaths and think about relaxing. Now that you feel very relaxed, I want you to visualize in your mind walking to the door and opening it."

Questions

1. What is the difference between a panic attack and Panic Disorder? What symptoms does Caroline have, and do they match the criteria for a diagnosis of Panic Disorder?

2. What is the usual onset of panic attacks and Panic Disorder? Is there a gender difference in the prevalence of panic attacks and Panic Disorder?

3. Caroline has Agoraphobia. What is Agoraphobia and what symptoms of this problem does Caroline exhibit?

4. How can Caroline's significant others (e.g., mother, boyfriend, roommate, classmates, and peers in group) best support her in dealing with panic attacks and Agoraphobia?

5. One of Caroline's group peers shares with the nurse that he thinks Caroline is psychotic and is paranoid and delusional about somebody putting a spell on her. If you were the nurse, how would you respond?

6. How would you respond if Caroline shares with you that she believes she has a fatal disease that no one has found and that someone is putting a spell on her or choking and putting pins in a voodoo doll that represents her?

7. Why did the nurse respond by encouraging relaxation and visualization when Caroline called to say she would not make it to the evening therapy program?

8. What teaching does the nurse need to do with Caroline in regard to the paroxetine (Paxil) she has begun to take for her Panic Disorder? What problem associated with paroxetine (Paxil) often causes clients, particularly men, to stop taking it, and what can be done about this? What assessments does the nurse need to do because Caroline is on paroxetine (Paxil)?

9. What medications have been found to be effective in reducing the number and/or severity of panic attacks?

10. What therapies other than medication are currently being used to treat Panic Disorder and Agoraphobia?

11. What nursing diagnoses would you write for Caroline?

12. Discuss some nursing interventions for at least one of the likely nursing diagnoses.

13. Carolyn's boyfriend asks: "What causes Panic Disorder?" How would you answer him? Why might he be concerned?

GENDER

Female

AGE

25

SETTING

■ General hospital

ETHNICITY

■ Central American

CULTURAL CONSIDERATIONS

■ Colombian

PREEXISTING CONDITION

COEXISTING CONDITION

COMMUNICATION

DISABILITY

SOCIOECONOMIC

SPIRITUAL/RELIGIOUS

PHARMACOLOGIC

■ Trazodone (Desyrl)

PSYCHOSOCIAL

■ Impaired social interaction
■ Situational low self-esteem

LEGAL

■ Confidentiality
■ Consent for release of information

ETHICAL

■ Client's right not to report a crime vs. nurse and health care team members' views

ALTERNATIVE THERAPY

PRIORITIZATION

DELEGATION

POST TRAUMATIC STRESS DISORDER (PTSD), ADULT

Level of difficulty: High

Overview: Requires the nurse to select therapeutic communication techniques to use with a client who has signs and symptoms of PTSD. The nurse must decide what action to take when the client reveals being raped in the past and asks the nurse to keep this information confidential. The nurse is challenged to do holistic nursing with this client who has psychological needs and sexual education and support needs as well as medical needs.

DIFFICULT

Client Profile

Claudia is a single, bright 25-year-old graduate student from a small town in the mountains of Colombia in Central America. She came to the United States to do her graduate work at a large state university. One night she decided to go meet friends at a local bar frequented by college students, locals, and tourists. Her friends did not show up. A nice-looking man bought her a few drinks and then offered to take her home. When she arrived home this man forcibly performed sexual acts and made her perform sexual acts on him. He then forced her to shower to "wash away evidence" and threatened to kill her if she reported the incident. She felt a great deal of fear and helplessness. Claudia thought perhaps this rape was her fault for dressing too sexy or going out unescorted. Almost immediately Claudia began to have a feeling of being numb and detached from everything and seemed to be in a daze, and she seemed to not be able to recall much of the incident at all. She continued her studies and moved in with her boyfriend, but did not tell him about the incident, and she has not told her family in Colombia that she has moved in with her boyfriend. She avoided the bar and the friends that she was supposed to meet. She decided she would move on with her life.

Eventually she started having trouble falling asleep and had nightmares, and her boyfriend recognized she was less interested in intimacy and had begun talking about never getting married or having children. She asked him not to wear a certain aftershave, which she had always complimented him on before.

Case Study

About a year after the rape episode, Claudia is admitted to the general hospital for an appendectomy. The night after surgery Claudia screams in the middle of the night and the night nurse finds her crying. The night nurse decides to sit with Claudia until she relaxes. The nurse offers to sit with Claudia and to listen if she wants to talk and then sits quietly.

Claudia is silent for a while, and then says: "I have had bad dreams almost every night for about a year, and I have bad memories come on me sometimes in the daytime. I have not told anyone about it, and I don't want to talk about it, but I was raped about a year ago and please do not put that in my chart. I am here to have surgery and not talk about the rape. That is in the past. Even my boyfriend does not know about it." The nurse notices that Claudia is hypervigilant, alert to every small noise and is easily startled.

Two days later, the health care provider gives Claudia a tentative diagnosis of Post Traumatic Stress Disorder (PTSD) and asks a psychiatric mental health nurse clinician employed by the hospital to work with the client and the medical team.

Questions

1. What communication techniques did the night nurse use that encouraged the client to reveal that her bad dreams had to do with being raped? Were these recognized therapeutic communication techniques? What other therapeutic communication techniques could the nurse use in response to the client saying she was raped a few months ago?

2. If you were the night nurse and the client asked you not to tell anyone about the rape, how would you respond, and what would you do with the information?

3. The client promises you she will talk with her doctor in the morning. What could you chart about the client's crying out?

4. If the client were to agree to let you call the health care provider in the middle of the night, what would you say to this provider?

Questions (continued)

5. The client is talking about the rape being all her fault for not using better judgment and dressing provocatively. Is this unusual behavior from a rape victim? How do you, as her nurse, respond?

6. Do you pass on this information about the client saying she had been raped in the report to the next shift? What sort of things do you consider in making your decision?

7. Looking at the information in the client profile and the case study, what signs and symptoms has this client had, and perhaps still has, that led the health care provider to a tentative diagnosis of PTSD? If diagnosed with PTSD, would this client likely be diagnosed as having acute, chronic, or delayed onset PTSD?

8. What events can place individuals at risk for PTSD, and which events have the highest risk?

9. What nursing diagnoses would you write for this client, given the limited amount of information that you have?

10. What are some of the current treatments for PTSD?

11. What teaching would you do about trazodone (Desyrl) with this client?

12. How can the primary nurse work with the client in regard to sexuality? How can the primary nurse teach the boyfriend ways to be supportive as well as to deal with his expressed concerns about the client's decreased interest in sexual intimacy?

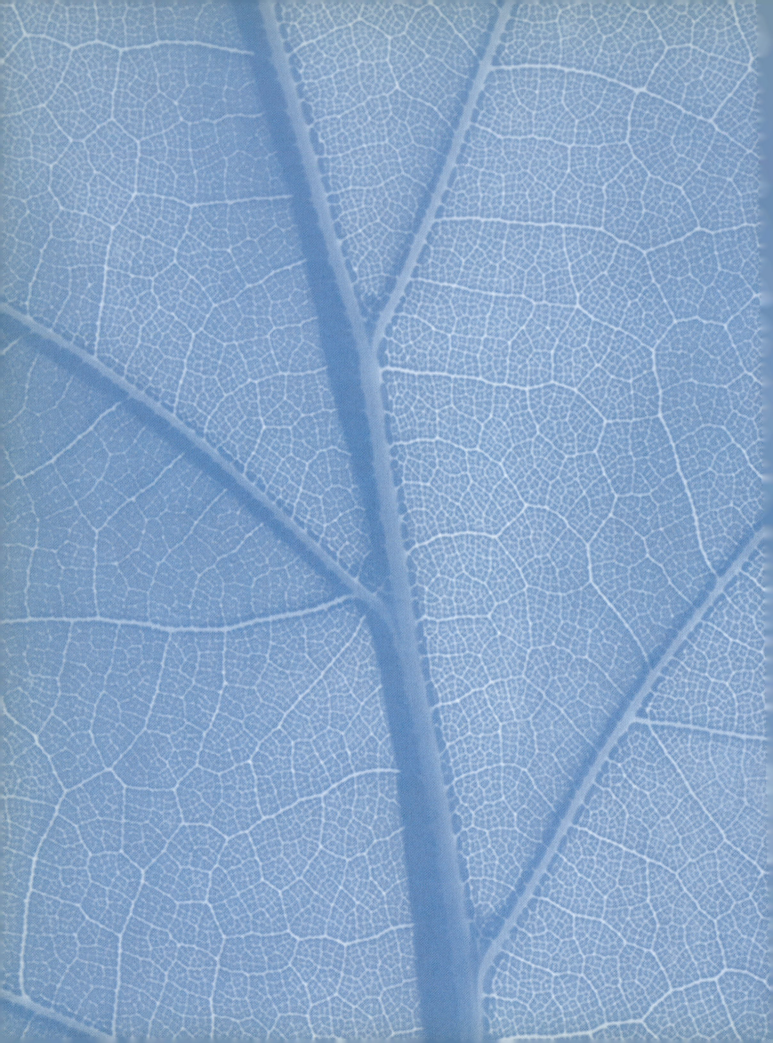

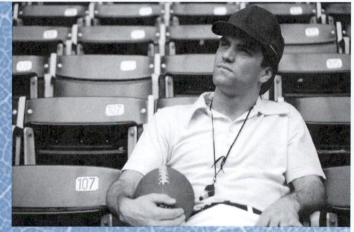

## PART THREE

The Client Experiencing Depression or Mania

John

GENDER

Male

AGE

14

SETTING

- Adolescent unit of a psychiatric hospital

ETHNICITY

- Black American

CULTURAL CONSIDERATIONS

PREEXISTING CONDITION

COEXISTING CONDITION

- Obesity Hypoventilation Syndrome

COMMUNICATION

DISABILITY

SOCIOECONOMIC

- Low-income family
- Public assistance
- Housing project

SPIRITUAL/RELIGIOUS

PHARMACOLOGIC

- Vitamins
- Sertraline (Zoloft)

PSYCHOSOCIAL

- Social relationships with peers limited due to obesity/depressed mood
- Low self-esteem

LEGAL

- Obtaining permission for a child or adolescent to take an antidepressant

ETHICAL

- Alternative therapy

PRIORITIZATION

- Addressing physical and psychological conditions while acknowledging self-esteem and identity-building needs

DELEGATION

- Delegation of crisis on unit to another team member

DYSTHYMIA

Level of difficulty: Easy

Overview: Requires the nurse to build a trusting relationship with a young client and his mother. The nurse must determine whether to respond to a unit crisis or delegate that task to a nurse colleague, so a promise to the client and mother can be kept. Challenges for the nurse also include making the mother part of the team identifying treatment goals and interventions. The nurse is called upon to describe current theories of treatment of dysthymia and to demonstrate understanding of a coexisting physical problem: Obesity Hypoventilation Syndrome.

Client Profile

John is a 14-year-old male who lives in urban public housing with his mother. John's father is not in contact. John has had a low level of energy and is described by his mother and teachers as looking sad and being somewhat irritable for the past eighteen months. His major activities outside of school are watching television, using the computer, eating, and attending the native Baptist Church with his mother. Peers in the housing project make fun of John for attending church with his mother, but he likes the church music and the church potluck suppers.

John resists joining activities. He declines peer activity and offers one or more reasons why the activity is not desirable. "I don't care" is a phrase he frequently uses (e.g., if he doesn't do his homework and is given a consequence, he says: "I don't care"). His teachers describe John as "easily distracted" unless he is doing something he is extremely interested in. He is morbidly obese and short of breath after walking a short distance. John is found on a routine school physical to be somewhat depressed and so overweight that it affects his breathing. The health care provider doing the physical refers John to an endocrinologist and a psychiatrist.

Case Study

John is admitted to the adolescent unit of a private psychiatric hospital by his endocrinologist and psychiatrist. The hospital is interested in receiving additional future admissions with similar psychiatric diagnoses and endocrine problems combined, and agrees to accept this case without payment.

On admission, the admitting nurse greets the client and his mother and introduces himself. The nurse interviews John's mother while John is given a tour of the unit. During the interview, a staff member comes and asks the admitting nurse to step out to discuss something urgent. The nurse tells John's mother he will be right back. The staff nurse describes an urgent situation on the unit and indicates the admitting nurse should take care of it; however, the admitting nurse delegates it to someone else and returns quickly to continue the interview. The mother is asked to describe a typical day in the family in chronological sequence and to write down what she and John had eaten at meals the previous day. Later, when the nurse interviews John alone, he asks John: "What do you like to do that you are good at?" John replies: "I can cook, do really cool magic tricks, and play computer games." John tells the nurse that other kids are mean to him and tell him he is too fat to play with them. He says he would like to be able to play football. John is shown a page of faces with various expressions and asked to pick out the way he feels most of the time. He picks out the sad face.

Just before mother leaves, she says to the nurse: "John's birthday is next week; I want to bring a birthday cake for him. Would that be all right if I brought a second cake for the other kids?"

John's tentative diagnoses are early onset Dysthymic Disorder and Obesity Hypoventilation Syndrome. He is admitted for professional help in safely losing weight, to begin medication for dysthymia, and to participate in group, family, and individual therapy. In addition to orders for these therapies, the admission orders include daily vitamins and a strict diet (e.g., protein diet drink to be mixed by the nutritionist and sent to the unit three times a day, one cup of salad, and a four-ounce skinless broiled chicken breast or broiled piece of fish at lunch and dinner). The orders also include nocturnal polysomnography testing in the sleep studies laboratory. Oxygen saturation levels are to be taken four times a day, and John is to wear a pulse oxymeter at night and recordings of the readings are to be made every hour. A $PaCO_2$ level is to be drawn during the day. In the progress notes, the health care provider writes: "Consider Sertraline (Zoloft)."

Questions

1. Discuss how John's observed behavior may or may not match a diagnosis of Dysthymic Disorder (DD). How do the criteria for a diagnosis of DD differ for adults compared to children and adolescents? What does the psychiatrist mean when he refers to John as having early onset Dysthymic Disorder (EODD)?

2. What is the risk for a person in a clinical setting with a diagnosis of Dysthymic Disorder to develop a major depressive disorder?

3. Is ethnicity a risk factor for Dysthymic Disorder? Are there other risk factors? What gender differences, if any, are there in the occurrence of Dysthymic Disorder in children and in adults?

4. Describe the usual course of Dysthymic Disorder.

5. Discuss what you know about Obesity Hypoventilation Syndrome from your reading on this subject.

6. When the staff member called the nurse out of the interview with John's mother, why do you suppose he delegated whatever needed doing and went right back into the interview?

7. The nurse asked John what he likes to do and what he is good at. What can the nurse and the treatment team use this information for?

8. Describe the possible reasons for John to go to individual, group, and family therapy sessions.

9. If you were the admitting nurse and John's mother asked you if she could bring him a birthday cake the following week, what would your response be?

10. From the limited information you have been given, what nursing diagnoses are most likely for this client?

11. Describe some interventions you would use for at least one of these nursing diagnoses.

12. What is the health care provider likely considering before starting sertraline (Zoloft)? What assessments need to be done prior to the client being started on sertraline, and what teaching needs to be done with the client and the client's mother? Who needs to sign permission for the client to take sertraline?

GENDER

Female

AGE

35

SETTING

- Inpatient hospital psychiatric unit

ETHNICITY

- Central American

CULTURAL CONSIDERATIONS

- Hispanic culture, rural Nicaraguan

PREEXISTING CONDITION

COEXISTING CONDITION

COMMUNICATION

- Speaks little English; Spanish preferred language

DISABILITY

SOCIOECONOMIC

- Raised by poor parents; now upper middle class

SPIRITUAL/RELIGIOUS

- Catholic

PHARMACOLOGIC

- Birth control
- Lithium carbonate (Eskalith)
- Olanzapine (Zyprexa)

PSYCHOSOCIAL

LEGAL

- Confidentiality
- Right to refuse medication

ETHICAL

- Birth control vs. Catholic teachings

ALTERNATIVE THERAPY

PRIORITIZATION

DELEGATION

- collaborating treatment planning with team
- collaborating management of lithium levels with team

BIPOLAR I MANIC EPISODE

Level of difficulty: Moderate

Overview: Requires critical thinking to therapeutically deal with the client's lack of judgment in areas such as spending, sexuality, and dress. Requires the nurse to consider how a client's culture and religion can affect treatment. The client's high levels of energy, activity, and distractibility require the nurse to develop strategies to get the client to eat, sleep, and attend to hygiene tasks. Requires management of the client's medication at a therapeutic level and to delegate this aspect of care at discharge.

Client Profile

Maria is a 35-year-old married female born and raised in a small village in Nicaragua, Central America. Her parents are poor. Her husband is a university professor who was serving as a Peace Corps worker when they met. She has been in the United States for two years and speaks a little English but requires Spanish for clear understanding. They have a 4-year-old daughter. Maria has been diagnosed with Bipolar I and takes lithium carbonate. Recently she stopped taking her lithium and has been staying up all night and eating very little. She is dressing and behaving in a sexually provocative manner and going on spending sprees buying things she does not need and cannot afford (e.g., a motorcycle that she does not know how to ride and a drum set that she does not know how to play). Her husband decides she is out of control and calls Maria's psychiatrist who suggests admission to the psychiatric unit of the hospital.

Case Study

During the admission process, the nurse observes that Maria is dressed in a short and tight-fitting dress. Her speech is clear but sprinkled with profanity as she moves rapidly from topic to topic. At the nurse's request, Maria sits down, then jumps up and moves about the room.

Maria's husband says that Maria has stopped taking her lithium and has not been sleeping or eating enough. He describes her extravagant purchases, some of which were returned or given away to strangers (e.g., Maria gave part of a drum set to a man she met in a bar). The husband explains that Maria has put the family in serious debt and states she is unfit to care for their child. With her husband translating for her, Maria objects to being admitted to the hospital, but then agrees to admission. The husband expresses concern about her sexually provocative behavior and states he fears that she will get sexually involved with other clients.

At the first meal after admission, Maria is in the dining room with the other clients. Instead of eating, Maria carries napkins to, and talks to, all the other clients and ignores the food. Staff members have told Maria several times to sit down and eat, and she has not complied.

The nurse asks the dietitian to prepare a sandwich and a banana for Maria. After the clients are finished with lunch, the nurse suggests Maria go to her room to wash her face and hands.

The psychiatrist-ordered pregnancy test comes back negative. The psychiatrist orders Lithium carbonate (Eskalith), olanzapine (Zyprexa), and birth control pills.

At medication time, the nurse gives Maria her medications and then examines Maria's mouth. The nurse does some teaching about the medications with Maria, who becomes upset when she learns she has been prescribed birth control and says she will not take it as it is not allowed in her religion.

The nurse notices that Maria is irritable and verbally hostile at times as well as inappropriate during her first days on the unit. During one encounter with Maria, the nurse senses great hostile energy coming from Maria, who says, "You think you so smart! You don't know nothing!" Sometimes Maria is demanding or threatening. For example, she demands that the nurse send someone to the store to pick up items for her and take her credit card to pay for them. Maria continues to dress and talk in a sexually provocative manner. She asks the male nurse, who passes medications in the early morning, to perform some sexual acts with her. At one point Maria is intrusive with another client in the day room and the client is threatening to harm Maria. The nurse observes that both clients are loud and their behavior is escalating.

After one month, during a meeting of the psychiatric health team, the psychiatrist discusses Maria's past psychiatric history, which includes two episodes of depression and one of mania. He offers a diagnosis of Bipolar I, Manic Episode for Maria. He orders that blood be drawn for a lithium level. The lithium level comes back at 1.5.

Questions

1. What criteria is essential for a diagnosis of Bipolar I? What would need to be different for Maria to have a diagnosis of Bipolar II Disorder? Which of Maria's behaviors are consistent with the criteria for a manic episode?

2. What would it feel like to be manic, and why would someone who is manic stop taking medication to bring their mood down to "normal"?

3. If you were Maria's nurse, what needs would you assess in relation to her culture and communication? What accommodations would you most likely try to make for her?

4. Why did the nurse ask the dietitian to prepare a sandwich and a banana for Maria, and why did the nurse take Maria to her room?

5. What is the most likely reason for the psychiatrist ordering a pregnancy test on admission? Why did he order birth control pills? The client has refused the birth control pills. How do you feel about this, and what action would you take if you were the nurse in this case?

6. What reason did the nurse have for inspecting Maria's mouth after giving her the medication?

7. What teaching did the nurse need to do about lithium for Maria? What is the significance of the lithium level, and what action(s) does the nurse need to take, if any?

8. What is olanzapine (Zyprexa), and what is the likely reason that Maria is being prescribed olanzapine?

9. What would you do or say if you were the nurse standing in front of Maria when she says: "You think you so smart. You don't know nothing"?

10. What strategies could a nurse use when Maria is demanding that a staff member be sent to shop for her using her credit card? Do strategies differ depending on whether the client has supportive family and/or friends, or not?

11. What might you say or do in response to the husband's expressed fear that his wife will become involved sexually with a peer on the unit?

12. How would you feel and what would you say or do if you were the male nurse passing medications and Maria was talking seductively and using profanity?

13. When the nurse finds Maria has been intrusive with another client and that both clients are escalating and threatening, what is the best response by the nurse?

14. What are some potential nursing diagnoses that you could likely write for this client?

15. What developmental stage is Maria in, and what behaviors, if any, does she have to match the tasks of this stage?

CASE STUDY 3

Candice

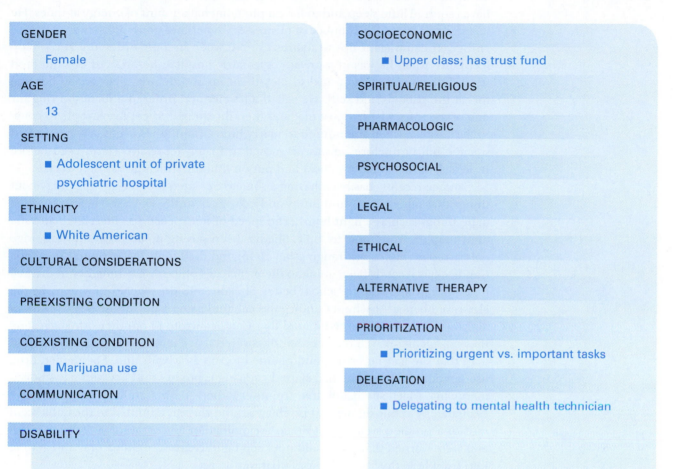

GENDER	**SOCIOECONOMIC**
Female	■ Upper class; has trust fund
AGE	**SPIRITUAL/RELIGIOUS**
13	
SETTING	**PHARMACOLOGIC**
■ Adolescent unit of private psychiatric hospital	**PSYCHOSOCIAL**
ETHNICITY	**LEGAL**
■ White American	
CULTURAL CONSIDERATIONS	**ETHICAL**
	ALTERNATIVE THERAPY
PREEXISTING CONDITION	
	PRIORITIZATION
COEXISTING CONDITION	■ Prioritizing urgent vs. important tasks
■ Marijuana use	**DELEGATION**
COMMUNICATION	■ Delegating to mental health technician
DISABILITY	

MODERATE

MOOD DISORDER IN A CHILD, BIPOLAR EPISODE

Level of difficulty: Moderate

Overview: Requires critical thinking to determine least restrictive yet effective interventions with an adolescent who has a family history of Bipolar Disorder (BPD) and symptoms of a Manic Episode. Requires therapeutic communication skills as well as empathy to help the client's parents understand treatment approaches and feel they are an essential part of the treatment team. Requires an understanding of the basic principles involved in seclusion and restraint.

Client Profile

Candice is a 13-year-old female whose grandfather made a fortune in the oil business and left her a trust fund when he died. Her grandfather was known to have required little sleep and to have a phenomenal amount of energy at times. He was said to have had a number of mistresses, sometimes gone on spending sprees, and given extravagant tips to waitresses even when he only ordered a cup of coffee. Once when he was in a private psychiatric hospital, he ordered two hundred steak dinners and called a taxi to pick them up and deliver them to the hospital for all the patients and staff. He called a jeweler and ordered a diamond ring for one of the nurses he had just met and then threatened to get five lawyers to come to the hospital when she refused to marry him. Grandfather eventually committed suicide, but not before he was diagnosed as manic-depressive (term used before Bipolar Disorder came into use) and put on lithium, which he refused to take.

Candice recently has been having a somewhat elated mood (e.g., giggling about things that others don't find funny and taking about the exquisite beauty in mundane things such as a light bulb). The speed of her speech has increased, and she jumps rapidly from topic to topic. She has been staying up all night drawing original cartoons and/or rearranging her room and the family living room. At school, Candice has recently been going to the principal's office or catching her in the hall to tell her how to run the school better. She also tells the teacher how to make the classroom better. At school Candice was caught kissing a boy in the boy's restroom and the teacher intercepted a note that Candice wrote to another boy suggesting they engage in sex. Candice's father discovered that she was e-mailing a 27-year-old man that she had never met and planned to run away with him. She denied drug use but admitted that she had started smoking cigarettes and occasionally smoked marijuana, which she had gotten from her father's desk. Candice's father had her evaluated by a child-adolescent psychiatrist, and she was admitted to the adolescent unit of a private psychiatric hospital for evaluation and treatment. Candice's parents were worried that they could not keep Candice from running away and getting into trouble so they agreed to pay whatever it cost.

Case Study

Candice has been admitted to the adolescent unit. The nurse notices that Candice is pacing rapidly in the day room and goes to talk to her. Candice talks rapidly, moving from topic to topic. One of her themes is getting out of the hospital to meet her "friend." As the nurse walks away, she hears one of Candice's peers on the unit tell her: "Back off; get out of my face." The nurse then sees Candice scratching and hitting the peer. When a male mental health technician tries to pull Candice away from the peer, Candice scratches him deeply with her long fingernails and kicks him. Other staff members, including the nurse, take Candice to the seclusion room. The nurse calls the psychiatrist for an order to seclude Candice, who is in the seclusion room scratching herself superficially with her nails and smearing blood on the walls. The mental health worker reports later that Candice is asleep in the seclusion room. When she awakes the nurse talks with her and decides to let her out of seclusion but not before cutting Candice's fingernails. When Candice's parents come to visit, they are very angry about her long nails being cut and about her being put in seclusion. They express concern about the possibility of sexual activity with boys on the unit and whether or not Candice is stopping her seemingly constant motion long enough to eat.

MOOD LOG

Name: _____

Month: _____ Year: _____

Rate mood
0 ——— 50 ——— 100
Dep   Normal   Mania

Days of Month →	1	2	3	4	5	6	7	8	9	10	11	12	13	14	15	16	17	18	19	20	21	22	23	24	25	26	27	28	29	30	31
Mania																															
Depression																															
Anxiety (1–10)																															

Medication

	1	2	3	4	5	6	7	8	9	10	11	12	13	14	15	16	17	18	19	20	21	22	23	24	25	26	27	28	29	30	31
Menses																																
Sleep																																

A mood log can be used to document periods of mania and depression

Questions

1. Should you, if you were the nurse in this case, have gotten an order from the physician before secluding the client? When secluding a client, is it ever correct to delegate all communication with the client to another team member such as a mental health technician?

2. Discuss safety precautions and tasks required of the staff when a child or adolescent is secluded. What needs to be documented? How would you decide when to release the client from seclusion?

3. Just as you pick up the phone to call the health care provider for orders for secluding Candice, another adolescent client comes running up to you and says: "I need to talk with you right now about something very important." Do you stop what you are doing and listen, get the orders first then listen, send this child to another staff member, or come up with another solution?

4. After the client is out of seclusion, you sit in on a debriefing with the seclusion team. Do you think that the situation in the day room that led to seclusion was handled well, or could seclusion have been avoided? Could the injuries have been avoided? What would you say or do in the briefing?

5. What behaviors do children and adolescents who are diagnosed with Bipolar Disorder exhibit? What diagnostic criteria would Candice, or other children and/or adolescents, have to meet to be diagnosed as having a Bipolar Episode or a Bipolar Disorder? Does her behavior match any of these criteria?

6. Describe why clinicians have difficulty diagnosing mood disorders in children and adolescents and why parents and clinicians confuse it with other disorders.

7. What do you think causes Bipolar Disorder? Does genetics play a role in the cause of Bipolar Disorder? What is the age of onset and the usual course of Bipolar Disorder? Is the course the same in children compared to adults?

8. What is your response to the parents' anger about Candice being in seclusion and having her nails cut? How would you answer the parents in regard to their concerns about their daughter's possible sexual activity while in the facility?

9. What nursing diagnoses are you likely to write for this client given what information you have? What are some tentative goals that you might develop with input from the client/family/colleagues on the unit? What interventions do you think would be necessary and/or helpful?

10. What medications and treatments are being used today for children and adolescents who are exhibiting signs of mood disorders, particularly signs of a Bipolar Disorder?

11. What research has been done, or is currently being carried out, with children and adolescents who have a diagnosis of Bipolar Disorder?

GENDER

Female

AGE

41

SETTING

- Psychiatric unit of a general hospital

ETHNICITY

- German

CULTURAL CONSIDERATIONS

- German
- Military

PREEXISTING CONDITION

COEXISTING CONDITION

COMMUNICATION

DISABILITY

SOCIOECONOMIC

SPIRITUAL/RELIGIOUS

PHARMACOLOGIC

- Citalopram hydrochloride (Celexa)

PSYCHOSOCIAL

- Isolating

LEGAL

- Confidentiality
- Client right to refuse treatment

ETHICAL

- Respect for confidentiality vs. informing neighbor to ensure client safely.

ALTERNATIVE THERAPY

PRIORITIZATION

- Safety issues

DELEGATION

MAJOR DEPRESSIVE DISORDER

Level of difficulty: High

Overview: Requires the nurse to identify symptoms of major depression, look at factors contributing to depression, and identify strategies to prevent suicide.

DIFFICULT

Client Profile

Elke, a 41-year-old female, came to the United States five years ago, shortly after marrying a career U.S. military soldier. Elke has two children: a 10-year-old from a previous marriage and a 6-year-old from the current marriage. Elke has been a meticulous housekeeper and has managed the family finances. Since arriving in the United States, she has not been back to Germany to see her parents and siblings. Although she would very much like to visit her family, she can't afford to do so.

Case Study

Elke is admitted to the psychiatric unit of the city's general hospital. Her husband had noticed that she was so depressed she no longer laughed or smiled. She had admitted to him that she had been having thoughts of killing herself. She was not eating or drinking enough, had lost fifteen pounds in three weeks, and was not attending to her hygiene. Elke seemed to have little or no interest in anything except sleeping or sitting in a chair. The client's husband accompanies her on admission and shares with the staff that he is afraid Elke will kill herself and he is unable to watch her around the clock. He says that he believes if she does not kill herself by some means such as hoarding pills and overdosing that she will deteriorate by not eating or drinking enough.

On admission the psychiatric nurse asks Elke about any prior episodes of depression. The client admits to having had a deep depression about a year prior. The nurse assesses Elke for suicide ideation and finds her describing feeling like she is in a deep dark hole with no way out and her life is hopeless. The nurse first assesses the client alone and then talks with the husband and client. At one point the nurse asks Elke to tell her what it means when someone says: "Don't cry over spilled milk." Elke says: "Don't cry when milk is spilled because you can buy some more at the store."

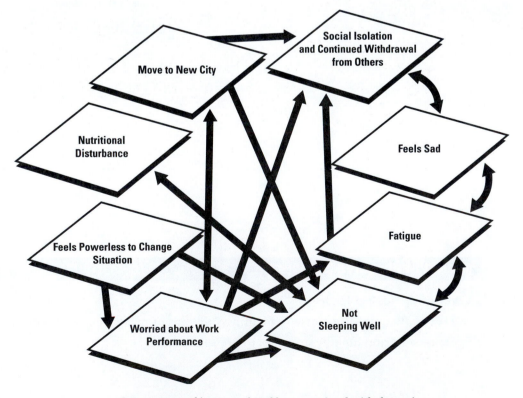

Concept map of issues and problems associated with depression

The nurse takes Elke's vital signs, weight, and height. Her vital signs are normal: height is 5 foot 5 inches and weight is 100 pounds.

The psychiatrist puts Elke on citalopram hydrochloride (Celexa), an SSRI. The nurse who admits Elke, and who continues to be assigned to her, notices that Elke isolates, verbalizes very little, and does little except when she is prompted and rewarded with points. Elke refuses to play volleyball or go to the movies with peers and staff. About five weeks after admission, Elke seems to be doing better. Her affect is brighter. She begins to play the piano in the dayroom. She asks the doctor for a pass to go home briefly to pay some bills and check on things there. Her children are now at her mother-in-law's home and her husband is away on military duty, and she has to take care of paying the bills.

Questions

1. Which signs and symptoms does Elke have that are consistent with those of a Major Depressive Episode?

2. What factor(s) do you think could have contributed to Elke's depression?

3. Why is the nurse interested in whether Elke has had prior episodes of major depression?

4. The nurse makes an observation that Elke had an episode of depression one year ago. What does the nurse need to learn from Elke and/or her husband, and what significance could it possibly have if Elke were depressed every year at the same time?

5. Why does the nurse ask Elke to interpret what is meant by "Don't cry over spilled milk"? What does the nurse learn from Elke's response?

6. What percentage of people with Major Depressive Disorder kill themselves? What could the nurse do to help keep Elke from killing herself?

7. How would you feel if you were Elke, and what would you need if you were Elke? What would it be like to be Elke's spouse or to be the spouse of any person with Major Depressive Disorder?

8. What interventions would you most likely initiate if you were writing a care plan for someone like Elke?

9. When Elke's mood seems to improve greatly and she wants to get a pass to go home and take care of some urgent business, would you support her having a pass? Why or why not?

10. The health care provider signs the pass allowing Elke to go home for four hours, provided an adult accompanies her, and she gets her neighbor to drive her home and back. What would you do if you were Elke's nurse?

11. What is a token economy or a point system, and how is this used to change behavior?

12. Is ECT used today for clients with depression? How do you feel about this?

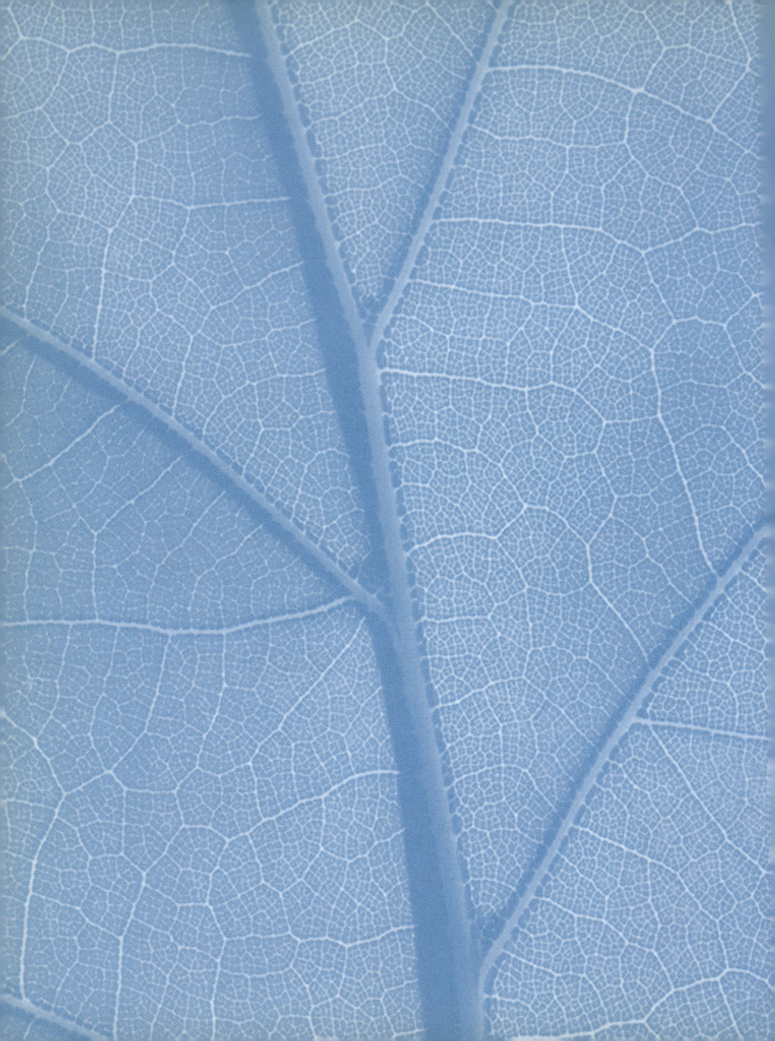

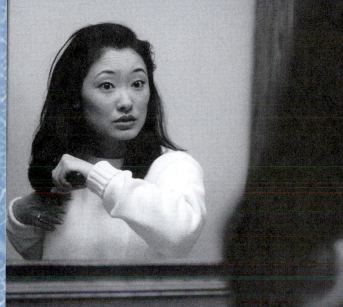

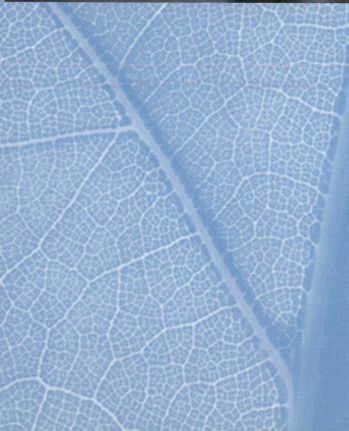

## PART FOUR

The Client Who Abuses Chemical Substances

Ron

GENDER

Male

AGE

42

SETTING

■ Hospital

ETHNICITY

■ White American

CULTURAL CONSIDERATIONS

■ "Hippie" culture

PREEXISTING CONDITION

COEXISTING CONDITION

COMMUNICATION

DISABILITY

SOCIOECONOMIC

■ Middle class

SPIRITUAL/RELIGIOUS

■ Buddhist

PHARMACOLOGIC

PSYCHOSOCIAL

LEGAL

■ Illegal drug possession and use
■ Charting must be factual
■ Possibility of nurse involvement in court proceedings

ETHICAL

■ Care based on client lifestyle

ALTERNATIVE THERAPY

■ Acupuncture

PRIORITIZATION

DELEGATION

CANNABIS ABUSE

Level of difficulty: Moderate

Overview: This case involves treating an illegal drug user with additional health concerns.

Client Profile

Ron is a 42-year-old high school teacher who smokes marijuana (Cannabis sativa) occasionally. He has been using marijuana with varying intensity since junior high school. His drug use prolonged his college education, but he did eventually earn a bachelor's degree and teaching certificate for high-school-level history, English, and science. The drug use also contributed to the dissolution of his first marriage. Since then he has become fascinated with Buddhist teachings and studies them often.

Ron continues to smoke marijuana "to relax," although it makes him anxious, paranoid, and impacts his short-term memory. He has to be particularly careful that none of his students or their parents see him, so he only smokes at his home or the homes of close friends, and never within several hours of teaching. The school has a zero tolerance policy on drug use.

After an argument, Ron's girlfriend, Patsy, hid some marijuana in his briefcase and then anonymously notified the principal of his school once Ron had gone to work. Due to the tip, the principal inspected Ron's briefcase, found the marijuana, and notified the police. Ron was suspended from his job, but after Patsy admitted to planting the marijuana, the school board agreed to give Ron another chance if he would complete a twenty-eight-day (two weeks inpatient and two weeks outpatient) treatment program and agree to abstain from marijuana or other illegal substance use following treatment. Ron consented to save his job. He has a court date in a month for a charge of marijuana possession.

Case Study

Ron decides to smoke a little marijuana to control his nerves and mellow himself out before going to be admitted to the drug treatment program. He also reasons that he should smoke the remainder of his marijuana rather than flush it down the toilet. On the way to the program he is in an automobile accident, is injured, and ends up being admitted to the orthopedic unit of a large medical-surgical hospital. Patsy arrives just as Ron is admitted and blurts out: "He was on his way to the outpatient treatment program to be treated for marijuana abuse when he had this accident. He is going to lose his job if he doesn't go for treatment. This is awful."

Questions

1. Why do you think Ron smoked the last of his marijuana before going to the first night of inpatient treatment for drug abuse? How did Ron's behavior demonstrate the difference between insight and judgment?

2. How would you respond if you were the nurse listening to the girlfriend comment about the client using marijuana before his accident and his need to complete the drug abuse treatment program in order to save his job as a teacher?

3. How would you feel if you were assigned to work with this client who has been abusing cannabis (marijuana) and teaching high school students and is now in need of medical care, possibly due to using cannabis (marijuana) then driving?

4. What are the criteria for cannabis abuse, and does this client appear to meet any of those criteria? What is the difference between someone who abuses marijuana and someone who is dependent on it?

5. Would you expect this client to have withdrawal symptoms if he does not have marijuana to smoke? How would withdrawal manifest?

6. What is/are the current treatment(s) for cannabis abuse?

7. You are to instruct Ron about harmful effects of cannabis, but he is skeptical and thinks there are no harmful effects. Has cannabis been shown to adversely affect the health of someone who abuses it?

Questions (continued)

8. Are there medical uses for cannabis, and is there a medical source or sources of cannabis?

9. Is marijuana use for medical purposes permitted in your state? If not, are there nearby states where it is?

10. Would you feel better caring for this client if he had a medical prescription for marijuana or if smoking marijuana for personal use were legal? If so, under what circumstances should a client smoke marijuana for personal use?

11. How does this client's belief in Buddhism impact or affect your care?

12. The client's mother comes to visit and you talk to her about the importance of support and compassion. She asks you to explain the difference between support and compassion and enabling. She tells you that she was told in the past not to enable Ron's abuse of marijuana.

13. If you were to write a care plan for this client, what assessment data would you like to have?

14. What nursing diagnoses would you write for this client? What goals are likely for this client?

15. What interventions would you likely write for this client?

Margaret

GENDER

Female

AGE

51

SETTING

- Home/visiting nurse

ETHNICITY

- White American

CULTURAL CONSIDERATIONS

- Appalachian/Northern European descent

PREEXISTING CONDITION

- Possible Alpha-1 Antitrypsin deficiency

COEXISTING CONDITION

- Chronic Obstructive Pulmonary Disease (COPD) related to Chronic Emphysema

COMMUNICATION

DISABILITY

- Disabled due to Emphysema and COPD

SOCIOECONOMIC

- Husband on social security; client receives social security disability payments; subsidized housing

SPIRITUAL/RELIGIOUS

- Used to attend church but now too tiring to attend

PHARMACOLOGIC

- Nicotine spray
- Bupropion (Zyban)
- Ipratropium bromide (Atrovent)

PSYCHOSOCIAL

- Decreased social life due to tiring easily because of COPD and Emphysema
- External locus of control

LEGAL

- Confidentiality

ETHICAL

- Should people have the right to smoke when it harms their health and that of others in their environment?

ALTERNATIVE THERAPY

- Hypnosis
- Acupuncture
- Guided imagery

PRIORITIZATION

DELEGATION

MODERATE

NICOTINE DEPENDENCE

Level of difficulty: Moderate

Overview: Requires critical thinking to come up with strategies to motivate a client, who is disabled due to Emphysema, to give up smoking. The nurse must get the client to move beyond her external locus of control thinking. The nurse must explore her own thinking about, and issues regarding, smoking in order to be effective with the client.

Client Profile

Margaret is a 51-year-old woman who smokes a package of cigarettes a day even though she has Chronic Obstructive Pulmonary Disease (COPD) from Chronic Emphysema. She has severe shortness of breath at times during the day. She cannot walk from the car to the house or carry her own groceries without tiring. Margaret's husband, John, smokes too, but just a cigar each day in the evening along with a glass of beer. Margaret has a "little glass of beer" with him. Margaret's daughter won't let her children go to Margaret's home because of the secondhand smoke and Margaret does not have the energy to climb the stairs to her daughter's home, so she has not seen her grandchildren for over a year. John does all the cooking, and the daughter takes Margaret's list and does the shopping. Margaret does not go to the church she has attended since she was a child because she does not want her many friends there to see her so short of breath and easily exhausted.

Sometimes Margaret cuts back on the groceries she puts on her list so she can have enough money for cigarettes and beer. Her daughter won't buy the cigarettes when she does the shopping, so Margaret calls the liquor store to deliver them along with a case of beer.

Margaret developed pneumonia recently and was hospitalized for treatment. The doctor mentioned to her on discharge that it would be a good idea for her to stop smoking and that he was sending the visiting nurse to work with her to quit smoking.

Case Study

The visiting nurse calls Margaret and tells her that the doctor has asked her to stop by for a visit. Margaret says she is doing OK and doesn't think she needs to see the nurse. The nurse replies: "I'd like to see you even though you are doing fine. Would you like me to come on Tuesday at 10 AM or Thursday at 4 PM?" Margaret agrees to the Tuesday visit. When the nurse arrives at Margaret and John's home, she visits a few minutes with Margaret and John and then checks Margaret's vital signs, listens to her lungs and heart sounds, does oxygen saturation, and draws some blood to send to the lab for CBC. She checks the capillary refill and then asks Margaret if they could have a cup of tea and just visit.

The nurse has brought some "special" tea bags. The nurse makes the tea and begins to discuss smoking with Margaret. The nurse asks Margaret how long she has been smoking, and the answer is: "Since I was 18 years old." The nurse asks her if she has ever thought about quitting, and she says: "No, I need it to calm my nerves." The nurse replies: "Perhaps the doctor can prescribe something to help you calm your nerves. While there are pros to smoking like increased alertness and relaxation, there are some cons to smoking like it increases the risk of serious illness and it makes your Emphysema worse." Margaret tells the nurse that she has known lots of people who smoked and none of them got Emphysema or pulmonary disease or cancer or lung problems: "It is just bad luck that I got this Emphysema, and I have hospital insurance and cancer insurance." Margaret tells the nurse that her father raised tobacco and tobacco is a good plant. She describes how she used to help her father by cutting the blooms out of the tobacco to keep them from sucking energy from the plant. Then Margaret asks: "Do you smoke or did you ever smoke, nurse?"

Before the visit ends, the nurse asks Margaret about her ancestry. Margaret says her father's parents came from Denmark and her mother's great-grandparents came from Finland. When the nurse reports back to Margaret's doctor, she tells him that it will be difficult to get Margaret to quit smoking but that she has some ideas, and she asks him about the possibility of Alpha-1 Antitrypsin (AT) deficiency.

Questions

1. Why do you think the health care provider wants Margaret to give up smoking? What would be some common feelings of nurses assigned to work with a client like Margaret?

2. If you were the nurse, how would you respond when the client asks if you smoke or ever smoked? Do you think a nurse who smokes can help a client successfully give up smoking?

3. Margaret's family asks: "What is Emphysema and what causes it?" How would you answer? What do you know about Alpha-1 AT deficiency as a cause of Emphysema, and what clues point to the possibility Margaret could have this deficiency?

4. Why would this client, or any client, refuse to have testing for Alpha-1 AT deficiency? Why would a client want to have the testing? What are the current treatments for Alpha-1 AT deficiency and for Emphysema?

5. What are the criteria for a diagnosis of nicotine dependence, and does Margaret appear to meet these criteria? Is there a measuring tool that measures the degree of nicotine dependency of clients?

6. What are the current theories on causation of nicotine dependence?

7. What are the current treatments for nicotine dependence? Would it be easy or difficult to get someone who is nicotine dependent to give up smoking, and what would help a person who doesn't want to give up smoking?

8. Is smoking more common among lower socio-economic groups or other groups? What general characteristics of individuals from Appalachia have been identified that might be helpful to keep in mind in designing interventions to help the client stop smoking?

9. What will you do to help this client maintain a nonsmoking status if she agrees to stop smoking? How will you feel and what attitude will you adopt if she relapses again?

10. What are the withdrawal symptoms this client will probably have?

11. What data do you want to gather on this client? What nursing diagnoses, goals, and interventions would you likely write if you were writing a care plan for this client?

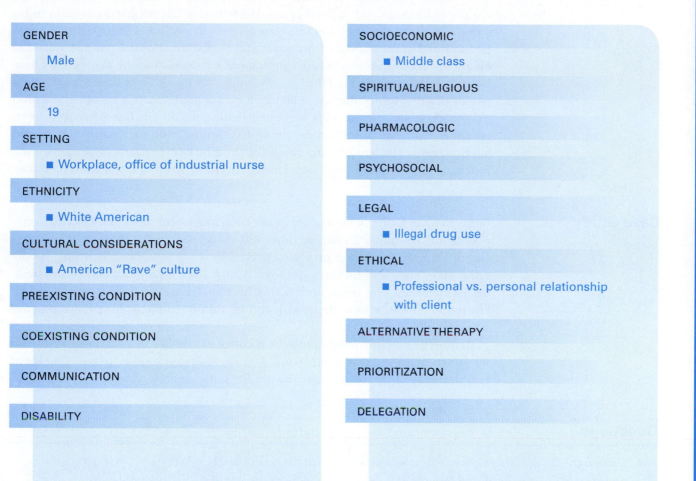

GENDER	**SOCIOECONOMIC**
Male	■ Middle class
AGE	**SPIRITUAL/RELIGIOUS**
19	
SETTING	**PHARMACOLOGIC**
■ Workplace, office of industrial nurse	
ETHNICITY	**PSYCHOSOCIAL**
■ White American	
CULTURAL CONSIDERATIONS	**LEGAL**
	■ Illegal drug use
■ American "Rave" culture	**ETHICAL**
PREEXISTING CONDITION	■ Professional vs. personal relationship with client
COEXISTING CONDITION	**ALTERNATIVE THERAPY**
COMMUNICATION	**PRIORITIZATION**
DISABILITY	**DELEGATION**

HALLUCINOGEN ABUSE

Level of difficulty: High

Overview: Requires the nurse to accept a young adult whose behavior is risky to his health and who is using the illegal stimulant/hallucinogen MDMA (Ecstasy) and has a lifestyle totally different from that of the nurse. The nurse must maintain professional behavior and help the client develop a trusting relationship before attempting to motivate a change in behavior in the client.

DIFFICULT

Client Profile

Bennie is a 19-year-old adopted male, who has worn leather and chains at times in the past couple of years. His hair has occasionally been spiked up the middle of his head and colored green. His behavior has attracted attention in his parents' conservative upper-middle-class neighborhood. In addition to his hairstyle he has stood in the middle of the street and cursed his adoptive parents, talked to neighbors about smoking "weed," and played his drums loudly. The parents have been concerned about his effect on a younger brother who is their natural child and involved in sports and not at all like their adopted son. Just before graduation from high school, the parents suggested Bennie move out. Bennie moved to an apartment with one of his friends, got a job designing computer games, and started going to raves. His passions are: raves, the drug MDMA (Ecstasy), Macintosh computers, computer games, and cars. His parents have asked him not to come home.

Case Study

Bennie comes to the nurse's office in the company where he works. His chief complaints are insomnia, feeling anxious and nauseated, and experiencing blurred vision. He wants his blood pressure checked to see if something is wrong. As the nurse takes his vital signs, the nurse finds Bennie has a rapid pulse of 124 and tremors in his hands. The nurse notices that his muscles are tense and he is sweating. His mood appears a little depressed, and he thinks people in his department are sabotaging his work.

Bennie tells the nurse he thinks she is cute and asks her to go out with him. The nurse's response is: "When you go out, Bennie, where do you like to go?" The client reveals he likes to go to raves and invites the nurse to go with him to a rave.

Questions

1. If you were the female nurse in this case, would it be acceptable for you to go out socially with this client? Why or why not? What developmental stage, according to Erickson, is this client in and how does that relate to the client's behavior? Could the nurse have professional reason(s) for asking Bennie what he really likes to do in his time away from work?

2. What does the client mean by a "rave"?

3. What is the most common drug used at raves and why? What other drugs are commonly found at raves? Is there drug paraphernalia associated with MDMA (Ecstasy)? Is the typical way of dressing at raves leather and chains, and if not, what is it?

4. What drugs are considered hallucinogens? How are hallucinogens usually taken, and how is Ecstasy taken? Have there been or are there currently any medical uses for hallucinogens?

5. What effect does MDMA have on the person taking it? Is the strength of the drug MDMA consistent, and what is the danger of receiving PMA (paramethoxyamphetamine) as a substitute for MDMA?

6. Does admitting attendance at raves affirm that the client does hallucinogenic drugs? The client admits taking MDMA. What action(s) do you take? What is your top priority with this client?

7. What are the criteria for Hallucinogen Intoxication? Does this client appear to meet those criteria?

8. What are the criteria for Hallucinogen Abuse, and does this client seem to meet the criteria for Hallucinogen Abuse? What diagnoses are associated with hallucinogens that are not associated with some other addictions such as alcohol, and what significance does this have for the nurse?

9. Has the use of Ecstasy increased or decreased in recent years? How is the prevalence of hallucinogen use, particularly that of Ecstasy, estimated?

10. What treatments are currently being used for clients who use or abuse Ecstasy?

11. What data would you like to have if you were the nurse writing a nursing care plan for this client? What nursing diagnoses and goals would you likely write for this client? What interventions could you write for this client?

12. What research is being conducted with hallucinogens?

GENDER

Female

AGE

13

SETTING

- School nurse called to the girl's restroom

ETHNICITY

- White American

CULTURAL CONSIDERATIONS

PREEXISTING CONDITION

- Neglect; physical, sexual, and psychological abuse

COEXISTING CONDITION

COMMUNICATION

DISABILITY

SOCIOECONOMIC

- Lower socioeconomic group; living below poverty line

SPIRITUAL/RELIGIOUS

PHARMACOLOGIC

PSYCHOSOCIAL

LEGAL

- Laws requiring reporting suspected child abuse
- Legal issues when child is truant

ETHICAL

- Question of when it is all right to plant an idea in the client's mind and when it is not

ALTERNATIVE THERAPY

PRIORITIZATION

- Nurse has several students needing care

DELEGATION

- Question of what to delegate to nonnursing personnel

INHALANT ABUSE

Level of difficulty: High

Overview: Requires perseverance and patience to work with a teenager who has been "huffing" gasoline and inhaling spray paint fumes. The nurse must use therapeutic communication skills, observational skills, and other means to discover what is going on with the client. The nurse is required to prioritize and delegate some tasks to others as there are other students seeking services at the same time this client is experiencing problems.

DIFFICULT

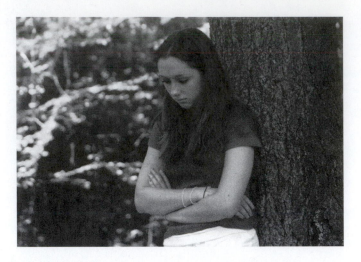

Client Profile

Pena is a 13-year-old girl whose parents are alcoholics. The family is below the poverty level in income and lives on social security disability and the food stamp program. They often sell or trade food they get with food stamps or from the WIC program to get alcohol and cigarettes, since food stamps are not accepted in payment for these items. The father tells Pena that she will never amount to anything and frequently tells her she is "stupid." Her parents don't like to ruin a good alcoholic "buzz" by eating, and they rarely prepare a meal for Pena. She eats whatever she can find in the refrigerator or cupboard. Her mother slaps Pena and yells at her. Her father sexually abuses her. Pena has learned to be as invisible as possible at home and school. She has begun to realize that some of her classmates make fun of her because she doesn't have clothes and shoes like they do and she always looks forlorn. Pena sometimes feels sorry that she is alive.

One of the neighborhood boys tells Pena she will feel better if she breathes some gasoline in a plastic bag. She has a supply of gasoline as her father keeps gasoline in a storage shed for an old lawn mower that he makes Pena use to mow the grass and weeds. She feels great for a short while after "bagging" gasoline fumes, then the old hopeless and worthless feelings return.

One day before school, after "bagging" gasoline, the boy who told her about the gasoline says he has something else they can use to feel better and gives her something else to breathe. He also touches her in some private places. Pena thinks about saying "no," but she does not care. She begins to feel euphoric. When she comes down from the high, she feels awful but goes to school because it is better than going home and she doesn't want the truancy officer visiting her home again. She hates to go to school because she can't concentrate and has little idea of what is going on in class. She is failing in school. Pena feels guilty about letting the boy touch her in private places, but he is the only one who talks to her and he has introduced her to inhalants that make her feel good, even if the feeling lasts only a short while.

Case Study

Pena passes out in the girl's bathroom at school. One of her classmates goes to get the school nurse. Pena has regained consciousness when the school nurse arrives. The nurse smells a chemical odor to Pena's breath. She seems lethargic, her movements are uncoordinated, her eyes are red, and her speech is slurred; however,

Pena does begin to respond to questions. The nurse says: "Tell me what happened." Pena replies: "I just passed out because I forgot to eat supper last night and I got up late and didn't have time for breakfast this morning." The nurse notices some gold paint on Pena's face and hands.

A student comes into the bathroom with a nosebleed, and another girl says she has just started her first menstrual period and needs a pad. It is nearly time for the nurse to begin teaching a health care class, and the truancy officer has sent word that he wants to talk to the nurse before he goes out to visit one of the families.

Questions

1. If you were the school nurse, would you say: "Tell me what happened"? Why or why not? What else would you say or do or avoid saying and/or doing when approaching this client initially? Based on the client's symptoms, what problem(s) could this client have instead of inhalant use? What are some clues that this student has been using inhalants?

2. What are the criteria for Inhalant Intoxication, and could Pena likely meet those criteria? What are the criteria for Inhalant Abuse, and does this client appear to meet any of those criteria?

3. You learn from one of Pena's classmates that several students are inhaling solvents. What are solvents? Are there different categories of inhalants that this client could have used? How are nitrites different from the other three types of solvents? Give some examples of nitrites. How are solvents used?

4. Two students (one with nosebleed and one starting a first menstrual period), the truancy officer, and a class that the nurse needs to teach compete with this client's needs for the nurse's attention. How would you prioritize and proceed, that is, what would you put on hold and/or delegate? Would you accompany Pena to the hospital if you were the nurse in this case?

5. Is it possible for the hospital emergency room staff to run a routine drug screen for inhalants on this or any client (i.e., does an inhalant like gasoline appear in the urine or blood)?

6. The client receives care at the hospital and returns to school. You ask the client to stop by your office each day and check in with you. You try to discuss the harmful effects of solvent inhalation. The client says: "I don't care." Is this a typical response from inhalant users? What are the harmful effects of solvent inhalation that you would like to discuss with Pena?

7. If you were provided training and assigned by the principal to do a support group for this client and other children who are having problems, what would be the expected benefits of this group?

8. Would you put together a homogenous or a heterogeneous support group for children? What circumstances would warrant breaking confidentiality, and who could receive the information? How would you prepare the students to know about and accept the situations that could not be kept within the group?

9. If you were the school nurse, would you educate children in the classroom about Inhalant Abuse and the dangers of using inhalants? What are the signs and symptoms you could teach parents to look for that would indicate their child might be inhaling solvents?

10. Would you expect this client to have withdrawal symptoms if she stops using inhalants? If so, what symptoms would you expect?

11. What are the current treatment(s) for Inhalant Intoxication and for Inhalant Abuse?

12. In writing a care plan for this client, what assessment data would you gather? What nursing diagnoses, goals, and interventions would you write for this client and share with the team mentioned above?

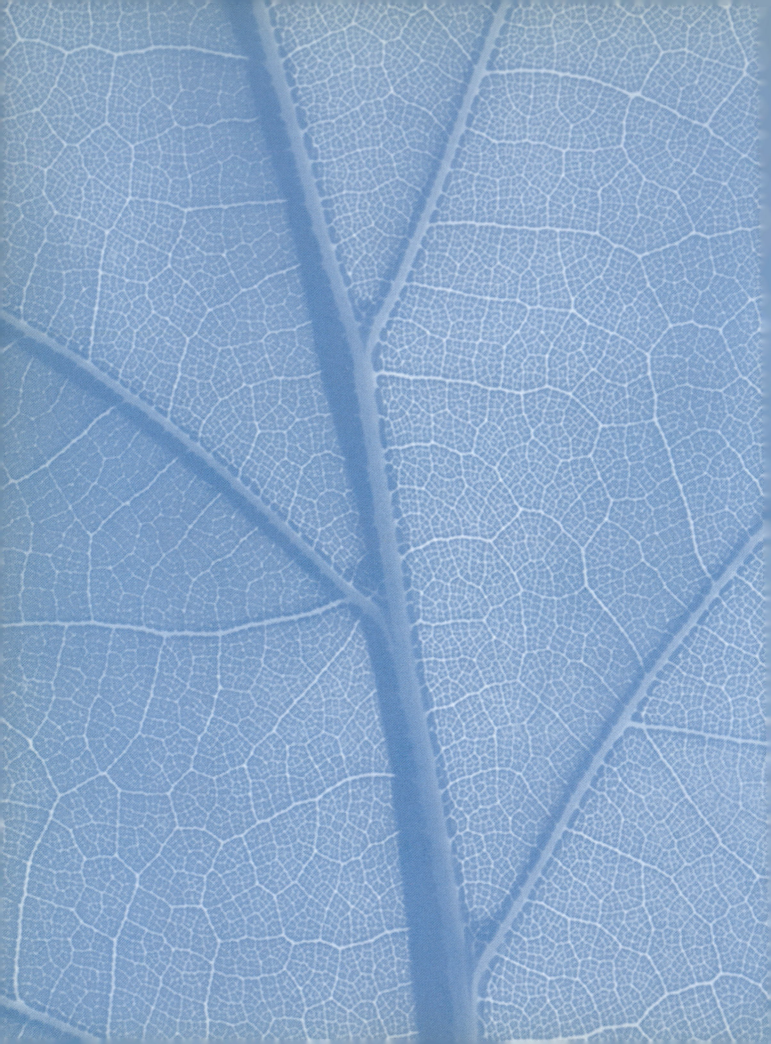

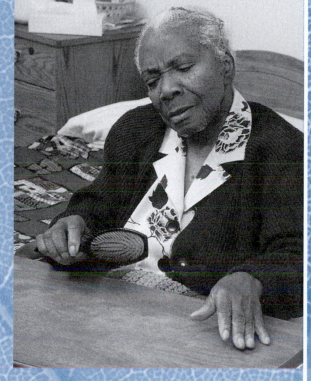

## PART FIVE

The Client with a Personality Disorder

Vicky

GENDER

Female

AGE

27

SETTING

- Company nurse's office

ETHNICITY

- White American

CULTURAL CONSIDERATIONS

- Midwestern farming culture; pioneer and Germanic influence

PREEXISTING CONDITION

COEXISTING CONDITION

COMMUNICATION

DISABILITY

SOCIOECONOMIC

- Upper-class professional

SPIRITUAL/RELIGIOUS

PHARMACOLOGIC

PSYCHOSOCIAL

- Desire for approval from father
- Perfectionism and control issues interfere with social relationships

LEGAL

ETHICAL

- Recommending one therapist: therapeutic or unethical?

ALTERNATIVE THERAPY

PRIORITIZATION

DELEGATION

OBSESSIVE-COMPULSIVE PERSONALITY DISORDER

Level of difficulty: Easy

Overview: Requires the nurse to use critical thinking to identify and understand the behavioral traits of Obsessive-Compulsive Personality Disorder (OCPD) and to determine effective therapeutic approaches. The nurse must differentiate OCPD from Obsessive-Compulsive Disorder. Requires the nurse to identify the role of the industrial nurse and to make decisions within that role.

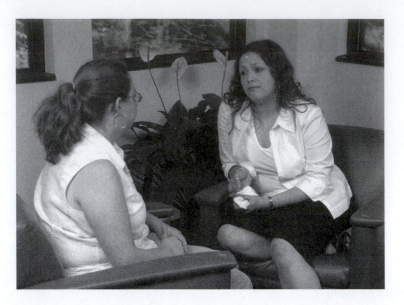

Client Profile

Vicky is a 27-year-old single woman who lives alone and works for a technology company. Vicky grew up on a midwestern small farm with frugal parents. An authoritarian father rarely said much to her except to criticize her behavior. She tried to be perfect at school, often recopying papers several times and thus failing to get them in on time, which meant only a B or C grade. Once when she got a 98 on a paper and was hopeful of getting praise at home, her father said: "What are you going to do about getting 100 next time?" By college Vicky was a straight A student, but her father still didn't praise her. Growing up, she was overly organized with everything in its place in her room and lists posted everywhere. Vicky resisted going to bed until work on the lists was done or she was exhausted and gave up. In the past few years, Vicky has had trouble getting rid of things. She tries to set things aside for charity, but eventually takes things out, one by one, and puts them back inside the house, thinking maybe she will use them some day. Although she is wealthy, she is frugal with her money.

Vicky spends hours trying to get projects at work perfect. When assigned to a project with a coworker, she does most or all of the work herself, because she thinks coworkers won't do it correctly. Sometimes she realizes coworkers are having fun on the weekend while she has no time for leisure activities. Once in awhile she misses a project deadline due to trying to perfect the work.

A former coworker and friend with a romantic interest in Vicky has repeatedly invited her to visit him in another city. Finally, Vicky accepts since she will have her own room and a housekeeper will be there. The friend takes her to a museum to see a European art collection on loan. Vicky insists on viewing the paintings starting at the entrance and going right to left, seeing each painting, reading each plaque, and making a note about it. By the time the museum closes, they have not gotten close to the collection they came to see. Before going out to eat, Vicky insists her friend change his shirt to match his pants and then change his tie. She organizes his ties by color and after some indecision selects one. Before Vicky leaves, her friend tells her he cares for her and gently asks her to see a therapist about her perfectionism and need to control.

Case Study

On Monday afternoon, Vicky presents in the nurse's office of the company where she works asking the nurse to take her blood pressure and complaining of feeling dizzy. The nurse notices that Vicky has rearranged the magazines in the office waiting area and has brought a large stack of what looks like work with her. The nurse asks her about the stack of papers. Vicky says she is behind schedule since she was out of town over the weekend. She shares that she thought maybe she would have time to do some work while waiting to see the nurse. Vicky's blood pressure is within normal limits, as are the rest of the vital signs. The nurse observes that the client looks thin and seems anxious. When the nurse assesses Vicky's heath practices and asks about diet, Vicky says: "Oh, I eat well, but sometimes I skip lunch to get some work done or I forget to eat breakfast when I get busy doing work before I come to work." She admits to getting four to five hours of sleep nightly. The nurse asks Vicky about turning some of this work over to her team members and going home to rest. Vicky seems anxious and even angry as she replies: "No one else can get it right." Then she bursts into tears and says: "A friend of mine says I am a perfectionist and controlling and I should get some help. He doesn't really understand. Do you think I should see a therapist? I really don't have time."

Questions

1. If you were the nurse talking with Vicky, how would you respond to her statements about her friend's thoughts on her perfectionism, need to control, and need to see a therapist, as well as her question to you on whether she should see a therapist or not?

2. What behaviors did Vicky exhibit in the waiting room and nurse's office that might clue the nurse to assess further for behaviors matching traits of Obsessive-Compulsive Personality Disorder?

3. If you were the nurse, what other assessments would you want to do at this time?

4. What are the traits of Obsessive-Compulsive Personality? What behaviors does Vicky have that match these traits? What are the criteria for a diagnosis of OCPD by a professional qualified to make a diagnosis?

5. Obsessive-Compulsive Personality Disorder sounds a lot like Obsessive-Compulsive Disorder. Are they two different disorders or not? Discuss how OCPD and OCD are alike and how they are different.

6. Is there any difference in the reported prevalence of this disorder in males compared to females?

7. If Vicky goes to a therapist, the therapist will probably ask about her family and her experiences growing up. Does childhood family environment possibly play a role in the development of Obsessive-Compulsive Personality Disorder? Was Vicky's father's behavior possibly culturally influenced in any way?

8. Are environmental factors the accepted cause of Obsessive-Compulsive Disorder?

9. Using Erickson's psychosocial development theory, what developmental stage is this client in and how could that play a role in her wanting to modify her behavior by working with a therapist?

10. What nursing diagnoses would you write for this client?

11. What interventions do professional counselors, therapists, or psychiatric nurse clinicians use in working with clients who have traits of OCPD or a diagnosis of this disorder? What interventions would be helpful on the part of the industrial nurse in this case?

George

GENDER

Male

AGE

39

SETTING

- Outpatient community mental health center

ETHNICITY

- White American

CULTURAL CONSIDERATIONS

- Girlfriend is Hispanic

PREEXISTING CONDITION

COEXISTING CONDITION

- Chronic depressed mood, possibly dysthymia

COMMUNICATION

DISABILITY

SOCIOECONOMIC

- Slightly above minimum wage

SPIRITUAL/RELIGIOUS

PHARMACOLOGIC

- Paroxetine (Paxil)
- Trasodone (Desyrel)

PSYCHOSOCIAL

LEGAL

- Legal obligation to provide secure e-mail if e-mailing with clients

ETHICAL

ALTERNATIVE THERAPY

PRIORITIZATION

DELEGATION

AVOIDANT PERSONALITY DISORDER

Level of difficulty: Easy

Overview: Requires recognition of the basic traits associated with Avoidant Personality Disorder and critical thinking to build a professional nurse-client relationship and keep the client engaged in treatment. Helping the client to slowly increase social contact requires careful planning, effective interventions, and patience.

Client Profile

George is a 39-year-old male who lives alone. He divides his time between work and being in his bedroom on the computer. He has rarely socialized with anyone because of a fear of being criticized or rejected. Recently George quit a day job because he thought the store owner was critical of him, when in reality the store owner wanted to promote him to day manager. George felt inadequate to be a manager, fearing he would embarrass himself in the job and be criticized more. George likes his new job better because he works nights at a convenience store and does not have to interact with many people. This job is also close to a bus stop; George cannot afford a car. He has difficulty sleeping whether he is working days or nights. When he can't sleep, he works on the computer.

George had one date with Maria, whose family is from Mexico. He went to pick her up and was greeted by her extended family. He felt totally inadequate around her family and felt he was embarrassing himself and Maria, especially after Maria told him she wanted to help him shop for clothes and offered him advice on losing weight. Now he only communicates with Maria by e-mail or telephone, telling her he is "resting up for work" or "busy" when she asks him to go somewhere with her. He fantasizes about relationships with Maria and with women he meets in chat rooms, but he does not meet with them except on the computer.

Members of George's own family criticize each other in a teasing but emotionally hurtful sort of way. He has always felt rejected and criticized by his family, but once or twice a year on special occasions, he attends a family gathering at the urging of his mother. George's father talked him into going to college, but George skipped many of the classes. His father thinks he is just a few hours short of a degree when in reality he has few credits.

Case Study

George comes to the community outpatient mental health center clinic saying his father asked him to see about an antidepressant because he is overweight and seems depressed. The nurse notices that George seems very shy, as evidenced by looking down, speaking softly, and blushing at times.

George is assessed for depression, and the nurse takes an extensive health history. George describes symptoms of a depressed mood nearly every day for several years with no episodes of deep depression or elevated mood. At one point, during the history taking, George says: "You seem busy today; perhaps I could come back another day." The nurse's reply is effective as George stays for the rest of the appointment.

During assessment, the nurse uncovers much of the information in the client profile above and does a complete review of systems and asks about past and current health problems. A head-to-toe physical assessment is postponed until the next visit. The nurse finds that in addition to being somewhat depressed in mood most of the time, George has some traits of Avoidant Personality Disorder. The nurse wonders if George has sufficient traits for a diagnosis of avoidant personality disorder

The nurse suspects that George could benefit from an antidepressant and consults with the community mental health center psychiatrist, who also talks with George and prescribes a two-week supply of samples of paroxetine (Paxil) and trasodone (Desyrel). The nurse does some education with George about the medications and gives George an appointment in two weeks' time. George responds: "My job keeps me pretty busy. I don't have much time off. Could I just e-mail and tell you how I am doing? You could mail the medication to me."

Questions

1. Discuss possible reasons for George saying to the nurse: "You seem busy today; perhaps I could come back another day." What would be a good response on the part of the nurse to this statement?

2. Why did the client receive only a two-week supply of paroxetine and trasodone instead of a month or three months supply?

3. Describe an acceptable response to George's suggestion that he could e-mail rather than keep a follow-up appointment.

4. What do you think was the rationale for delaying a head-to-toe physical assessment? Discuss the value of doing the physical examination versus delaying it.

5. The nurse observed some client behaviors that suggest this client might have Avoidant Personality Disorder. What traits does George have that match this disorder? What percentage of clients in the outpatient mental health clinic would likely meet the criteria for a diagnosis of Avoidant Personality Disorder?

6. What approach or approaches by the nurse would most likely work best with this client?

7. What cause(s) of Avoidant Personality Disorder?

8. Will paroxetine and/or trasodone change the traits of Avoidant Personality Disorder as well as the symptoms of depression?

9. What education does the nurse need to do with George in regard to paroxetine (Paxil)?

10. What is the most likely reason that this client stopped seeing Maria, the girl he once dated and now only e-mails? Would her Hispanic culture present any special challenges/problems in a relationship with George and his Avoidant Personality Disorder traits?

11. What treatment(s) has been found to be helpful to the client with Avoidant Personality Disorder?

12. What nursing diagnoses would you write for this client? What goals would you likely write in collaboration with the client? Describe one or more interventions and identify how you would apply the evaluation part of nursing process.

Jim

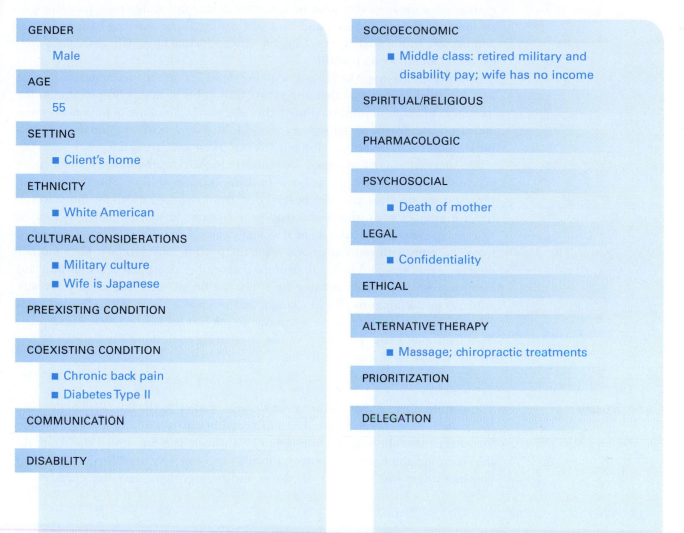

GENDER

Male

AGE

55

SETTING

- Client's home

ETHNICITY

- White American

CULTURAL CONSIDERATIONS

- Military culture
- Wife is Japanese

PREEXISTING CONDITION

COEXISTING CONDITION

- Chronic back pain
- Diabetes Type II

COMMUNICATION

DISABILITY

SOCIOECONOMIC

- Middle class: retired military and disability pay; wife has no income

SPIRITUAL/RELIGIOUS

PHARMACOLOGIC

PSYCHOSOCIAL

- Death of mother

LEGAL

- Confidentiality

ETHICAL

ALTERNATIVE THERAPY

- Massage; chiropractic treatments

PRIORITIZATION

DELEGATION

DEPENDENT PERSONALITY DISORDER

Level of difficulty: Easy

Overview: Requires identification of effective ways to work with an individual who not only has traits of Dependent Personality Disorder, but also has chronic pain. Requires critical thinking to determine what culturally influenced behaviors of the spouse are enabling the husband's dependence and how to work with the spouse to modify her behavior.

Client Profile

Jim is a 55-year-old male who has both psychological and medical problems. He sees a nurse psychotherapist, goes to a pain clinic, a massage therapist, and a chiropractor for help with what he describes as uncontrollable back pain; he sees an internist for his diabetes; and he has a visiting nurse working with both him and his wife with a goal of increasing his independence in activities of daily living, exercises, and diabetes control.

In individual therapy Jim reveals a nanny cared for him for six months when he was separated from his mother at age two, due to his mother's hospitalization for treatment of major depression. Jim's father was overly protective as Jim was adopted and his father feared social services would find a reason to take Jim away. When Jim's mother returned home, Jim felt anxious when away from her.

Jim married young and joined the army. He turned every responsibility he could over to his wife whether he was home on leave or away on duty. Shortly before he retired from the army, his wife "burned out" from doing so much for him and left him for another man who paid attention to her needs. Jim immediately married Mari, a Japanese woman who seemed willing to take care of him. He then separated from the army with retirement and disability pay for a back injury. Jim's mother died two years ago, and he is still depressed about her death. He fears his wife and caregivers will reject him because he is not worthy of their attention. Jim's wife wants to go to Japan to visit her family, but when she mentions it, Jim becomes "clingy." Jim says he can't make a trip due to his bad back, which gets worse when Mari mentions a trip. Jim won't let her go, fearing something will happen to her and he'll have no one to care for him.

Case Study

The visiting nurse arrives at the client's home. Earlier in the day, the client's wife had called the nurse and described Jim becoming dizzy while shopping with her. She shared that she is now pushing Jim in a wheelchair. She stated she could do the shopping alone, but her husband insists on going with her. She said Jim often becomes angry with clerks in the stores and berates them, and this embarrasses

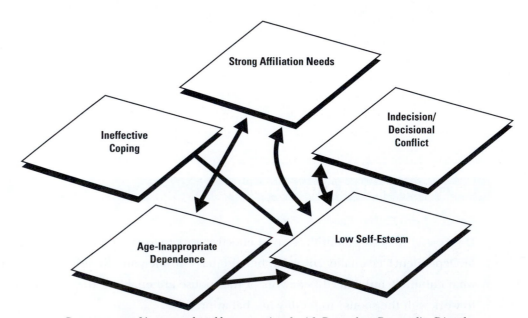

Concept map of issues and problems associated with Dependent Personality Disorder

her. She thinks he is on too much pain medication and it is causing him to be forgetful and dizzy at times. Mari said that Jim won't make decisions, has her pick out his clothes for the day, and won't do any tasks on his own initiative. She has to remind him to do his blood sugar testing and then he wants her to do it. Before the conversation ended, Mari added: "Jim needs constant care. I am getting tired. I am worried that he will get worse."

Jim greets the visiting nurse and says he needs help deciding what to do about his back pain. It is not getting better, and he has to take more pain medication and anti-anxiety medication. He can't do the exercises the doctor prescribed because it hurts too much; maybe if she would give him a massage and help him exercise, he could do a little exercise. He asks the nurse: "Would you also check my blood sugar before you do the massage?" The nurse recalls that Jim has been taught to check his own blood sugar.

Questions

1. Why would the visiting nurse need to discuss this client's case with his other care providers as well as Jim and his wife? Does the nurse need to get a release of information signed by the client before discussing his case?

2. What is a person with Dependent Personality Disorder like?

3. If you were the visiting nurse and had all the information available about Jim from other health care providers, as well as your own observations, what traits of Dependent Personality Disorder would you identify in this client?

4. What causes Dependent Personality Disorder?

5. What would be a helpful response on the part of the visiting nurse when Jim asks her to check his blood sugar?

6. What nursing diagnoses would you write for Jim if you were the visiting nurse?

7. The visiting nurse and others caring for the client, including the spouse, are scheduled to meet for a planning conference. What goals or outcomes do you think the team might come up with? Should Jim meet with the team?

8. Would Mari's cultural background have an impact on how she relates to Jim's dependency needs? How would you work with her in terms of culturally generated behavioral tendencies?

9. What general approaches do you think might be helpful for the nurse to use in working with Jim or any other client with Dependent Personality Disorder? What types of treatment modalities have been found to be helpful in working with clients with Dependent Personality Disorder?

10. What interventions would you write and utilize in regard to one or more of this client's nursing diagnoses?

11. Is Dependent Personality Disorder common in clients with medical disorders in general and with chronic pain specifically?

12. Do clients with Dependent Personality Disorder seek treatment, and if so, under what conditions?

Brad

GENDER

Male

AGE

62

SETTING

■ Private psychiatric hospital outpatient clinic

ETHNICITY

■ White American

CULTURAL CONSIDERATIONS

PREEXISTING CONDITION

■ High blood pressure
■ High cholesterol

COEXISTING CONDITION

COMMUNICATION

DISABILITY

SOCIOECONOMIC

■ Affluent
■ Professional

SPIRITUAL/RELIGIOUS

■ Attends a church with prestigious upper-class members

PHARMACOLOGIC

PSYCHOSOCIAL

■ Seeks relationships with people viewed as special or important

LEGAL

■ Keeping information provided by a spouse confidential from the other spouse

ETHICAL

ALTERNATIVE THERAPY

■ Chiropractic
■ Massage therapy
■ Health club workouts with trainer

PRIORITIZATION

■ Needs of client with Narcissistic Personality Disorder vs. needs of partner

DELEGATION

NARCISSISTIC PERSONALITY DISORDER

Level of difficulty: Moderate

Overview: Requires knowledge of Narcissistic Personality Disorder and the use of therapeutic communication skills to work with the client. The nurse will need to help the client identify the needs he has to meet for himself and those that cause distress in his relationships.

Client Profile

Brad is a 62-year-old married male whose recall of growing up includes a feeling of feast or famine in terms of attention or lack of attention by his mother. She either smothered him with too much attention or was too busy to give him any attention. His father's business was also unpredictable, resulting in the family having lots of money most of the time with occasional periods of having to move to less pretentious housing or change from private school to public school for a semester or two, both traumatic events to a young boy. When Brad started high school, he was back in private school and his father had bought a boat. Having a boat made Brad popular with the girls, and he learned the importance of having special possessions that would attract desirable people into his company and make him feel important. He went to law school and became a lawyer. He studied finance and became a stockbroker and later began managing large financial portfolios. All these activities helped lessen his fear of losing special status and brought him into contact with prestigious people.

Brad married Mary, a girl with money and family prestige. After many years, Mary has developed health problems and is concerned that Brad had no empathy for her health situation. She is irritated at Brad frequently asking her to drop whatever she is doing and meet him somewhere or do something for him. She suspects he has had a number of affairs. After a trip to a local prestigious private psychiatric outpatient clinic, Mary tells Brad she expects him to get therapy at the clinic or she may divorce him.

Case Study

On hearing from Mary that she has been to the outpatient clinic and is thinking about divorce, Brad agrees to go alone and do a preliminary intake meeting with the staff nurse. The threat of Mary leaving him, rather than him leaving her, distresses him. Brad presents himself at the outpatient clinic. He is well-dressed and well-groomed and appears somewhat arrogant and haughty in wanting to check the credentials of the staff and dropping some names of important doctors that he knows. He states that he expects to be seen on time, as time is money in his business. He wants to use the center telephone to make some important business calls even though a sign says the telephone is for staff use only. He displays a money clip with a large number of bills and flashes a large diamond ring. He gives the impression that he is someone important and is entitled to special privileges. He calls and has a large gift basket delivered to the health care provider's home.

As the staff nurse begins the intake process, she recalls that Brad's wife, Mary, described Brad as lacking empathy and consideration and probably having affairs in the past, but the nurse is determined to keep an open mind as she gathers data from Brad. The nurse notices that Brad answers questions briefly, then asks questions about the nurse's qualifications. Brad seems to know a lot about the medications he is taking for elevated blood pressure and cholesterol and tests the nurse's knowledge about these medications and seems to enjoy any time the nurse knows less than he does about the medication.

Brad manages to mention that he owns a vacation home in an exotic location. He describes important people that he has taken there and mentions he might take the nurse to his vacation home. The nurse replies: "Let's get back to the questions on the assessment" and asks about Brad's relationship with his wife. Brad paints a picture of being very generous with his wife and her being stubborn, unloving, and unappreciative. Brad does not reveal a series of affairs throughout the years or that there is a woman he fantasizes about as an ideal lover and mate. The nurse notes that Brad seems concerned that he is aging, and this seems to be a major stressor for him. He reveals he is spending time and money seeing chiropractors and massage therapists and working out in the most prestigious health club in town. At the end of the session, the nurse suspects Brad meets a number of the criteria for Narcissistic Personality Disorder. Before Brad leaves, he says to the nurse: "I would love to know what my wife told you about me." The nurse will present the intake information to the team, and a therapist or therapists will be assigned to Brad and his wife, Mary.

Questions

1. When the nurse hears Brad say he might take her to his vacation home, she replies: "Let's get back to the questions on the assessment." What technique is she using, and what is a rationale for this reply? What is a likely rationale for Brad suggesting the trip to the nurse and for sending the health care provider a large gift basket?

2. What are the criteria for a diagnosis of Narcissistic Personality Disorder (NPD), and which criteria does Brad seem to meet?

3. Most persons with a diagnosis of Narcissistic Personality Disorder are of what gender? How often are persons diagnosed with Narcissistic Personality Disorder hospitalized specifically for treatment of this disorder?

4. Describe Kohut's and/or Kernberg's theory of causation of Narcissistic Personality Disorder.

5. What possible motivation is behind Brad calling Mary to meet him at a moment's notice? How would you feel and what would you need if you were Mary?

6. What would it feel like to be Brad? How would Brad and others with NPD likely react to changes associated with aging?

7. What will the nurse therapist most likely need to do to keep Brad engaged in couples therapy? Would there be any advantages to the nurse therapist bringing in a second therapist or cotherapist to work with this couple? What does Brad need to gain from therapy?

8. What will the therapist most likely need to do to help Mary get her needs met in this relationship?

9. How does the staff nurse need to respond to Brad's statement: "I would love to know what my wife told you about me"?

10. If you were a nurse in a health care provider's office or on a medical unit in the hospital and your assessment of a client revealed some narcissistic personality traits, would you plan your care differently to work more effectively with this client, and if so, how?

Leah

GENDER

Female

AGE

22

SETTING

■ University health center

ETHNICITY

■ White American

CULTURAL CONSIDERATIONS

■ Sorority house culture

PRE-EXISTING CONDITION

CO-EXISTING CONDITION

COMMUNICATION

DISABILITY

SOCIOECONOMIC

■ Affluent

SPIRITUAL/RELIGIOUS

PHARMACOLOGIC

PSYCHOSOCIAL

LEGAL

■ Providing female nurse presence during physical examination of female client by male health care provider to avoid a false claim of sexual misconduct.

ETHICAL

■ Protecting female client from misconduct by male physician during physical examination.

ALTERNATIVE THERAPY

PRIORITIZATION

■ Nurse decision to accept phone call versus remaining present during physical examination.

DELEGATION

■ Male nurse delegates assisting male health care provider with physical exam to female nurse peer.

Level of difficulty: Easy

Overview: Requires understanding of Histrionic Personality Disorder (HPD). Requires critical thinking to avoid legal ramifications for the professional staff, especially for the male health care provider and male nurse. The nurse must also identify effective techniques for working with the client with HPD.

Client Profile

Leah is a 22-year-old female college student who has always seemed to be the center of attention in her family, in school, and in her peer group. Although Leah's sister has many material things from their affluent family, she can't seem to get any attention from their parents. When Leah enters a room, it is with great dramatic flair. She spends a great deal of energy, time, and money on her appearance and dresses seductively. Leah has been known to fish for compliments. She is flirtatious and sometimes insinuates that she is intimate or close to important males when there is not a close relationship at all. Leah appears uncomfortable when she is not the center of attention and goes to great lengths to regain status. Leah says things like "He is such a difficult person." She gives no details and leaves the recipient of this statement wondering what she meant. Leah frequently goes through a variety of emotions rather quickly.

Case Study

Leah comes to the student health center seeking care for the "very worst cold" she has ever had. She tells the male nurse that it may be pneumonia or worse. She wonders if she should get an important close friend to fly her to Florida in his private plane. She says she feels like she will die if she does not get some sun. Later Leah mentions she might need to go to the Mayo Clinic and see the chief of the medical staff who is a close friend of her father's.

The male nurse asks the health care provider to wait a few minutes before the physical examination on Leah. He asks a female nurse peer to assist the male health care provider. The female nurse is with the health care provider when he examines Leah. The nurse thinks Leah is engaging in seductive behavior around the health care provider. Leah suggests she might need the health care provider to make a house call. Leah has obviously spent a lot of time grooming for the occasion but says to the health care provider. "I am so sick. I must look awful. Do you think I look dreadful?" The female nurse receives a message that she has an urgent telephone call, and she wonders if she can leave the examining room. The health care provider is almost finished with the examination and ready to tell Leah to get dressed.

Before Leah leaves the clinic, she dramatically approaches the male nurse saying that she is horribly depressed and maybe that is why she got a cold. Her boyfriend broke up with her and she is "just devastated." She then says: "Maybe, darling, you would be willing to make a house call to my sorority house?" The nurse responds: "I would be glad to sit and talk with you for a few minutes here at the clinic." Leah responds: "Oh well, if you don't make house calls, perhaps you would take me to the football game. I think you could make me feel much better."

Leah goes to the football game with a friend and tells the friend that "Bill" the health care provider at the clinic wanted to take her to the game, but he had to work. She suddenly yells out a girl's name and runs down the steps in the middle of the ballgame, struggles across a row of people, and hugs a girl in the middle of the row. Leah then turns to the crowd during a play that most people are trying to watch and yells out dramatically, "This is my old roommate and I haven't seen her for a month."

Questions

1. What personality trait of a person with a diagnosis of Histrionic Personality Disorder is usually most noticeable? Which of Leah's behaviors make you suspect she has this personality trait?

2. Could Leah or anyone else have personality traits of Histrionic Personality Disorder and not have the disorder itself? If yes, what behaviors would Leah have to have to get this diagnosis and does she have these behaviors?

3. Why did the male nurse delegate the task of assisting the health care provider with the physical examination to a female nurse? If you were the female nurse in the examining room with the health care provider while he examined Leah, what would you do if someone came and told you that you had an urgent telephone call? Give a rationale for your decision.

4. Did the male nurse respond appropriately when Leah suggested he make a house call? Why or why not?

5. If you were the male nurse, how would you have responded when Leah asked you to take her to the football game?

6. Based on your limited knowledge of Leah's behavior, what nursing diagnoses do you suppose would most likely apply in her case?

7. What nursing interactions might be of help to Leah?

8. What treatment interventions are currently being used in the treatment of Histrionic Personality Disorder?

9. Do clients with Histrionic Personality Disorder get better?

10. What causes Histrionic Personality Disorder?

Howard

GENDER

Male

AGE

36

SETTING

- Emergency room

ETHNICITY

- White American

CULTURAL CONSIDERATIONS

PREEXISTING CONDITION

COEXISTING CONDITION

- Fractured arm

COMMUNICATION

DISABILITY

SOCIOECONOMIC

- Low-paid, white-collar government worker with good health benefits

SPIRITUAL/RELIGIOUS

- Is not a "joiner"
- Prefers to worship alone

PHARMACOLOGIC

PSYCHOSOCIAL

LEGAL

ETHICAL

- Nurse's spouse has relationship with client
- Nurse has potential for dual relationship with client
- Strict confidentiality vs. selective breach to nurse's spouse

ALTERNATIVE THERAPY

PRIORITIZATION

DELEGATION

DIFFICULT

SCHIZOID PERSONALITY DISORDER

Level of difficulty: High

Overview: Requires critical thinking to assure confidentiality in a situation in which the nurse and the nurse's spouse each have a professional relationship with the client and the nurse has potential for a dual relationship. Requires critical thinking in determining effective means of communicating with a client who prefers to be alone and does not enjoy interacting with others.

Client Profile

Howard is a 36-year-old male who was raised by his father after his mother died when he was 6 months old. The father was absent a lot from Howard's life due to his work and dating the same woman for twenty years before he suddenly died. Howard only met the father's girlfriend a handful of times and was raised by a strict grandmother. Howard stayed away from grandmother as much as he could so he would not be punished.

As Howard grew up, he became fascinated with computers and now calls himself a computer "geek." He works in a remote office inputting computer data and doing research for a state agency. He keeps track of the milk production of cows by county throughout the state. The pay is fairly low, but he does not have to go to meetings or interface with anyone except for meeting twice each month with his supervisor. Howard's work earned an award in his state agency, but he would not go to the dinner to accept the award. His supervisor picked the award up for him.

Howard is described by others as pretty much a "loner": living alone, never trying to make friends, and never joining any group. He does not attend a church, preferring to read the bible and pray alone. A first cousin and childhood playmate of Howard recalls that Howard has stayed away from family activities ever since he was old enough not to require a babysitter. Once in awhile the cousin goes to visit him, but Howard never initiates a visit to the cousin. The cousin recalls that Howard's facial expression has always been somewhat flat, and as a child he did not mimic her when she would smile or make faces. The cousin has never noticed any behavior that would indicate Howard is interested sexually in women or perhaps men. A neighbor once tried to start a relationship, but she noticed that Howard became anxious whenever she came near him and he was somewhat cold and aloof.

Case Study

Howard has been brought to the emergency room by EMS. The emergency medical technician (EMT) reports that Howard had apparently been riding his bicycle to work when the driver of a car, claiming to have been blinded by the sun, hit him. The EMT further reports that Howard wanted to go home when he talked with the policeman on the scene, but finally agreed to come to the ER to get checked out for injuries.

When the ER receptionist asks Howard if she can call any of his family or a friend for him or if he would like to call them, he responds: "No." He hides behind a book in the corner of the ER until the x-ray technician comes to x-ray his arm, which he has said hurts and has some pins-and-needles-like feeling.

When the health care provider views the x-ray, it is clear that the ulna is broken. The provider shares with the emergency room nurse that he wants to reset the broken bone, cast the arm, and keep Howard overnight. The nurse goes to tell Howard what the provider plans to do.

After surgery, Howard is taken to his room. It is late in the evening shift when he arrives at his room. When the nurse gets her assignments and receives report, she goes to do the initial assessment on Howard and finds him wide awake. She introduces herself. Howard says: "That is an interesting and unusual last name. My supervisor at work must be related to you. His name is Mark." The night nurse realizes that Howard's supervisor is her husband and that she may see Howard in the future when she attends activities at her husband's workplace.

Questions

1. Does Howard demonstrate traits of Schizoid Personality Disorder (SZPD), and if so, what traits?

2. Can a person described as a "loner" with all or most of the traits of Schizoid Personality Disorder still not meet all the requirements for a diagnosis of SZPD? If so, what additional requirement has to be met?

3. Looking at Howard's behaviors, what makes you more certain they are those associated with SZPD and not those of Avoidant Personality Disorder?

4. If you were the female nurse going to tell Howard about the health care provider's plans to set his arm and cast it and keep him overnight, what would you keep in mind as you plan your approach? What would you say to this client, and how would you say it?

5. If you were the female nurse ready to do the initial assessment of this client and he discovered that you were the wife of his supervisor, what options would you have and which one would you select?

6. What nursing diagnoses, in addition to acute pain and impaired skin integrity for his broken arm, would you write for this client in relation to traits of SZPD?

7. How would you go about writing goals for this client, and what goals might you write if the client is to stay in the rehabilitation hospital for several days or weeks?

8. What interventions might the nurse implement?

9. What are some theories of causation of Schizoid Personality Disorder?

10. What is the current treatment for Schizoid Personality Disorder?

GENDER

Male

AGE

32

SETTING

■ Outpatient mental health center clinic

ETHNICITY

■ Black/White American

CULTURAL CONSIDERATIONS

■ White American father, Black American mother

PREEXISTING CONDITION

COEXISTING CONDITION

■ Hypertension

COMMUNICATION

DISABILITY

SOCIOECONOMIC

SPIRITUAL/RELIGIOUS

PHARMACOLOGIC

■ Captopril in combination with hydrochlorthiazide (Capozide)
■ Lorazepam (Ativan)
■ Olanzapine (Zyprexa)

PSYCHOSOCIAL

■ Paranoia limits and distorts interactions with others

LEGAL

ETHICAL

ALTERNATIVE THERAPY

■ Over-the-counter vitamins, minerals, and enzymes

PRIORITIZATION

DELEGATION

PARANOID PERSONALITY DISORDER

Level of difficulty: High

Overview: Requires critical thinking and decision making in regard to who is going to be most effective in interacting with the client when the client's paranoia worsens. The nurse is required to work collaboratively with other team members and to provide supervision for the client's nonnurse case manager who works with the client in his independent living situation. The nurse is required to work with physical problems as well as mental health problems and to look at possible connections between psychological and medical problems and the medications used to treat them.

DIFFICULT

Client Profile

Stan is a 32-year-old single male. Stan lives alone in a government-subsidized apartment and receives social security disability income (SSDI). He says he stays away from his neighbors, as they are not to be trusted and could turn against him for no reason at all if he were to let them into his apartment.

Stan holds grudges against his mother and has not attempted to contact her for a couple of years. He talks about his mother trying to control his mind and his life and working against him to get him into treatment when he did not want or need it. He carries a grudge over his mother not giving him a birthday party ten years ago when his brother got a party: "Not that I wanted one, but it just was not fair of my mom to do that." Stan is also angry at his mother for giving him a White American father so Black American peers did not accept him and for her being Black American and causing him not to be accepted by White American peers when he was growing up. He was married briefly to Yvonne, a Black American woman he met in group therapy. He was extremely jealous of Yvonne talking to other people and thought she was unfaithful when he heard her talking to a "Bobby" on the phone. Bobbie was a girl his wife had met when she was an inpatient in the psychiatric hospital. This prompted him to follow his wife everywhere she went and to try to keep her home whenever he could to prevent her from meeting this "other man." Stan was verbally hostile to his wife at times, thinking she was criticizing him when in fact she was complimenting him. Stan was jealous every time Yvonne went for psychiatric treatment. He thought she was "hogging all the therapy" (i.e., getting more than her share of psychiatric care).

Stan gets psychiatric care through the county outpatient mental health center clinic. He has a nonnurse case manager who takes vital signs, supervises him in taking his daily medication, helps him with managing his money, and transports him to appointments at the clinic where he sees a psychiatric mental health nurse for all his medication reviews and health assessments. He sees the psychiatrist only if the nurse refers him, and this usually happens only if he is experiencing a significant change in his mental health, has medical problems or problems with his medications, or needs to have additional medication prescribed. Stan currently has prescriptions for two medications: a pill for hypertension (captopril [Capozide 25/15]) and a multivitamin. His medicine cabinet is full of various kinds of vitamins, minerals, and enzymes.

Case Study

Stan reports in at the reception desk at the mental health center clinic. The nurse is walking out to call him into her office about the same time he notices two women talking across the waiting room. He calls out a derogatory name and tells them to stop talking about him. When he sees the nurse, he puts his hands on his hips in a threatening kind of stance and says: "You think you are so smart, but I know what you put in those pills. Don't think you fooled me. And don't put that in my chart." The nurse feels a great deal of energy coming from Stan and feeling threatened; she senses she needs to back away from him. The nurse says gently: "Please sit down and rest for just a few minutes. I'll have your caseworker sit with you, and in a little while when you are ready to talk she can come and get me."

The nurse alerts the psychiatrist that she is going to try to talk with Stan about his medication, but that if Stan is too paranoid, she may need the psychiatrist to discuss his medications with him. The nurse knows from working with Stan for a while and reading his chart that he has a diagnosis of Paranoid Personality Disorder.

When the psychiatrist sees Stan he notes that Stan's blood pressure is still elevated and that he is paranoid and somewhat psychotic. The psychiatrist continues the Capozide and vitamin and orders lorazepam (Ativan) and olanzapine (Zyprexa).

Questions

1. How would you feel and what would you think if you were assigned to work with Stan or any client has Paranoid Personality Disorder?

2. If you were the nurse and Stan said to you: "You think you are so smart," and you felt threatened, what would you think is going on with Stan?

3. What concept or rationale did the nurse possibly have in mind when she alerted the psychiatrist that she might need to have him go over Stan's medications?

4. What behaviors does Stan have that match those of someone with Paranoid Personality Disorder?

5. Is Paranoid Personality Disorder apparent in childhood and adolescence, and if so, what behaviors would clue the family and/or clinicians that a child has this disorder?

6. Some of the behaviors that qualify a person for a diagnosis of Paranoid Personality Disorder seem similar to other personality disorders. How can a person differentiate between PPD and other personality disorders, especially Schizotypal Personality Disorder (SZPD)?

7. How does Paranoid Personality differ from Schizophrenia, Paranoid Type?

8. What is the current treatment for Paranoid Personality Disorder?

9. What does the nurse need to know about the antihypertensive, antianxiety, and antipsychotic medications the client is on? Is there any connection between the client's race and taking one or more of these medications? What do these three medications have in common?

10. What assessment would you want/need to do if you were the nurse in this case? Given the information you have on this client, what nursing diagnoses would you write?

11. What goals would you write for this client? What interventions would be helpful?

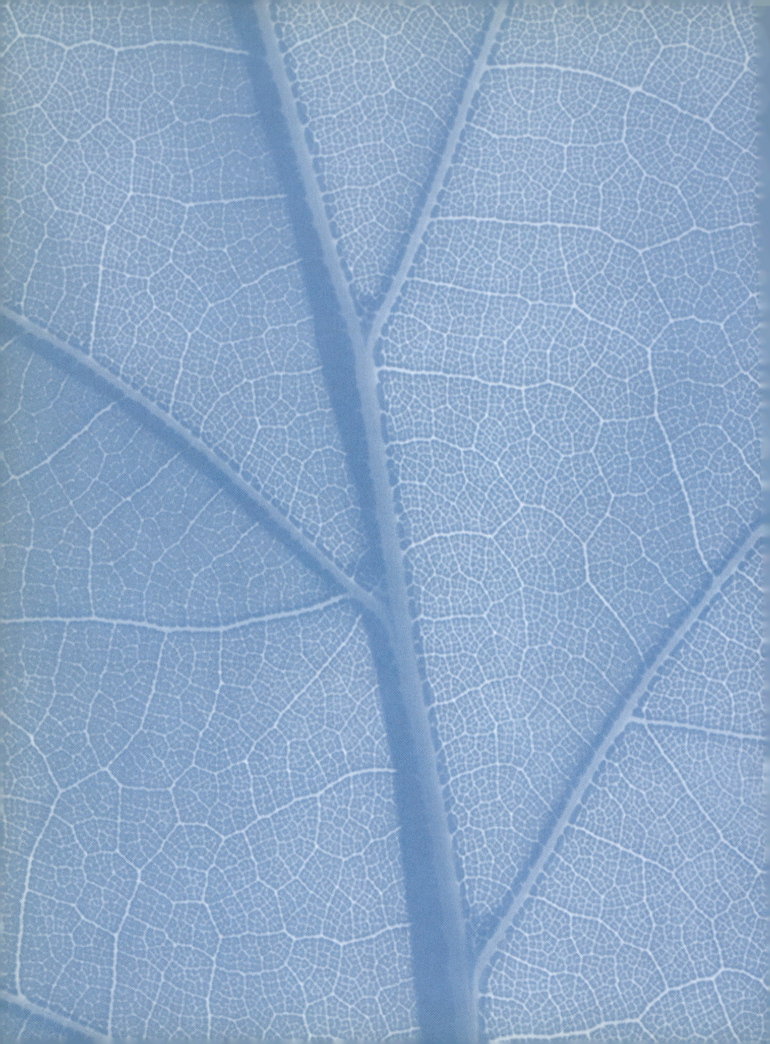

PART SIX

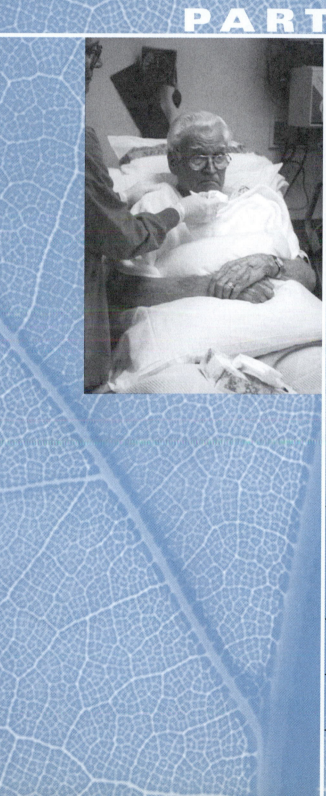

*The Client
Experiencing
a Somatoform,
Factitious, or
Dissociative
Disorder*

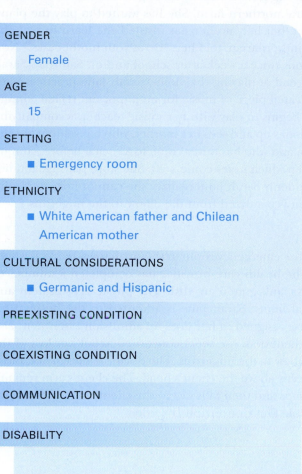

GENDER

Female

AGE

15

SETTING

■ Emergency room

ETHNICITY

■ White American father and Chilean American mother

CULTURAL CONSIDERATIONS

■ Germanic and Hispanic

PREEXISTING CONDITION

COEXISTING CONDITION

COMMUNICATION

DISABILITY

SOCIOECONOMIC

SPIRITUAL/RELIGIOUS

PHARMACOLOGIC

PSYCHOSOCIAL

LEGAL

■ Possible lawsuit if Conversion Disorder is misdiagnosed and treated in error as a medical or neurological condition

ETHICAL

ALTERNATIVE THERAPY

PRIORITIZATION

DELEGATION

CONVERSION DISORDER

Level of difficulty: Easy

Overview: Requires realization that Conversion Disorder results from a subconscious defense mechanism and is not something within the client's control. Effective interventions will need to convey caring and empathy for the client without alienating the client's parents. Requires anyone working with the client to set aside any negative feelings or desire to confront the client.

Client Profile

Sarah Jane is a 15-year-old adolescent whose mother was born and raised in Chile and whose father's family was from Germany three generations back. She and her parents live on a small rural northern farm. She has wanted to play the piano like her paternal grandmother, but her mother has insisted she learn to play the violin. Her father, who is very authoritarian, told her: "Do as your mother asks." Now after eight years of violin lessons twice a week after school and on Saturday, Sarah Jane believes she is not very good at playing the violin. Sarah Jane practices hard to learn a lengthy and complicated piece of music for an important recital coming up. At the recital, Sarah Jane begins to play with her music teacher accompanying her on the piano. Sarah Jane looks up and sees her mother, who has seldom left the house because of agoraphobia and who has never come to a recital before, coming in late. Sarah Jane has forgotten which notes come next. She stops playing, and her teacher has her start over. Suddenly Sarah Jane realizes she cannot hold the violin up with her left hand. Her arm is paralyzed from the elbow to the fingertips.

Case Study

Sarah Jane has been taken to the emergency room in the small town hospital where she was playing her recital. The health care provider has completed a number of neurological tests, taken x-rays, and gotten an MRI. The physical assessment and vital signs were within normal limits. Sarah Jane is admitted to the hospital for observation. The primary nurse assigned to her does an admission assessment and finds it remarkable that this client does not seem concerned about her loss of the use of her left arm from the elbow to the fingertips. The doctor comes in and raises the client's paralyzed arm directly above the client's head. The client's arm remains above the head for a few seconds and then falls out to the client's side. The doctor writes in the client's chart: "Rule Out Conversion Disorder."

Questions

1. What is Conversion Disorder? What symptoms does this client have that are consistent with Conversion Disorder?

2. What are the current theories about what causes Conversion Disorder?

3. If this client had symptoms of Conversion Disorder, why did the health care provider order more tests? Why did the provider put the client's affected arm above her head and leave it unsupported?

4. Do people with Conversion Disorder deliberately produce the symptoms for secondary gain?

5. What subtypes of Conversion Disorder are there? Which subtype of Conversion Disorder does this client seem to have? Does this subtype always produce symptoms of paralysis, or could other symptoms be produced instead? If so, what symptoms?

6. Does this client's onset of symptoms fit within the general onset of Conversion Disorder? What will be this client's course if she follows a typical course associated with Conversion Disorder?

7. What stage of development, according to Erickson, is this client trying to master? What roles might stage of development and culture play in this client's development of Conversion Disorder?

8. What information in data gathering or assessing would be helpful to the treatment team as well as the nurse?

9. What nursing diagnoses would you likely write for a client with Conversion Disorder?

10. What treatment goals would you likely write for this client? What interventions do you think would likely work well with this client?

11. What treatment approaches are reported in the literature?

GENDER

Female

AGE

51

SETTING

- Home with visiting nurse

ETHNICITY

- African

CULTURAL CONSIDERATIONS

- African

PREEXISTING CONDITION

COEXISTING CONDITION

COMMUNICATION

DISABILITY

SOCIOECONOMIC

SPIRITUAL/RELIGIOUS

PHARMACOLOGIC

PSYCHOSOCIAL

- Socialization altered by client's focus on physical symptoms

LEGAL

- Possible lawsuit for unnecessary surgery, especially if complications from surgery or if an actual medical problem occurs and is missed

ETHICAL

ALTERNATIVE THERAPY

PRIORITIZATION

DELEGATION

SOMATIZATION DISORDER

Level of difficulty: Moderate

Overview: Requires critical thinking and decision making about when to listen to symptoms and when to refocus the client on the task at hand. Involves critical thinking in terms of assessing and identifying problems that are current and need to be the focus of interventions.

Client Profile

Melba is a 51-year-old married female of African birth who immigrated to the United States with her parents when she was 15 years old. She has a history of numerous physical complaints and several surgeries. She is presently recuperating at home from exploratory surgery. She had complained of abdominal pain, changes in bowel habits, abdominal bloating, nausea, and vomiting, and after numerous trips to a variety of health care providers who prescribed a number of medications for the pain, nausea, and constipation, she found a surgeon who thought an exploratory laparotomy was warranted. No pathology was found during this surgery. Melba's hospital stay was extended due to an infection at the incisional site and then she was sent home on antibiotics and wet to dry dressings. On discharge, instructions included no sexual intercourse until the incision heals. Her husband's response to the nurse was, "My wife has not thought about sex in years." Melba is to have home visits from a registered nurse.

Case Study

The home health agency nurse arrives at Melba's home. After introducing herself, the nurse begins to take Melba's vital signs, but finds it hard to concentrate as Melba wants to talk about her prior health problems and surgeries. Melba describes a series of surgeries and complaints going back several years beginning at age 26 with back surgery, although she is somewhat lacking in details of what was found or done in the surgery. Then there was the time she could not seem to empty her bladder: "It would fill up with nearly a gallon before I could get somewhere to be catheterized." Melba describes excruciating pain when urinating, bladder infections, and high fevers off and on for several years. Her health care provider has not diagnosed any bladder problems. She also talks about years of impaired coordination and balance keeping her from being able to work. Melba says sometimes she can't sleep at night because it feels like ants are crawling under her skin. She currently complains of knee pain keeping her from walking. X-rays and an MRI of the knee were negative. From Melba's story, the nurse feels certain that there have been few or no periods of time in Melba's life that she has been symptom-free. The nurse finishes the vital signs, which are normal, and suggests Melba learn to do the wet to dry dressings for her abdominal incision. Melba says her husband will do the dressings and to teach him. The nurse recalls an old lecture from nursing school and realizes that some of Melba's behavior sounds like it matches what she learned about Somatization Disorder.

Questions

1. What is Somatization Disorder? What symptoms does Melba have or has she had that caused the nurse to think she might have Somatization Disorder? Could a person have some symptoms of this disorder and not meet the criteria for the diagnosis?

2. How do you think you might feel if you were working with Melba or a client with a similar history of physical complaints for which no medical explanation can be found?

3. What are the current theories about the causation of Somatization Disorder?

4. What is the incidence of Somatization Disorder?

5. Do nurses other than psychiatric nurses need to know about this disorder, and if so, where would nurses encounter a client with this diagnosis or some of the traits of this disorder?

6. If you were Melba's nurse, how would you respond when she tells you that she is not going to learn to do the dressing change and that you can teach her husband to do it?

7. What assessment areas would you like to assess if you were this client's nurse?

Questions (continued)

8. What impact might culture have on a client's symptoms?

9. What nursing diagnoses would you most likely write for this client? What would be some treatment goals of the nurse and client? What interventions

would seem indicated for this client and possibly for the majority of clients with Somatization Disorder?

10. What are current treatment approaches to clients with this disorder?

Amanda

GENDER

Female

AGE

34

SETTING

- Adult psychiatric unit

ETHNICITY

- White American

CULTURAL CONSIDERATIONS

- Rural southern farming and strong churchgoing culture
- Culture of abuse

PRE-EXISTING CONDITION

CO-EXISTING CONDITION

COMMUNICATION

DISABILITY

SOCIOECONOMIC

- Raised poor then lower middle class when married

SPIRITUAL/RELIGIOUS

- Subconscious resistance to church related to abuse history.

PHARMACOLOGIC

PSYCHOSOCIAL

- Alternates between being withdrawn and uninhibited based on what alternative personality ("alter") is in charge.

LEGAL

- Need to avoid causing false memories of abuse
- Confidentiality

ETHICAL

- Is it educational or is it inappropriate, exploitive, and unethical to ask a client with Dissociative Identity Disorder (DID) to appear in public to discuss or demonstrate alternative personalities?

ALTERNATIVE THERAPY

PRIORITIZATION

DELEGATION

DIFFICULT

DISSOCIATIVE IDENTITY DISORDER (FORMERLY MULTIPLE PERSONALITY DISORDER)

Level of difficulty: High

Overview: Requires knowledge of DID and critical thinking to respond therapeutically to the client and any "alters," which present with a variety of behaviors and attitudes. Requires critical thinking to avoid letting personal attitudes or feelings get in the way of working effectively with the client and to avoid leading the client to false memories.

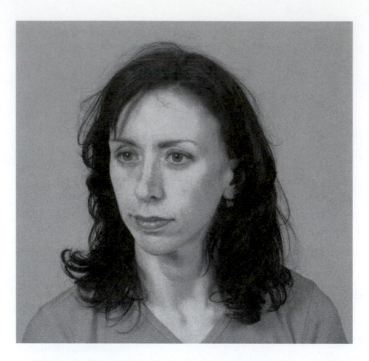

Client Profile

Amanda is a 34-year-old married female who was raised in a strong church-going family on a rural southern Bible Belt farm. Her grandfather as well as her father sexually, physically, and mentally abused her as a child. Each of them told her it would kill her mother if she found out and not to tell anyone or they would punish her. Her father, a deacon in the church, routinely abused her on Sundays after church and Sunday dinner when other family members took a nap. At first Amanda screamed, but no one seemed to hear. She began to dissociate: to mentally float above what was happening and feel like an observer. Her grandfather and her father died before she was 10 years old. Amanda repressed the abuse in her subconscious mind. At age 19 Amanda married Fred, a long-distance truck driver, who was kind to her but not often home. The marriage provided a means to get away from her mother who wasn't kind or supportive and who had actually known about the abuse and done nothing.

Recently Amanda noticed what she calls "trashy" clothes in her closet. She thought her husband had bought the seductive dresses until she found a charge receipt with her signature on it. Amanda has found herself in a store temporarily unable to recall what she came to buy or who she is. She has found herself talking in a strange childish voice or in a sultry seductive way: not like her real self at all. Amanda suspects she has different personalities within herself: one (Audrey) who likes to dress "trashy," tease men, and control; a small playful bear ("Bear"); "Sissy," age 5, who likes to play but is afraid of adults; Tom, who knows about "Sissy" and wants to protect her. Neither Tom nor Sissy know about Audrey, who seems to know everyone except Butch, who is angry about the abuse and wants Amanda to cut her arms. Amanda never has felt connected to the world and other people. She has little recall of her childhood and tries to deny flashbacks of the abuse.

Case Study

Amanda is admitted to the adult psychiatric unit. Her husband tells the nurse he fears his wife is " going crazy." Fred describes Amanda cutting her arms and having periods of time for which she has no memory. He relates that Amanda became very upset when he asked her to go to church with him. After the husband leaves, the psychiatric technician goes through the things Amanda brought to the hospital and removes items that she might hurt herself with, inventories them, and locks them up. The admitting orders provide a diagnosis of Dissociative Identity Disorder. The psychiatrist's history and physical on Amanda states she has had one previous admission to the facility. The nurse orders and reads the old chart from medical records and becomes aware of some of the alters (alternative personalities) Amanda has revealed to her psychiatrist and therapists. The nurse offers to play checkers with Amanda after the evening meal. During the checker game one of the alters comes out and says in a child's voice, "I don't want to play with you."

Questions

1. If you were the nurse on the unit, what would you say to the husband when he says that his wife (your client) is "going crazy"?

2. Why is the diagnosis of DID controversial? Is this a real disorder, or do mental health professionals and clients misapply and misuse this diagnosis?

3. What is the culture of abuse? What role did the southern, rural farm, Bible Belt culture possibly play in the abuse and dissociation?

4. Are all clients who are diagnosed with DID survivors of sexual abuse, and are all sexual abuse survivors likely to have or to develop DID?

5. Discuss some characteristics and behaviors of a person with Dissociative Identity Disorder. What are the criteria for a diagnosis of DID, and does Amanda meet the criteria for this diagnosis?

6. What is the cause of DID? What are the risk factors for DID?

7. If you were the nurse playing checkers with Amanda and she said in a childlike voice, "I don't want to play with you," what therapeutic response would you make and why?

8. What should the nurse do if the treatment team doesn't want staff nurses to interact with the client's alters?

9. Are alters real people within one person's body?

10. Why do people who have DID self-mutilate? If you were Amanda's nurse, how would you respond to this client or any client who is thinking of hurting herself, threatening to hurt herself, or has hurt herself?

11. What nursing diagnoses and treatment goals might the nurse write for this client?

12. What are some of the nursing interventions and professional treatment approaches to DID?

13. What additional research is being done in the area of DID?

GENDER	**SPIRITUAL/RELIGIOUS**
Female	
AGE	**PHARMACOLOGIC**
31	
SETTING	**PSYCHOSOCIAL**
Physician's office	
ETHNICITY	**LEGAL**
White American	■ Need to avoid libel or slander
CULTURAL CONSIDERATIONS	**ETHICAL**
	■ Refusing to treat client or alienating client so she goes to another health provider is questionable from an ethical standpoint
PREEXISTING CONDITION	
COEXISTING CONDITION	**ALTERNATIVE THERAPY**
	■ Getting a pet
	■ Volunteer work
COMMUNICATION	**PRIORITIZATION**
DISABILITY	**DELEGATION**
SOCIOECONOMIC	
■ Has a trust fund and is upper class without having to work	

DIFFICULT

FACTITIOUS DISORDER

Level of difficulty: High

Overview: Requires keeping an open mind while carefully observing and assessing client's behaviors and sharing findings with team members who must be consistent in their responses to the client. The nurse must control any negative thoughts or reactions and select an appropriate professional attitude and behaviors. Knowledge of transference and countertransference is useful. Avoidance of defamation of character by libel or slander is essential.

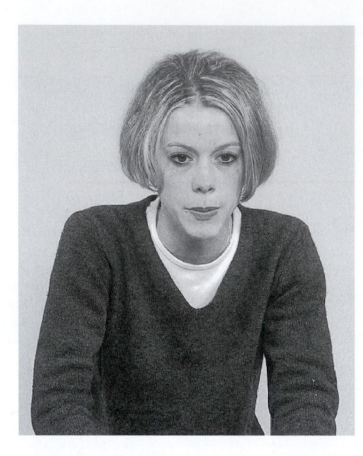

Client Profile

Linda is a 31-year-old single female who does not have to work as she has a trust fund left to her by a grandfather. A lawyer manages the trust fund and approves requests from Linda for money. Linda has lived in her own home, but is currently living with her parents because she says she is too ill at times to care for herself.

Linda has recently begun to frequently complain of seeing blood in her urine and having chills, fever, and bladder pain. She has been seeing a health care provider who is puzzled by her symptoms because the urinalyses are almost always normal with an occasional urine infection that responds to antibiotics. The client has a fever at each visit and looks pale and uncomfortable. On the first visit with the bladder-related symptoms, she provided a story about having extra pockets in her bladder wall that fill with urine and get infected; when they don't have urine in them, they have air, which is painful and requires hospitalization. In trying to verify this strange condition, the health care provider sought to find the name and address of the provider who identified it. The client was evasive, complaining of not remembering and providing a long involved story of earlier treatment by a urologist in a famous university hospital without supplying any real details.

Case Study

The office nurse goes to the waiting room to get Linda, weighs her, and takes her vital signs and a short history in preparation for seeing the health care provider. The nurse puts a glass thermometer in Linda's mouth and leaves the room to get a drink for the client who has complained of being thirsty. After the nurse closes the door, she remembers she forgot to remind the client to keep the thermometer under her tongue. As she opens the door, she thinks she sees the client take the thermometer from under the water faucet. The client quickly tells a story of needing to wash her hands. Linda's temperature is 101.8.

Although she cannot be sure the client had the thermometer under the faucet, the nurse mentions her suspicions to the health care provider. The provider does not say anything to the client but goes ahead with his assessment, and examination and orders a urinalysis. He tells the client he will be back after she is dressed. The doctor tells the nurse to recheck the temperature and stay in the room while it is being taken. The temperature is 98.4 on rechecking it. Neither the nurse nor the health care provider questions the client about this temperature. It is simply noted. The client is to drink at least six glasses of water a day and two glasses of cranberry juice and return in one week for further testing.

Later the health care provider mentions to the nurse in private that he suspects this client has Factitious Disorder. The provider tells the nurse he would like her to get some medical history on the client from the parents. The nurse recalls that she overheard the client tell the parents that the provider said he would have to run more tests and she was lucky to have parents to take care of her since she was so ill.

Questions

1. What is Factitious Disorder (FD), and how does this disorder differ from the somatoform disorders?

2. What do you suppose the nurse was thinking when she opened the door and thought she saw the thermometer being held under the faucet water by the client? What emotions might this observation arouse in the nurse?

3. Do you agree with the nurse's actions to say nothing of her suspicions about the thermometer being under the faucet to the client, but to then share her possible observation with the health care provider in private? Give a rationale for your answer.

4. If you were the nurse working with this client, how would you handle the situation if the provider asked you to recheck the client's temperature?

5. Does this client have any signs and/or symptoms that match the criteria for Factitious Disorder?

6. What is thought to be the cause of Factitious Disorder?

7. Why is the true incidence of Factitious Disorder in the general population unknown?

8. In what settings would a nurse encounter a client with Factitious Disorder?

9. If you were the nurse in this case, what additional assessments would you like to do? What nursing diagnoses would you likely find in this client or other clients with Factitious Disorder? What goals would you likely write for this client or other clients with Factitious Disorder?

10. What interventions would you likely write for this client or another client with a similar situation?

11. One of your peers asks you to explain Munchausen's Syndrome by Proxy. Give a brief explanation.

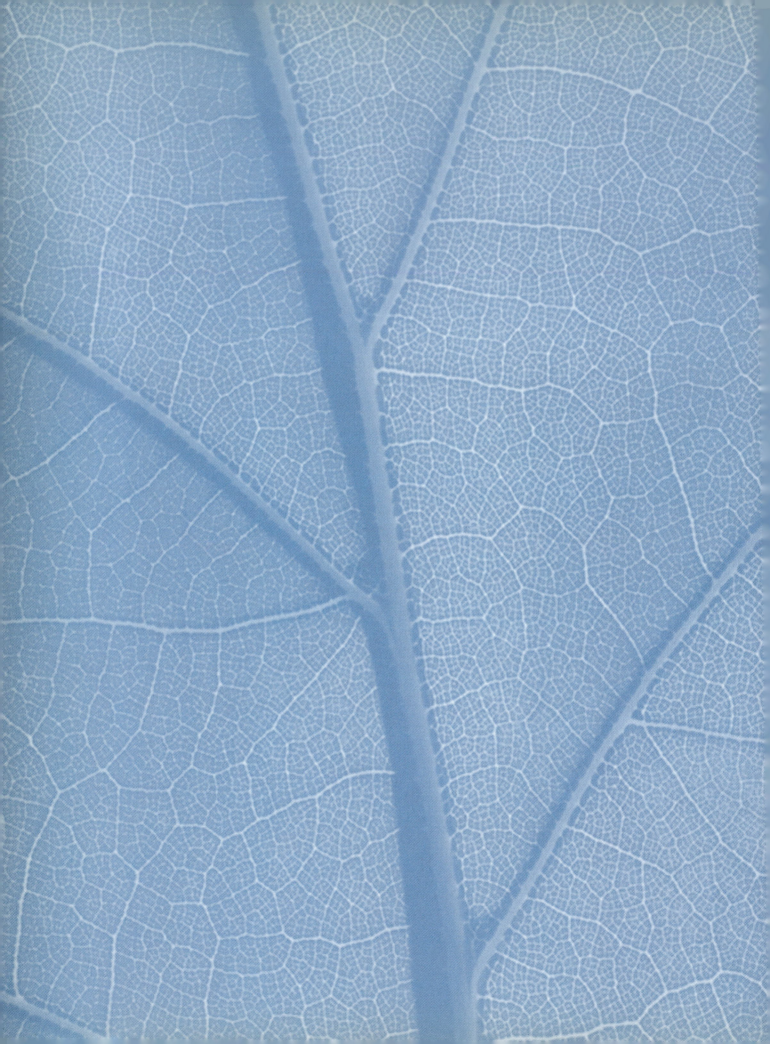

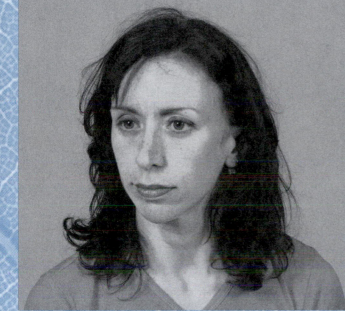

PART SEVEN

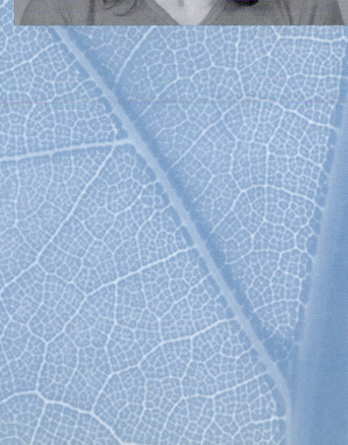

The Client with Disorders of Self-Regulation

MODERATE

GENDER

Female

AGE

26

SETTING

- Eating disorders unit of a private psychiatric hospital

ETHNICITY

- White American

CULTURAL CONSIDERATIONS

PREEXISTING CONDITION

COEXISTING CONDITIONS

- Nicotine abuse
- Alcohol abuse
- Depressed mood

COMMUNICATION

DISABILITY

SOCIOECONOMIC

- Upper middle class

SPIRITUAL/RELIGIOUS

- Connecting with a higher power to deal with abuse of food and alcohol and as a means of dealing with anxiety

PHARMACOLOGIC

- Buproprion hydrochloride (Wellbutrin, Zyban)

PSYCHOSOCIAL

- Socialization impaired by need to hide eating behavior

LEGAL

ETHICAL

ALTERNATIVE THERAPY

- Twelve-step program of AA for alcohol abuse and abuse of food
- Hypnosis for smoking

PRIORITIZATION

DELEGATION

BULIMIA NERVOSA, PURGING TYPE

Level of difficulty: Moderate

Overview: Requires knowledge of the signs and symptoms and behaviors associated with Bulimia Nervosa in order to identify clients who may have this disorder early on. Critical thinking is necessary to identify therapeutic approaches to clients with Bulimia Nervosa and to help them change harmful behaviors associated with binging and purging. Knowledge of the disorder is necessary in order to educate clients about the disorder.

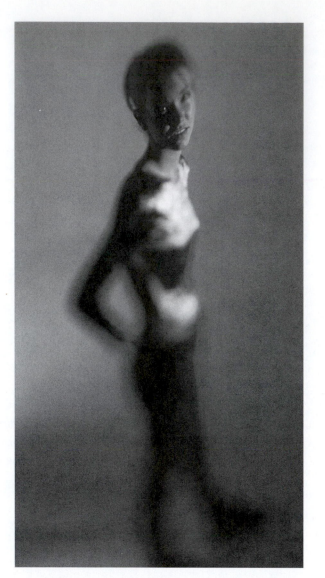

*Sabine has a distorted body image because of
her eating disorder.*

Client Profile

Sabine is a 26-year-old single woman who grew up in an urban upper-middle-class family in a western state. Her parents both worked and gave her whatever she wanted except their time, so she soothed herself with food. Sabine was a cheerleader in junior high school but failed to make the team in high school due to being overweight. Currently she is living alone in an apartment complex. She has a master's degree from a major university and earns over $100,000 a year managing a software development team. Sabine wants an attractive figure and will do almost anything not to be overweight like she was as a teenager. For the past four months, four or five times a week, she has been stopping at night at the grocery store on the way home from work and buying foods she has been denying herself in her previous dieting phase—donuts, cookies, potato chips, and ice cream bars—which she eats as fast as she can in the car on the way home. When she gets home she goes to the bathroom and makes herself vomit. She feels guilty after the binging and vows she won't do it again, but within a few days she finds herself binging again. She also eats excessively at all-you-can-eat buffets, then goes home and takes an excessive amount of laxatives and prune juice. Sabine feels guilty about her binging and purging, abuses alcohol to make herself forget, then feels guilty about drinking too much, and eats some more. She smokes from one to two packages of cigarettes a day. Sometimes she feels "depressed."

Sabine began to have abdominal discomfort and pain in the middle of her chest (esophageal area). She went to see a nurse practitioner, who noticed that she had enlarged parotid glands and eroded teeth enamel. When questioned about her eating habits, Sabine admitted to binging and purging. The nurse practitioner convinced Sabine to get treatment at an inpatient eating disorder program. Sabine went home, called work to arrange time off, drank a few drinks, packed a couple of suitcases, and called a taxi to take her to the eating disorders unit.

Case Study

Sabine is admitted to the eating disorders unit. During the initial assessment by the primary nurse, Sabine describes bowel irregularities and says she will need the laxatives she brought with her. The nurse advises Sabine that all the laxatives she has will have to be turned in and any she takes will have to be ordered by the doctor and dispensed by the nurse. Sabine becomes very upset and says: "I will talk to the doctor about this. I will just leave if I can't have my laxatives that I need."

The nurse reviews Sabine's chart and the CBC report, and during the initial assessment notices the client's affect is somewhat blunted. The nurse notices the client's enlarged parotid glands and the erosion of dental enamel. The nurse looks at Sabine's hands and asks: "Are you left-handed or right-handed?" Sabine answers: "Left-handed."

The nurse finds that Sabine weighs 142 pounds and is 5 foot 5 inches tall. Sabine sees herself in the mirror and says: "I look like a beer barrel." A psychiatrist, who examines Sabine, makes a diagnosis of Bulimia Nervosa. He orders individual and group therapy, a 12-step program, and buproprion hydrochloride (Wellbutrin). She asks for hypnosis to help with smoking cessation, and the psychiatrist orders it. After a few days, Sabine is offering to help on the unit.

Questions

1. What signs did the nurse practitioner and the nurse find that would lead any health care professional to suspect an eating disorder? What signs and symptoms suggest Sabine has Bulimia Nervosa and not Anorexia Nervosa? How do these eating disorders differ and how are they similar?

2. The psychiatrist gave Sabine a diagnosis of Bulimia Nervosa, Purging Type. What criteria does she have to meet to receive this diagnosis? Does she appear to meet these criteria?

3. Why was the nurse interested in knowing whether the client was left-handed or right-handed? When the nurse reviews the lab tests, which tests are likely to be abnormal in this client because of purging by self-induced vomiting?

4. What two screening questions could the nurse practitioner have used to screen this client for Bulimia? What other screening(s) might the nurse have done?

5. What possible reasons could the nurse practitioner have had for referring the client to an inpatient eating disorders clinic rather than an outpatient program?

6. What items might Sabine have brought with her to the hospital that would have to be inventoried and locked up? Can the nurse delegate these tasks to ancillary staff? How can the nurse deal with Sabine's threat to leave if she is not allowed to keep her laxatives?

Questions (continued)

7. Sabine offers to help the nurses with little tasks and in general tries to please the nurses on the unit. Is this common behavior of someone with Bulimia Nervosa, and what must you and other nurses keep in mind when this occurs?

8. You are teaching a class on the eating disorders unit. Sabine wants to know if males ever suffer from Bulimia Nervosa. She has observed that all the clients on the unit are female. Peers ask about the usual onset of Bulimia and the cause of Bulimia. How would you answer these questions?

9. Clients with Bulimia who are in the education class about the disorder, learn about medical problems that arise from their binging and purging. What medical problems associated with Bulimia Nervosa do these clients, nurses, and other health care professionals need to be aware of?

10. When assisting in gathering data on this client, what information would you especially be interested in gathering?

11. What nursing diagnoses would Sabine likely have that are related to her diagnosis of Bulimia Nervosa? What goals would you likely write for this client?

12. What interventions would you need to write and implement for this client? What interventions would you need to be sure and include with this client. What nonpharmaceutical interventions are commonly used with clients who have Bulimia Nervosa? Are medications used to treat Bulimia Nervosa? What are the likely reasons for the health care provider ordering buproprion hydrochloride (Wellbutrin, Zyban)?

CASE STUDY 2

Deidre

GENDER

Female

AGE

21

SETTING

- General hospital

ETHNICITY

- East Asian American mother and White American father (deceased)

CULTURAL CONSIDERATIONS

- Eastern value of honesty conflicts with need to hide and lie about hair pulling

PREEXISTING CONDITION

COEXISTING CONDITION

- Depressed mood

COMMUNICATION

DISABILITY

SOCIOECONOMIC

- Low-income college student with scholarship and part-time job with little or no help from family

SPIRITUAL/RELIGIOUS

PHARMACOLOGIC

- Fluoxetine (Prozac)

PSYCHOSOCIAL

- Prior sexual abuse
- Isolates herself to pull hair

LEGAL

- Adult client reveals sexual abuse as a child

ETHICAL

ALTERNATIVE THERAPY

- Marjoram Leaves
- Aromatherapy
- Acupuncture
- Hypnosis

PRIORITIZATION

DELEGATION

IMPULSE CONTROL DISORDERS: NOT ELSEWHERE CLASSIFIED TRICHOTILLOMANIA

Level of difficulty: Moderate

Overview: Requires knowledge of impulse control disorders, understanding of the client's background and personal situation, empathy and rapport with the client, and understanding of the impact of traditional and alternative medications and therapies.

437

Client Profile

Deidre is a 21-year-old student at a large university, on scholarship and part-time work with little financial help from her family. When she was seven, her mother went into the psychiatric hospital for depression. Her father had been killed in an accident when she was a toddler so a grandfather cared for Deidre and her brother. The grandfather sexually abused her, and by the time her mother came home Deidre literally was pulling her hair out. She would pull first one hair and then another from the top of her head and then eat the hair. Deidre also pulled out eyelashes at times and began to pull out pubic hair, thinking no one would see that area and she could better hide her hair pulling. She did not tell her mother about the sexual abuse because her grandfather said her mother would either go away again or die if she found out. Deidre isolates herself, choosing not to date or go places with other girls. She tries hard not to pull her hair out and may go several days without pulling, but always begins again. Her habit is to carefully choose a hair, twirl the hair, pull it in such a way as to remove the hair bulb with the hair, rub the hair between her fingers, and then eat it.

Case Study

Deidre has been eating marjoram leaves and doing aromatherapy in an effort to stop eating hair. She experiences a loss of appetite, weight loss, weakness, diarrhea, nausea and vomiting, increased white blood cells, and fever. She has resisted going to see a health care provider, but finally allows her mother to take her to the provider's office. The provider notices Deidre has a strange pattern of baldness on her head. He asks her if she pulls her hair, but she denies it. Deidre is admitted to the hospital for observation prior to possible exploratory laparoscopy. The primary nurse assigned to Deidre does a head-to-toe assessment and makes a note of the bald spot at the top of Deidre's head. Later the nurse forgets to knock before entering Deidre's room, and just as she is getting ready to apologize for not knocking, she sees Deidre, with her eyes closed, put what looks like a hair in her mouth and swallow it. During the hospitalization, Deidre undergoes an exploratory laparoscopy. The surgeon finds a trichobezoar. When the surgeon confronts Deidre about the trichobezoar, the mother becomes angry with Deidre for insisting on the first visit to the health care provider and thereafter that she was not eating her hair. Deidre's mother demands that Deidre stop eating hair and stop lying immediately.

The health care provider diagnoses Deidre with Trichotillomania, suggests acupuncture and hypnosis, and prescribes fluoxetine (Prozac).

Questions

1. Why do you suppose Deidre denied pulling her hair when the health care provider asked her? Is it common for people who pull their hair out to deny it?

2. What is Trichotillomania, and what are the essential features of Trichotillomania? Describe some common behaviors carried out by individuals with Trichotillomania.

3. You have entered the client's room without knocking. You are pretty sure that the client is not aware that you entered the room and saw her eating a hair. What will you do now? If you confront the client and she says: "You must be mistaken. I would never think of doing such a thing," what do you say or do?

4. Is there a relationship between Trichotillomania and self-esteem and/or body image?

5. What is a trichobezoar? Is the response of the mother, to the news that Deidre has a trichobezoar, helpful or not? How will you respond to the client and her mother in regard to what the mother has said to the client?

Questions (continued)

6. Deidre's mother asks you, "What causes Trichotillomania?" and "What are the complications of Trichotillomania?" What is your response?

7. What happens when people with Trichotillomania try to just stop pulling their hair as Deidre's mother suggests?

8. The client asks you if you think munching marjoram leaves and some aromatherapy will calm her enough to stop the impulses to pull out her hair. What will you tell her? What type of treatment has been found to work for people with Trichotillomania? Discuss acupuncture and hypnosis as treatments for Trichotillomania.

9. What teaching will you do on fluoxetine (Prozac)? What response will you give to the client sharing her fear she cannot afford the Prozac?

10. What is your response to the client's revelation that she was sexually abused when she was seven years old and she wants to keep it a secret?

11. What do you think is the primary nurse's role in caring for this client?

12. Based on the information you have, what nursing diagnoses, goals, and interventions would be appropriate for this client?

GENDER

Male

AGE

25

SETTING

Pediatric unit then local jail

ETHNICITY

- White American

CULTURAL CONSIDERATIONS

- Small town, large family

PREEXISTING CONDITION

COEXISTING CONDITION

COMMUNICATION

DISABILITY

SOCIOECONOMIC

- Lower middle class

SPIRITUAL/RELIGIOUS

PHARMACOLOGIC

PSYCHOSOCIAL

- Isolation due to stigma and fear of being found out
- Stress on marital relationship due to past and current sexual contact with children

LEGAL

- Reporting requirements in regard to a child telling about sexual activity with an adult
- Acting on sexual urges with children is a crime and punishable by law

ETHICAL

- Do Pedophiles deserve treatment and compassion or just punishment such as incarceration, probation, lifelong tracking, and ostracism?

ALTERNATIVE THERAPY

PRIORITIZATION

- Safety of the child
- Safety of other children (future victims)
- Need for psychological and medical help for child as victim as well as for child's family
- Psychological and other treatments for the client as perpetrator
- The perpetrator needs to be kept safe from hurting others and safe from suicide attempts

DELEGATION

PEDOPHILIA

Level of difficulty: High

Overview: Requires the ultimate in professionalism to help a person who has Pedophilia learn to control their sexual urges and to live in society without being sexually involved with children. Involves reporting to a state agency any information provided by children who have been the subject of sexual acts or personal knowledge of sexual activities between a child and an adult. Requires ability to assess for suicidal ideation and to "anchor" a person who has suicidal potential.

DIFFICULT

Client Profile

Edgar, a 25-year-old married male with a stepdaughter and a natural daughter, grew up the youngest child in a large family. The family lived in a small town where everyone knew everyone, but there were secrets in Edgar's family. Edgar's father drank a lot and talked about sex a lot, and something did not seem right when he was around small children. A couple of his grown children would not trust him alone with their children.

When Edgar graduated from high school, he moved into his married sister's home. In the car one day, her 6-year-old son said something that caused her to suspect sexual activities between her brother and her son. She had no proof, but she asked Edgar to leave. Edgar immediately moved in with his brother's family. He shared a room with the brother's 5-year-old boy. Edgar's brother had no idea of what had transpired in the sister's home. Not too long after Edgar moved in, his brother was playing with his son and the son asked if he wanted to play "tiger bellies" like Uncle. When he was asked what that was, the boy's father was shocked to hear it involved some genital stimulation. Edgar admitted to his brother that he had experienced fantasies and sexual urges about sex with children since he was 16 years old. Edgar was asked to leave and told by his brother to get counseling. Edgar did not go to counseling, but instead found himself another place to stay and a well-paying job. Within a couple of months, he married an attractive woman who had a 3-year-old daughter and a year later they had another child.

Case Study

Edgar's 5-year-old daughter, Mindy, is in the hospital for treatment associated with her diabetes. The hospital is in the closest city to the small town where the family lives. Edgar is going to stay all night on the cot in the child's room while his wife stays at home with the other daughter. The night nurse makes rounds and finds Mindy sleeping on the cot with Edgar. The night nurse did not think too much about this as children often feel insecure in the hospital and want their parents close by. The next day Mindy says to her primary nurse: "Don't touch me down there. Only my daddy can touch me there. Oops, I am not to tell anyone. Don't tell anyone, please."

Edgar finds himself in jail waiting to see the judge in regard to child sexual abuse charges. His wife has threatened divorce. He has begged her not to divorce him. He has agreed to go into treatment, yet he is afraid he will be sent to prison and lose his wife, his job, and all respect from any source due to the stigma attached to sexual preference of children and child molestation. The nurse working at the jail makes rounds. The nurse is to do a brief check on this new inmate.

Questions

1. What actions had to taken in response to Mindy's revelation that her daddy is the only one who can touch her "down there" (her genitals) in a certain way?

2. Does Edgar's behavior match the diagnostic criteria for Pedophilia? Does a person who meets these criteria have to experience distress in some area of functioning to have the diagnosis of Pedophilia? Do most Pedophiles abuse only children in their family or belonging to friends or neighbors?

3. Are some Pedophiles attracted only to children of a certain age? Do most Pedophiles begin to have sexual urges, fantasies, or activity with children in adolescence like Edgar? What justification do people with Pedophilia use when they have sexual activity with a child or children?

4. Is it unusual that this client is married, has sex with his wife, and has a second child? Are all Pedophiles male like the client in this case?

Questions (continued)

5. What are the current beliefs about the cause(s) of Pedophilia? Are all child abusers Pedophiles?

6. What did you think or feel when you read that Edgar had sexual activity with two of his nephews and then his stepdaughter?

7. Edgar was advised by his brother to go into counseling for his unacceptable behavior with children. Were you surprised that he didn't go to counseling? Why or why not?

8. If you were the nurse working in the jail, what would you ask Edgar and/or tell him when you go to do a brief check on him?

9. Will Edgar go to prison and/or to treatment, and will he have to register as a sexual offender?

10. Can Pedophilia be treated, and if so, what kinds of medications, therapy, and other treatments are being used today to treat Pedophiles?

11. Where will nurses encounter and care for people with Pedophilia in addition to pediatric units and the jail, and what will their role be?

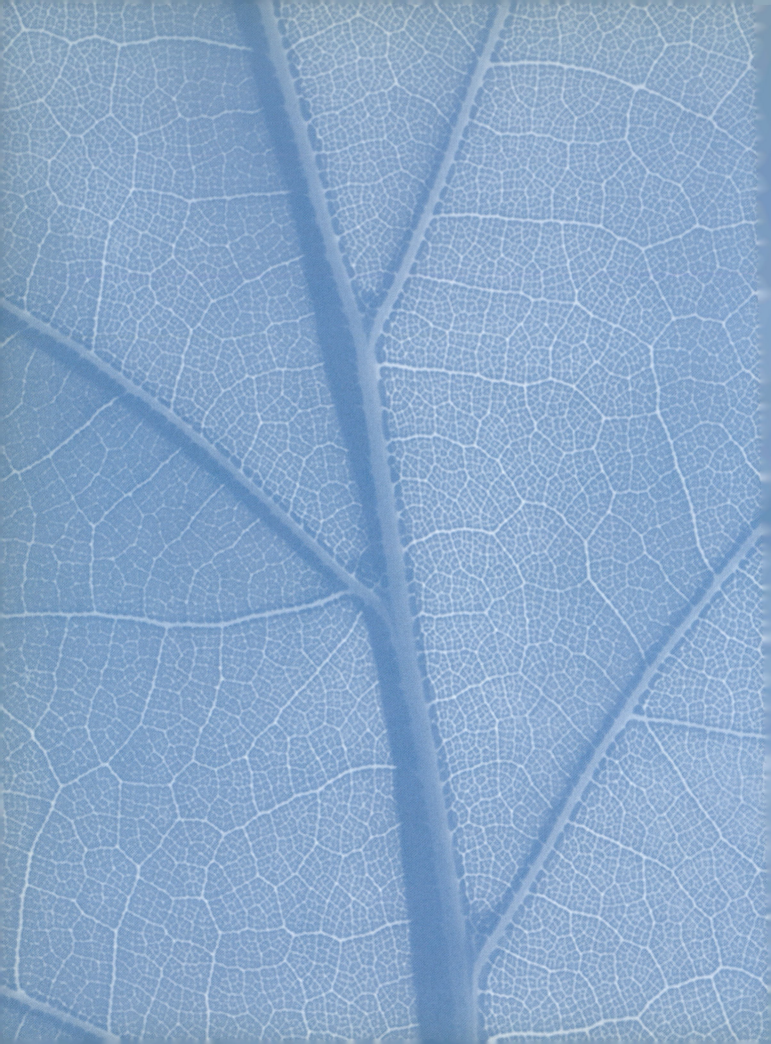

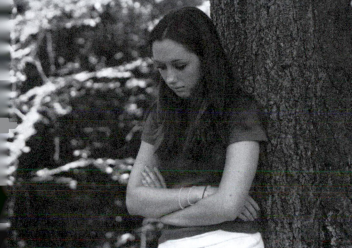

## PART EIGHT

Special Populations: The Child, Adolescent, or Elderly Client

GENDER

Male

AGE

13

SETTING

- Residential treatment facility for adolescents

ETHNICITY

- White American

CULTURAL CONSIDERATIONS

PREEXISTING CONDITIONS

COEXISTING CONDITIONS

COMMUNICATION

DISABILITY

SOCIOECONOMIC

- Parents divorced; mother is low income and father is middle income

SPIRITUAL/RELIGIOUS

PHARMACOLOGIC

PSYCHOSOCIAL

- Priority is being seen as tough by male acquaintances
- Difficulty establishing peer relationships

LEGAL

- History of sneaking out past legal curfew and drinking with older boys
- Found in neighbor's house uninvited; neighbor could press charges if Len leaves treatment early
- History of tardiness and skipping school

ETHICAL

ALTERNATIVE THERAPY

PRIORITIZATION

DELEGATION

MODERATE

OPPOSITIONAL DEFIANT DISORDER

Level of difficulty: Moderate

Overview: Requires working collaboratively as part of a multidisciplinary team, including client and client's family, to change the behavior of the client (a child) who has difficulty with authority figures. The nurse must be able to set limits consistently and help the client's family to recognize the need for, and to set, consistent limits for the child.

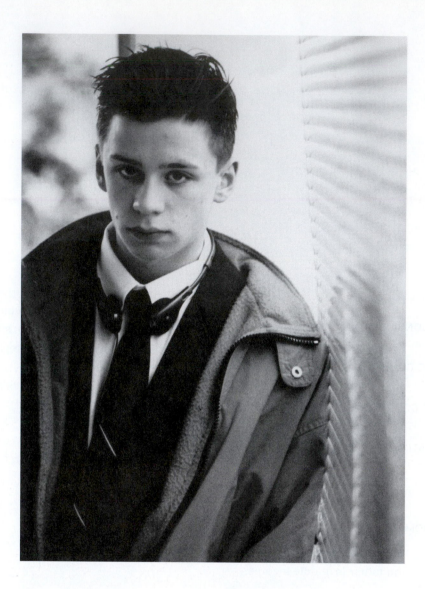

Client Profile

Len is a 13-year-old boy whose parents are divorced. Len's father is remarried and has two children by his second wife. The father is a truck driver and home only periodically. Len's mother tries to compete with his father in giving Len and his younger brother Nathan (Nate) material things. The mother recently bought Len some outrageously expensive tennis shoes that he demanded she buy. The mother doesn't work and has been buying things for Len and his brother on her brother's credit card. She is running up a large credit card debt on her brother's account and refuses to let him look at the bills that come in the mail. The boys and their uncle live with their mother, who is not good at setting limits. Their uncle and their father are also poor at setting limits.

Len has been in and out of trouble at school for the past year. He curses in class and is argumentative with teachers and the vice principal of his middle school. His mother takes Len's side in any disagreement between Len and authority figures. Len tells her that these adults are unfairly picking on him or they are stupid, and his mother believes him or at least she seems to when she goes to the school to "straighten the school people out." Recently a neighbor returned home to find Len in his house with some bizarre story of why he was there. The neighbor called the police who took Len into custody. The neighbor dropped charges when he learned that a deal had been worked out for the school system and Len's father's insurance to pay for Len going into residential psychiatric treatment.

Case Study

Len is admitted to a unit for adolescent boys at a residential treatment center by the nurse on duty. The nurse shows Len and his mother around the unit and gives both of them a copy of the unit rules. The nurse goes over the rules and has Len sign a statement that he has read, understands, and will abide by the rules. Consequences of breaking various rules are on the document. The unit is on a level system in which residents are promoted to a higher level and granted more privileges as they comply with rules and treatment. The nurse notices Len crossing his fingers, rolling his eyes, and then winking at his mother before signing the document.

Len and his mother are introduced to a nurse clinical specialist in child and adolescent mental health (certified by the American Nurses Association and prepared at the master's level in nursing) who will be Len's case manager, individual therapist, and the family therapist. Case managers in this facility can be nurse clinical specialists, master's prepared social workers or psychologists, or licensed professional counselors. The treatment plan is managed by the case manager but is developed, implemented, and evaluated by the treatment team members, from various disciplines, at formal meetings at designated time intervals.

Mother says to the nurse clinical specialist and the unit nurse: "I hope you will fix him so I can take him home soon. How soon can I visit?"

During the next few days, Len tests the staff by refusing to comply with unit rules, such as refusing to get out of bed and refusing to complete hygiene tasks without several prompts and using cuss words. Len loses his temper with peers and staff. Peers accuse him of hiding their belongings and playing pranks on them, which he denies and blames on someone else.

At a meeting of the staff in which Len's case is discussed, treatment team members from the various disciplines offer input about Len's behavior since admission. The psychiatrist suggests a diagnosis of Oppositional Defiant Disorder. Len and his mother meet with the treatment team. Len is given his diagnosis, and it is explained to him. His input and his mother's input are sought in regard to treatment goals and interventions. Len's response to the team is: "I am not oppositional and I am not defiant. You are all wrong and stupid."

Questions

1. If you were the nurse admitting Len to the unit, how would you respond to Len when he crosses his fingers, rolls his eyes, and winks at his mother before signing the rules agreement form? Give a rationale for your response.

2. How could you as a staff nurse develop some rapport with Len? How would you develop rapport and a trusting relationship with the client's family?

3. You are assigned to have a one on one with this client and he says he has nothing to say and you cannot make him talk. How would you react to this?

4. The health care provider asks you and the rest of the staff to identify behaviors in this client that match the diagnosis of Oppositional Defiant behavior. Does the client have behaviors that match the criteria for this disorder?

Questions (continued)

5. What if you as a staff nurse decide you don't like some of the interventions that the team has implemented and you would like to try something different? Can you do this?

6. One of the staff asks you: "What causes Oppositional Defiant Disorder?" What would you reply?

7. What nursing diagnoses would you write for this client? What goals would you write for this client?

8. Would you expect this child to be on medication to treat Oppositional Defiant Disorder? What

interventions do you think would work with this client?

9. The client talks with his mother on the phone and convinces his mother that he is better and asks her to come get him. He has not been discharged. How would you convince the mother that her son is not ready to be discharged?

10. Is there a link between Oppositional Defiant Disorder and Conduct Disorder and is there a link between ODD and ADHD?

Brandon

GENDER

Male

AGE

14

SETTING

- Pediatric unit of hospital

ETHNICITY

- White American

CULTURAL CONSIDERATIONS

PREEXISTING CONDITION

COEXISTING CONDITIONS

- Seizure disorder and mild mental retardation

COMMUNICATION

DISABILITY

- Impaired social interaction

SOCIOECONOMIC

- Middle to upper-middle income family

SPIRITUAL/RELIGIOUS

PHARMACOLOGIC

- Carbamazepine (Tegretol)
- Vicodin

PSYCHOSOCIAL

- Withdraws from others
- Limited speech
- Poor social skills
- Dependent on parents for help with activities of daily living

LEGAL

- Need for informed consent to gather information from health care providers and others outside the hospital system

ETHICAL

ALTERNATIVE THERAPY

PRIORITIZATION

DELEGATION

AUTISTIC DISORDER

Level of difficulty: High

Overview: Requires using the usual caregiver as a resource in planning and implementing care for a child who has Autistic Disorder and does not relate well to people. Requires prioritization of clients and determination of tasks to be delegated.

DIFFICULT

Client Profile

Brandon is a 14-year-old boy who was diagnosed with Autistic Disorder just before his third birthday. His older sister Anne also has Autistic Disorder. Three other siblings do not have the disorder. As a toddler Brandon would go off by himself and when people tried to get near him, he would make flapping motions and strike out at them. He has always been sensitive to clothing touching him, refusing to wear any rough feeling or new clothing. When seasons change his mother has to hide Brandon's old clothes or he would insist on wearing winter clothing in summer and summer clothes in winter. Brandon loves to put pebbles or marbles in a container then take them out and put them back one by one. He plays with a piece of string, a rubber band, or a small stick for hours. Brandon did not have very many words or sounds until he was enrolled in an early childhood education program prior to going to preschool. The speech therapist and teachers' aides worked very hard with him until he had sufficient vocabulary to make some of his needs known and to communicate in simple words and to give a hug to people who are familiar to him. He can use a message board if someone holds his elbow in a certain way. He exhibits echolalia. Brandon does not make eye contact with others, and sometimes people say he looks like he is in his own world. The teachers and mother get his attention by holding his face up or pinching his arm and using behavior modification rewarding techniques for his doing or saying what they are asking of him. Brandon sometimes rocks his body in a stereotypical fashion. He gets very upset when things are moved around in his room, his home, or in the classroom. Brandon plays tee-ball in a special league for kids with special needs, and he is very proud of his tee-ball uniform. He collects baseball cards and has them in a certain order. If they are out of order, he works hard to get them back in order. He often uses headphones and listens to music.

Brandon is a big boy for his age, nearly 6 feet tall, 200-plus pounds, and muscular. He is difficult to handle when he is upset. His mother is a petite women, and she has gotten a few bruises when interacting with Brandon and has had to stop the car sometimes when Brandon was pulling her hair or throwing things in the car. Brandon's father helps with Brandon when he is home, but the father travels with his job and is often away from home for several days.

Case Study

Brandon was practicing playing ball at home in the yard. His sister threw the ball in the street, and Brandon ran after it with his mother close behind yelling at him to stop. Brandon was hit by a car and taken by ambulance to the emergency room where he had a seizure and was moved to ICU for observation and treatment with Valium and an anticonvulsant. After about twenty-four hours he was moved to the pediatric unit of the hospital and admitted for further observation. He has a fractured radius, and his arm is scheduled to be casted in the morning. The pediatric nurse assigned to care for Brandon and admit him to the pediatric unit observes that he is clearly upset as he makes all kinds of sounds and is flapping his arms. Brandon won't let anyone come near him. This is problematic as the health care provider wants Brandon's forearm in a splint wrapped with an ace bandage, the lower arm elevated in a sling, and an ice pack applied. The provider also orders carbamazepine (Tegretol) two times a day, Vicodin for pain as necessary, and bed rest.

Brandon's mother is near hysterical and crying. She tells the pediatric nurse that the ambulance personnel did not want her to ride in the ambulance with Brandon, although she advised the ambulance personnel that they would soon wish she were with Brandon. She relates that the same thing happened in ICU at the hospital. The

ICU nurse did not want to have Brandon's mother stay with him in ICU without documentation she was the legal guardian. Within minutes of asking the mother to leave ICU, the ICU nurse assigned to Brandon came to get the mother to help her with Brandon. The mother did have to telephone Brandon's father and ask him to fax proof she is a legal guardian.

The pediatric nurse assigned to Brandon has been listening to Brandon's mother tell her story, but realizes that there are three other assigned clients as well as Brandon. The nurse is to give two pediatric clients their 9 A.M. medicines that are ordered and do a specific gravity on the urine of the third client. It is now 8:55 A.M. A preoperative medication must be given to a burn client at 9 A.M. prior to going to a whirlpool treatment. Brandon still needs his forearm wrapped and elevated in a sling with an ice pack. He gets upset and strikes out at the nurse (but misses) when the nurse tries to give him a hospital gown and asks him to put it on.

Questions

1. What is going on with the mother that she is near hysterical and crying, and what would be a good response if you were the nurse in this case?

2. Assuming you were the nurse in this case and looking at the clients assigned to you and their needs, what would be your first and second priorities? What sort of things would make Brandon's care a first priority to you? Could you delegate some of the tasks that you have to do, and if so, what and under what circumstances?

3. What is Autistic Disorder (AD), and does Brandon have behaviors that meet the criteria for AD? Do all children with AD have the same symptoms as Brandon?

4. How would you approach getting Brandon to wear the hospital gown and stay in bed? How would you get Brandon's splint on his arm and get it wrapped and put ice on it?

5. How would you figure out when Brandon is in pain and in need of a pain pill?

6. Brandon needs to urinate, and his mother wants to take him to the bathroom. She insists he will be upset if he urinates in the bed, and he won't understand the urinal. Brandon is on bed rest. How would you handle this situation?

7. Brandon's parents ask you several questions including: "What are the current theories about the cause of Autism?" "What is the prevalence/incidence of Autism, and is it more prevalent in one gender compared to the other or not?" "What is the usual onset of Autistic Disorder?" and "What disorders or medical problems are commonly associated with Autism?" What would you include in your answer?

8. Discuss any assessments you need to do. What nursing diagnoses and goals would you write for Brandon, and what interventions would you include in the plan of care?

9. What would you need to know, and want to make sure the mother knows, about carbamazepine (Tegretol)?

10. What research is being done in the field of Pervasive Developmental Disorders including Autism and Asperger's Disorder/Syndrome? Is there research into families in which than one child has an Autism Spectrum Disorder?

Christine

GENDER	**SPIRITUAL/RELIGIOUS**
Female	
AGE	**PHARMACOLOGIC**
8	
SETTING	**PSYCHOSOCIAL**
■ School nurse's office	■ No close relationships with peers due to fear something will happen to mother if not near mother
ETHNICITY	
■ White American	**LEGAL**
CULTURAL CONSIDERATIONS	■ School attendance
■ American culture values independence	**ETHICAL**
PREEXISTING CONDITION	■ Forcing child to work through anxiety and go to school versus homeschooling and not distressing child
COEXISTING CONDITION	
	ALTERNATIVE THERAPY
COMMUNICATION	
	PRIORITIZATION
DISABILITY	
	DELEGATION
SOCIOECONOMIC	

SEPARATION ANXIETY DISORDER

Level of difficulty: Moderate

Overview: Requires awareness of behaviors associated with Separation Anxiety Disorder in order to identify children at risk for this disorder The nurse must work cooperatively with the parent, teacher and others, as well as the child, to plan and utilize interventions to resolve issues associated with separation anxiety.

Client Profile

Christine is an 8-year-old female who becomes very anxious when separated from her mother. She refuses to go to school or to stay there. Christine clings to her mother and cries and begs her not to leave her in the morning when she takes Christine to school. Christine has not made friends with peers. Christine recently tried to stay overnight at the house of a girl who wants to be her friend. Within an hour of arriving at the girl's home, she began describing fears that something bad was going to happen to her mother, so she was permitted to call home several times. Each time she learned that everything was fine. She did not eat much at dinner, complaining she was allergic to everything or did not like it. At bedtime, she began to cry because she had forgotten her pillow from home and she wanted her mother to bring it or to go home and get it. About 2 A.M., when she called home again, her mother came to get her. Christine's mother describes her as like a shadow, saying that Christine won't let her out of her sight at home. Most nights she comes and gets into the parents' bed because she is fearful of not being close to mother. She hears a siren in the dark and thinks the ambulance is coming for her mother.

Case Study

Christine comes to the school nurse's office complaining of a stomachache and wanting her mother to come and get her and take her home. When the nurse calls the home, no one answers the phone. The school nurse offers to call the father at work and have him come and take her home. Christine says, "No, I don't want my father to come for me." Christine seems very upset until she recalls her mother was going to the dentist. The school nurse is aware that Christine has been falling behind her class in schoolwork due to having her mother come and get her and take her home from school two or three times a week. Christine asks the school nurse: "Would you please call the dentist's office to see if my mother is there and if she is all right? Could you ask her to come get me and take me home when she is finished at the dentist's office?" The nurse makes the call and then asks Christine if there has been a time in which her mother was sick or a time in which she worried about mom.

When the mother arrives at the school, she tells Christine that she can't keep taking her out of school and that she must learn to stay in school. When the nurse says: "It sounds like you are concerned that Christine stay in school," the mother replies: "Why wouldn't I be with the school truancy officer calling and coming to the house? Besides that she won't pass this grade if her attendance does not get better."

The mother asks the school nurse if she thinks Christine could have school phobia and wants to know if she should homeschool Christine.

When the nurse asks Christine's mother whether there was a time when she was sick and Christine worried about her, the mother shares that two years ago when Christine's sister was born, she was in labor for an extended time and then had to have a caesarian section. The sister was premature and had to remain in the hospital for a month. The mother had a number of complications, almost died, and also was in the hospital for three weeks. The nurse asks how long Christine has been like a shadow to her and worried about her. The mother answers that it has been about two years, although it has been worse since summer vacation ended six weeks ago.

Questions

1. What could you do instead of calling the mother to come get Christine? What would you do if you could not reach the mother?

2. Christine's mother has asked if Christine could have school phobia. How would you answer, and what is your rationale?

3. Could Christine have Separation Anxiety Disorder? Does her behavior match any of the criteria for Separation Anxiety Disorder?

4. Why does the nurse ask Christine and then her mother if there was a time when the mother was sick and Christine was worried about her mother?

5. What causes Separation Anxiety Disorder? What is the usual course of Separation Anxiety Disorder?

6. Christine's mother asks: "Are there many other children who have difficulty separating from their mothers at school age?" How would you answer her?

7. At what developmental stage (according to Erickson) is Christine, what are the tasks of this stage, and is she mastering these tasks? Christine's mother asks the school nurse if she should home-school Christine. What would you say to her if you were the school nurse?

8. What treatments have been found to be successful in reducing separation anxiety from major attachment figures?

9. From the information you have about Christine, what nursing diagnoses would you write for her? What are some reasonable goals for Christine?

10. What interventions do you think would work for this client, and how could you go about getting the mother and teacher(s) invested in initiating these interventions? How would you evaluate success of interventions?

Phyu

GENDER	**DISABILITY**
Female	**SOCIOECONOMIC**
AGE	■ Middle class
7	**SPIRITUAL/RELIGIOUS**
SETTING	
■ School nurse's office	**PHARMACOLOGIC**
ETHNICITY	
■ Asian American (Myanmar, formerly called Burma)	**PSYCHOSOCIAL**
	■ Shy and selective mute
CULTURAL CONSIDERATIONS	**LEGAL**
■ Military culture and Asian (Myanmar)	
	ETHICAL
PREEXISTING CONDITION	
	ALTERNATIVE THERAPY
COEXISTING CONDITION	
■ Possible Social Phobia	**PRIORITIZATION**
COMMUNICATION	
	DELEGATION

MODERATE

SELECTIVE MUTISM

Level of difficulty: Moderate

Overview: Requires enlisting the cooperation of the client's family, teacher, and peers to work together to help the client feel safe and motivated to talk out loud in a variety of settings and to a variety of people.

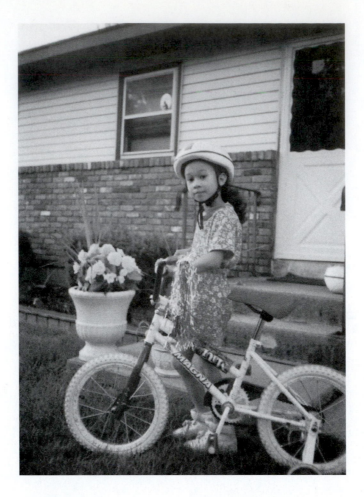

Client Profile

Phyu (pronounced Pee You) is 7 years old and lives with her mother and stepfather and an older sister. Her biological father lives in Myanmar (formerly Burma). Phyu's stepfather is a career military officer and currently on duty away from the family. The mother is from Myanmar. Phyu's mother and stepfather met in Bangkok where her mother had a job and the stepfather was on leave from the service. Phyu has moved frequently with her family, living first in Myanmar until her mother remarried, then on two different military bases in Asian countries. Recently the family moved to a small town in the Northwest near Phyu's stepfather's relatives while her stepfather was away on active duty.

Phyu has always been shy around distant relatives, strangers, and in strange situations. At 5 years old, she was talking to her sister in both English and the Myanmar language, but would not talk to anyone else. The parents and teacher did not worry about it the first month of school because they thought she was just shy and would start talking as soon as she got used to being in a different country and being at school. After the second month of not talking at school, the parents took Phyu to a pediatrician who diagnosed Phyu as having Selective Mutism. The parents thought Phyu would grow out of this problem, but it has persisted and now she is in the second grade and still does not talk in school.

Case Study

An older sister has brought Phyu to the school nurse's office. Phyu looks serious and somewhat sad. When the nurse asks her a question, Phyu plays with her hair, looks at the floor, and says nothing. The older sister talks for Phyu, saying that Phyu came to school this morning even though she was not feeling well and that she is now feeling worse and wants to go home. The school nurse starts to talk to Phyu, and her sister says: "She doesn't talk." The school nurse takes Phyu's temperature, and it is normal. Talking through the sister to Phyu, the school nurse learns that Phyu does not hurt anywhere but is "feeling bad." The school nurse asks Phyu and her sister to remain in the office and goes to talk briefly with the teacher. The teacher explains that the children in Phyu's class were going to be doing oral presentations, and a peer had teased her about her inability to talk in class and said: "I bet you won't give your report because the cat has got your tongue." Phyu was diagnosed with Selective Mutism when she was 5 years old, the teacher explains to the school nurse. The teacher says: "I would really appreciate it if you would work with me to find ways to help Phyu succeed at school. Perhaps you could get her mother involved in working with us. So far I have not had any luck getting the mother to participate in anything at school or to talk with me about Phyu on the phone."

Questions

1. If you were the school nurse, how would you respond to Phyu's request to go home?

2. You are the nurse in this case, and you decide to call the mother to come in and talk with you and the teacher. What action will you take if Phyu's mother offers a number of excuses for not coming to school to meet with you? What could be going on with the mother if she refuses to come to school for a discussion?

3. What is Selective Mutism? Which of the diagnostic criteria of Selective Mutism does Phyu meet?

4. When one of Phyu's teachers asks: "What causes Selective Mutism?" and "How common is Selective Mutism?" what will you tell him or her?

5. Does this client fit the usual pattern for age of onset of Selective Mutism? Is Selective Mutism found equally in boys and girls or not? What other disorders are frequently diagnosed concurrently with Selective Mutism?

6. What are children with Selective Mutism like?

7. What role do you think culture might play in this case?

8. What additional data would you like to gather on this child? What tentative nursing diagnoses would you likely write for this client? Working with Phyu's teachers and hopefully Phyu and her mother, what goals would be reasonable for Phyu?

9. What approach/interventions would you suggest to Phyu's mother, family, and teachers?

10. Why do you suppose some parents whose children have Selective Mutism don't want to get professional help for their children? Why do experts urge early diagnosis and treatment for children with Selective Mutism rather than waiting it out to see if it disappears?

11. In a conversation with the mother, she asks: "Is medication ever used to treat Selective Mutism, and if so, what medications?" How would you respond? What are the treatment approaches in addition to or instead of medication that are currently being used with children and adolescents?

CASE STUDY 5

Theera

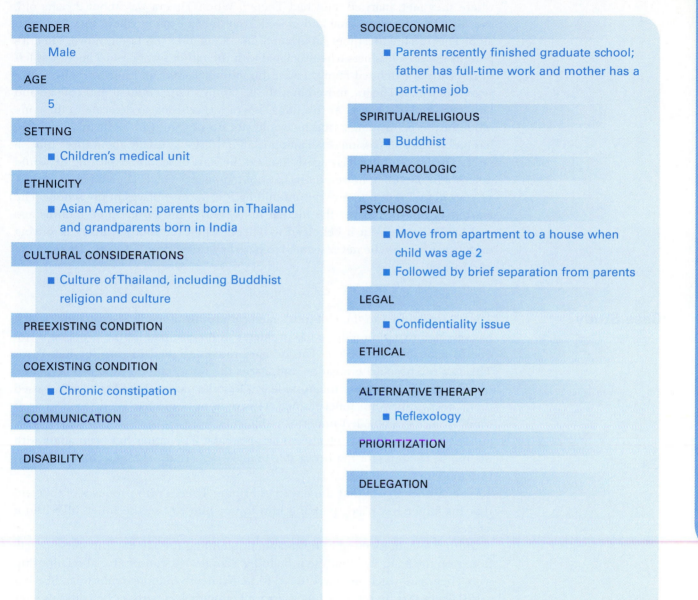

GENDER

Male

AGE

5

SETTING

- Children's medical unit

ETHNICITY

- Asian American: parents born in Thailand and grandparents born in India

CULTURAL CONSIDERATIONS

- Culture of Thailand, including Buddhist religion and culture

PREEXISTING CONDITION

COEXISTING CONDITION

- Chronic constipation

COMMUNICATION

DISABILITY

SOCIOECONOMIC

- Parents recently finished graduate school; father has full-time work and mother has a part-time job

SPIRITUAL/RELIGIOUS

- Buddhist

PHARMACOLOGIC

PSYCHOSOCIAL

- Move from apartment to a house when child was age 2
- Followed by brief separation from parents

LEGAL

- Confidentiality issue

ETHICAL

ALTERNATIVE THERAPY

- Reflexology

PRIORITIZATION

DELEGATION

MODERATE

ENCOPRESIS

Level of difficulty: Moderate

Overview: Requires critical thinking/problem solving to develop rapport with a 5-year-old client and get him to voluntarily give up defecating in his underwear and to use the toilet for this purpose. Requires supporting not only the client but his parents, who are frustrated, angry, and embarrassed at times.

Client Profile

Theera is a 5-year-old boy who was born in the United States to parents from Thailand. His parents came to this country to attend graduate school, and that is where they met, married, and had Theera. When Theera was about 2 years old, they purchased a new home and moved from the apartment where they had lived all of Theera's life to a quiet suburban home. Soon after this family move, Theera's parents left on a business trip associated with the father's work and Theera was left in the care of extended family. Later, the mother's sister and her son, who is two years older than Theera, moved in with the family so she could attend college and help take care of Theera. At this time Theera was refusing to defecate in the commode in the bathroom, saying he would not do this until he went to school. He has had periods of passing small amounts of hard stool, usually about three times a week. Theera's mother has eagerly awaited the start of school, expecting he would defecate in the toilet; however, this has not happened. Once Theera began school, he started soiling his underwear and hiding it in various places in the school. The teacher began to discover the hidden underwear a little over three months ago and finally figured out it belonged to Theera when the mother, tiring of buying underwear because he never seemed to have any clean, decided to put labels in the underwear.

Case Study

Theera is admitted to the children's medical unit for a medical evaluation, which has revealed that although he has problems with constipation, the problem is not due to a medical condition. The primary nurse assigned to care for him reads Theera's psychosocial evaluation and learns the information in the profile above. In talking with the mother the nurse learns that the parents have been embarrassed that Theera still is not toilet trained. His room at home has been so odorous at times from hidden soiled underwear that they were embarrassed to have guests, and the cousin made fun of Theera being a baby. The father has been angry with the mother at times for not being able to make Theera use the toilet and "babying" him too much.

The mother shares that she has tried bribing Theera with promises of toys and that his father has tried spanking him to get him to use the toilet, all without success.

During a team meeting to do treatment planning for Theera, the nurse practitioner on the team says that she is building a somewhat conspiratorial relationship with Theera in which she has offered to help Theera hide his underwear. She has told Theera that he is not hiding them well enough and perhaps he could use her help to hide them better.

The nurse practitioner also shares reading about a social worker who has had good luck working with children with Encopresis to get them to not let the "poop" be the boss, much in the way children learn not to let bullies get the best of them. Some of the team members tell the primary nurse that they think these ideas are crazy and what this child needs is laxatives, suppositories, and/or enemas followed with bowel training as well as limit setting.

Questions

1. What are some common feelings nurses might have when working with a child who soils his underwear and hides it in inappropriate places like under his bed or in the dresser drawers? What are some responses that parents might have to a child with Encopresis?

2. What rationale could the nurse practitioner have had for offering to help Theera hide his underwear?

3. What are the criteria for a diagnosis of Encopresis, and do you think Theera meets these criteria?

4. You are teaching an in-service education on Encopresis for your peers. How would you respond to questions regarding the cause and incidence of Encopresis and how Encopresis relates to constipation and soiling?

5. What kinds of varied treatments are being utilized to treat children with constipation, and what treatments are used for Encopresis?

6. Define and discuss reflexology as a treatment for Encopresis.

7. Theera's Aunt comes to visit him. She asks you to tell her what the doctor has said about Theera's problem. She also tells you that she wants to give you some information about Theera and the family. What is your response to her request for information and her offer to give you information?

8. What do you think about the social worker's idea of talking to the child about being boss over the poop?

9. The mother mentions that she has gone to the Buddhist temple to take food and robes for the monks, light incense, and get a wish about Theera offered up to Buddha. She says she thinks this problem with his not going to the toilet may have something to do with Theera's past lives. What would be an acceptable response given that you are not of the Buddhist religion?

10. What nursing diagnoses and treatment goals would you likely write for Theera? What interventions do you think would be helpful for this child and his family?

GENDER

Female

AGE

7

SETTING

- School nurse's office

ETHNICITY

- White American

CULTURAL CONSIDERATIONS

PREEXISTING CONDITION

COEXISTING CONDITION

COMMUNICATION

DISABILITY

SOCIOECONOMIC

SPIRITUAL/RELIGIOUS

PHARMACOLOGIC

- Desmopressin (DDAVP) tablets or spray

PSYCHOSOCIAL

- Does not accept invitations for overnight stays from peers due to bedwetting

LEGAL

ETHICAL

ALTERNATIVE THERAPY

- Alarm to alert of wetness at night and behavior modification
- Relaxation therapy

PRIORITIZATION

DELEGATION

ENURESIS

Level of difficulty: Moderate

Overview: Requires an understanding of Enuresis and its possible causes. Requires patience, empathy, and ability to use creative thinking to develop interventions utilizing a knowledge of the way children think and behave according to their developmental level.

Client Profile

Penny is a 7-year-old girl who wets the bed at night, nearly every night, and has done so since she was a baby. Her father is upset with her because he says he is tired of the smell of urine-soaked sheets and her mother having to get up at night to help her change her bed. The father often drinks several beers after work at night. He tends to be angry with her when he is drinking. When he is drinking too much, he makes Penny get out of bed at night and wash her own wet bedsheets. Penny's father calls her lazy and stupid and says she will never learn to get out of bed and go to the bathroom at night and she won't ever have a boyfriend or a husband because no one wants a bed wetter.

Penny is upset with herself not only because of what her father says to her but also because she cannot stay overnight with anyone from school or have anyone stay overnight with her until she stops wetting the bed. Her self-esteem and confidence in herself is so low that she never tries to make friends. Penny stays dry during the day, but at night she awakes with her pajamas and bedsheets wet. Penny's mother wet the bed when she was Penny's age, but she has not talked with Penny about it as she is embarrassed and is afraid of her husband being angry. She feels guilty and ashamed about this secret.

Case Study

In school one day, Penny asks the teacher if she can go to the bathroom and the teacher asks her to wait until she finishes a spelling test. Penny wets her underpants and is sent to the school nurse's office to get cleaned up. The school nurse encourages Penny to talk about how she feels about wetting her underpants and then asks her if she realizes that this happens to lots of other children. The school nurse reveals that when she was a child, she wet her own bed at night for several years. Penny replies that this is the first time that she has wet her underpants in the daytime but that she does wet her bed at night too. She wishes that she could stop doing this, but she says she will probably wet her bed all her life because her father said she would. The school nurse offers to talk to Penny's parents and to try to get them to help her stop wetting the bed at night: "Please let me talk to them about helping you stop bedwetting. I believe you can stop the bedwetting. It may take some time and some work, but it can be done."

Questions

1. What is Enuresis? Are there subtypes of Enuresis?

2. If you were the school nurse and you had wet the bed as a child, would you share with a child that you had also wet the bed?

3. If you were the school nurse, how would you approach getting the parents to discuss what to do for Penny?

4. If Penny's parents refuse to meet with you and refuse to get her treatment, will her bedwetting at night resolve itself? What can Penny's parents and others like them try in order to resolve their child's bedwetting? Will this take a commitment on the part of the parents and mean a change in their behavior?

5. What is the usual course of Enuresis?

6. Does Enuresis typically run in families, and does it occur equally in both genders or in one more than the other? What is the incidence of Enuresis?

7. The parents do meet with you, and the father asks you "What causes bedwetting? Is it laziness?" What would you tell the father?

Questions (continued)

8. The mother asks if it is possible that Penny's bedwetting is due to a medical cause. How would you respond if you were the school nurse?

9. The parents would like to know if there is some treatment for bedwetting. The mother has heard that one of the neighbor children took some pills to stop it. What are the current treatments for Enuresis?

10. What assessment information would you like to have in order to write a nursing care plan on this client?

11. What nursing diagnoses and goals would you likely write for this client and her family? What nursing interventions would you likely initiate?

GENDER

F

AGE

89

SETTING

- Home of client's daughter

ETHNICITY

- Black American

CULTURAL CONSIDERATIONS

PREEXISTING CONDITION

- Pernicious anemia

COEXISTING CONDITION

COMMUNICATION

- Requires hearing aides to hear

DISABILITY

- Difficulty hearing

SOCIOECONOMIC

- Upper middle class

SPIRITUAL/RELIGIOUS

- Methodist

PHARMACOLOGIC

- Anticholinergic medication
- Donepezil (Aricept)

PSYCHOSOCIAL

- Sits with old friends in Sunday school and with daughter in church: cannot recall events of the past or read bible verses but sings old familiar songs of her childhood

LEGAL

- Claiming power of attorney for a parent or declaring parent incompetent and getting guardianship

ETHICAL

- Ethical issue around making decisions for grown parents

ALTERNATIVE THERAPY

- Music therapy

PRIORITIZATION

DELEGATION

DEMENTIA OF THE ALZHEIMER'S TYPE

Level of difficulty: Moderate

Overview: Requires the nurse to be knowledgeable about Alzheimer's Disease and its stages. Nurse must do more explanations and teaching with the client's caregiver since the client has difficulty understanding or recalling what the nurse has explained to her. The nurse needs to determine when and if it is appropriate to see that the caregiver gets information about declaring the client incompetent or getting the power of attorney and about respite care.

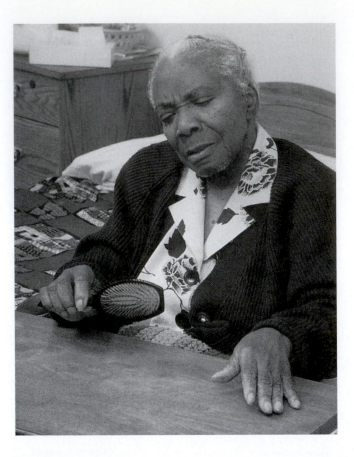

Client Profile

Hannah is an 89-year-old woman who had been living in her own home for years and fiercely protecting her independence from her five grown children. Hannah drove her car until she was 87 and did her own cooking, but had a cleaning woman come once a week. Women friends came on Sunday to take her to Sunday school and church. Hannah had been married three times, and one day in Sunday school she was asked to tell about her last husband who was now dead. She could not recall anything about him, including his name, so she said to a friend: "You tell about him." She did enjoy singing old familiar hymns and being with her women friends of many years. Hannah began to get even more forgetful, frequently forgetting the names of the grandchildren and her own children and covering this by calling them all "sugar." She began to pay some of her bills more than once, and when the daughter, Jean, found this out, she hired someone to live in with her mother and took over the bill paying. Jean decided to let her mother keep her car keys, but secretly took the battery out of the car. Hannah tried to start the car every day and would call Jean to tell her the car wasn't working, and Jean would say she had called someone to come repair it. The next day Hannah would forget that the car wasn't working and would try to start it again.

Within a week of Jean hiring someone to live with her, Hannah fired the woman. Jean decided to take her mother to live with her, about a ninety-minute drive from Hannah's home. Jean works out of her home and believed she could work and look after her mother without any problem; however, problems started as soon as Hannah arrived at Jean's home. Hannah begged people who called or came to visit her daughter to take her home. She would offer them money and say she was kidnapped. She fell and decided to stay in her bed and refused to get up. The daughter was unsure if her mother had broken her hip or not. Jean was concerned that her mother might be anemic because she had been diagnosed with pernicious anemia and was receiving B12 injections monthly before coming to live with Jean. Hannah lost five pounds after moving in with her daughter Jean. The weight loss was puzzling since her mother had a voracious appetite and seemed to eat enough for two people, demanding food several times a day in between meals and telling people "that woman is starving me." Jean decided to call a home health service that would send a home health nurse and a health care providers to the home and would draw blood for lab tests and send a mobile x-ray unit.

Case Study

A home heath agency nurse has come to visit Hannah at her daughter's home. Hannah offers the nurse a hundred dollars to take her home. Hannah whispers to the nurse that if she had car keys, she would drive herself home. The nurse fluffs up Hannah's pillows and chats with her awhile about her little dog. The nurse talks Hannah into letting him look at her hearing aids and check the batteries and into agreeing to wear the hearing aides. Hannah tells her daughter that she will wear the hearing aides "because that nice nurse wants me to wear them." After awhile the nurse gets Hannah to agree to have blood drawn for CBC, HIV, and thyroid tests. A portable X-ray technician is called to come and get an X-ray of Hannah's hip.

The nurse asks Jean if she has any old pictures of Hannah's parents or siblings and discovers a wedding picture of the parents. Hannah immediately identifies her parents. The nurse tests Hannah's orientation and finds she does not know the year, month, or day. Hannah thinks it is 1941. She refers to her daughter as "that woman who kidnapped me." The nurse does a Mini Multi-State Examination (MMSE).

The nurses talks to the client before leaving and tells her that a "nice doctor" will read the X-ray and review the results of the lab tests and make a home visit to see her. The nurse adds: "You will like the doctor."

In private, Jean shares with the nurse that her mother has been demanding and is wearing her down. Jean says her mother sleeps until noon, but stays up until dawn watching television, which she misinterprets because she can't hear it (e.g., Hannah thought the television said that local onions were poisoned and then she accused Jean of poisoning her). Jean describes efforts to be nice to her mother. She took her out to eat, but the next morning the mother did not recall going out to eat and accused Jean of starving her and holding her "prisoner in a dark place."

Hannah's son comes to visit, and in a moment of clarity she calls him by name and says, "Oh my, that woman in there must be your sister and she is trying to help me." Later Hannah refers again to Jean as "that woman" and does not seem to know her.

After reviewing the X-ray and lab tests, as well as the Mini Multi-State Examination and the past health history, and examining Hannah, the health care provider decides Hannah's hip is not broken and notes that she has a history of pernicious anemia and probably has Alzheimer's Disease. He writes orders for a B12 injection every week for three weeks, then every month; a home health aide for assistance with hygiene tasks; and prescribes 5 mg of donepezil (Aricept) daily.

Questions

1. Why did the nurse take time to chat with Hannah about her dog and fluff up her pillows? Why did the nurse check the batteries of the hearing aides and want her to wear hearing aides? What else does the nurse need to do at this point?

2. Why could the client identify her parents from an old picture and not recall the names of her children or grandchildren or the day, month, or year? Why can she recall words of songs, and what implications does this have for interventions?

3. Why did the nurse make a point of telling Hannah that the health care provider who would come would be very nice? What would you do or say differently if you were the nurse in this case? What in particular are the provider and nurse hoping to learn from the CBC, thyroid, and HIV laboratory tests?

4. The health care provider has diagnosed pernicious anemia for this client. Do you have reason to believe that pernicious anemia is the cause of this dementia? What is pernicious anemia?

5. What do you think of Jean's idea of taking the battery out of the car and letting Hannah try to start it every day?

6. If you were the nurse, would you mention to Hannah's daughter the possibility of having her mother declared incompetent in court at some point and becoming her mother's legal guardian?

7. The client's daughter asks you to explain what Alzheimer's Disease is. She also wants to know about the stages and incidence of Alzheimer's Disease. How would you respond to these questions?

8. What are the diagnostic criteria for dementia of the Alzheimer's type, and do you think this client matches those criteria?

9. Is there a definitive test for Alzheimer's Disease? What is the Mini Multi-State Exam that the health care provider ordered for Hannah?

10. What are the current theories of causation of Alzheimer's Disease?

11. What treatments are currently being used with Alzheimer's clients?

12. If you were the nurse in this case, what teaching would you do with the client and her daughter about donepezil (Aricept)? What do you need to know about the drug? If the client refuses to take her Aricept when offered by her daughter, what would you recommend?

13. The client's daughter says she has a fear and a reoccurring nightmare that she will eventually need to place her mother in a facility that cares for people with Alzheimer's, but she wants to keep her at home. Keeping in mind Black American culture, what questions, comments, or suggestions would you have for Jean at this time? Do you think Jean needs support, and if so, what kinds of support would you suggest?

14. What assessment data would you like to have if you were the nurse writing a nursing care plan for this client? What nursing diagnoses, goals, and interventions would you likely write for this client?

Elias

GENDER

Male

AGE

15

SETTING

- Alternative high school health classes with school nurse

ETHNICITY

- White American and Black American

CULTURAL CONSIDERATIONS

PREEXISTING CONDITIONS

- Learning disabilities

COEXISTING CONDITIONS

- Alcohol abuse

COMMUNICATION

DISABILITY

SOCIOECONOMIC

- Ward of state; qualifies for free school lunch

SPIRITUAL/RELIGIOUS

PHARMACOLOGIC

PSYCHOSOCIAL

- Current: sexually aggressive with girlfriend
- Early childhood: Father in prison
- Mother charged with neglect
- Multiple foster care situations

LEGAL

- On probation after serving sentence in juvenile justice system

ETHICAL

- Nurse contemplating adoption of client

ALTERNATIVE THERAPY

PRIORITIZATION

DELEGATION

DIFFICULT

CONDUCT DISORDER

Level of difficulty: High

Overview: Requires adhering to mental health principles that all people have worth and that all people can and do change. Requires maintaining a professional and helping therapeutic manner without losing sight of the need for setting consistent limits.

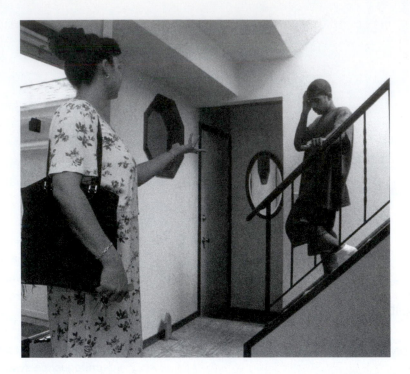

Client Profile

Elias is a 15-year-old male. His father is white American and his mother is black American. His father suddenly left the family when Elias was 7 years old. He later learned his father is in prison. Elias's mother tried to raise him and work two jobs. Elias started hanging out with a group of boys with a reputation for skipping school and drinking when he was 12 years old. A neighbor accused him of trying to drown her cat. He denied this, saying he was only trying to see if the cat could swim. The neighbor reported Elias's mother for neglect based on this and other instances of Elias getting into trouble while his mother was working. Elias became a ward of the state and was placed with a series of foster families. He has a reputation for starting fights and cutting a boy's face with his ring. The school expelled him because an ex-girlfriend accused him of threatening to hurt her if she didn't come back to him and have sex with him. The previous year a male student had killed his ex-girlfriend under similar circumstances, and the school was not about to risk a reoccurrence. In the past Elias has done some minor shoplifting without getting caught. About a year ago, he and some of his friends stole a car and decided to put on masks and costumes and rob people at knifepoint on Halloween. However, he chose an off-duty policeman to rob, and this ended in his being overpowered and arrested. He went to a state prison facility boot camp and a halfway house, then was placed with another foster family and returned to the public school system. He was not in the juvenile prison system long enough to get a GED and job training, but he did learn to live in a very structured system. Although he has learning disabilities, he made some progress in the prison education system in his reading skills.

Case Study

Elias is taking classes at an alternative high school with more flexible hours and programs for high school students who need to work, who have children, or who have been discipline problems and respond better in a structured, goal-oriented environment. Elias is taking a health course from a school nurse. The schools nurse gives Elias extra duties in the classroom and extra homework projects. He willingly completes the tasks. The school nurse tells Elias she is interested in his reading progress and offers to help him in reading or to assign a student with good reading skills to help him. The school nurse experienced trouble reading when she was a child, but received a lot of help and managed to compensate for some learning difficulties.

The school nurse receives a notice that she needs to come to a meeting of Elias's teachers and support staff. Elias has been having some discipline problems in one of his classes. The school nurse is surprised to hear this as Elias behaves well in health class.

In the faculty lounge waiting for the meeting about Elias to begin, the school nurse supervisor overhears two teachers talking about Elias. The general theme of their conversation is that they read his school records from the state juvenile corrections system and discovered that he has a diagnosis of Conduct Disorder (CD). One of the teachers says Elias is never going to amount to anything because he has Conduct Disorder. The other teacher says Elias is draining resources from other students as he will eventually go to prison. When the school nurse tries to talk with the teachers about Elias's good qualities, one of them suggests the school nurse adopt Elias if she likes him so well. The school nurse is not sure if the teacher is serious or not and begins to think the idea over.

Questions

1. If you were the school nurse in this case, would you have difficulty relating to Elias if he had been in prison for robbing someone at knifepoint? Would you treat him any differently if he had been imprisoned for doing or selling drugs? Describe an attitude and approach you and other nurses need to take with an adolescent like Elias.

2. Was the nurse's approach consisting of asking for assistance and offering to help with learning to read an acceptable approach or not? Provide a rationale for your answer. If you were the nurse in this case, how could you begin to work on developing empathy for Elias?

3. What criteria did Elias have to match to be diagnosed with Conduct Disorder? What behaviors does he have that match this diagnosis? Is it possible to have a mild case of Conduct Disorder, and what are the subtypes of Conduct Disorder?

4. Describe what keeps Elias from being diagnosed with Oppositional Defiant Disorder or Antisocial Personality Disorder instead of Conduct Disorder.

5. What are some theories about the cause of Conduct Disorder? What is the prevalence of Conduct Disorder?

6. What are learning disorders? Are learning disorders more common in adolescents with Conduct Disorder?

7. What data do you think would be most helpful to gather on this client? What nursing diagnoses and goals would you write for this client? What interventions would be helpful? Who do you need to work with in carrying out interventions?

8. What therapies are currently being used to treat Conduct Disorder? What is the likelihood that treatment of Conduct Disorder will have success?

9. Where would nurses encounter children and adolescents with diagnoses of Conduct Disorder other than the public school system?

10. Why is it important to care about and for children and adolescents who have a diagnosis of Conduct Disorder or who have traits of the diagnosis?

11. What do you think about the nurse's thought of adopting this client? What would you do in her place?

Martin

GENDER	**SOCIOECONOMIC**
Male	
AGE	**SPIRITUAL/RELIGIOUS**
7	
SETTING	**PHARMACOLOGIC**
■ Community mental health center	■ Methylphenidate hydrochloride (Concerta)
ETHNICITY	**PSYCHOSOCIAL**
■ White American	
CULTURAL CONSIDERATIONS	**LEGAL**
PREEXISTING CONDITION	**ETHICAL**
COEXISTING CONDITION	**ALTERNATIVE THERAPY**
COMMUNICATION	**PRIORITIZATION**
DISABILITY	**DELEGATION**

ATTENTION-DEFICIT/HYPERACTIVITY DISORDER

Level of difficulty: High

Overview: Requires the nurse to keep an open mind about whether a child with Attention-Deficit/ Hyperactivity Disorder (ADHD) might benefit from stimulant medication. Requires the nurse to discipline herself to neither advise for or against the medication, but to use the nursing process to assess an individual child's behavior, determine the child's problems (nursing diagnoses), and intervene in appropriate ways. Critical thinking is required to come up with creative ways to keep the child and others around him safe and to help him succeed in school when he has impulsivity, hyperactivity, and a short attention span.

DIFFICULT

Client Profile

Martin (Marty) is a 7-year-old boy who has a history of being so active that his family and others describe him like he is battery or motor-driven. He lives with his divorced father, two uncles, an aunt, and grandparents. His mother was given custody in divorce proceedings, but she changed her mind about caring for him as a single parent and left him with the father. Since that time Marty has only seen his mother once. The father intends to go to court for custody when he has money to pay the lawyer and court costs.

Marty has gone nonstop from the time he gets up until he goes to bed at night since he was a toddler. Marty seems to have no concern for safety. At age four he bit into a live lamp cord, resulting in a serious burn and scarring of his lip. This condition was corrected by plastic surgery. On a walk with a cousin, he suddenly climbed over the fence around an electrical transformer station and refused to get out. His attention span is short, and he goes from activity to activity quickly. One minute he is pointing a bow and arrow at a family member and the next jumping on the furniture. When he was four years old, he discovered the fun of doing somersaults in the tub, and those supervising him fear he is going to hit his head on the faucets. The family takes turns watching him as he quickly tires a person out. Family members have noticed when they send him to get something he forgets to bring it back.

His teacher at school has sent notes home and had conferences to communicate his behavior at school, including interrupting others, not wanting to wait his turn, and not following directions like other children. His hand is frequently up, and he has something to say whether it is relevant or not. When other children are finishing work, he is doing something else. He gets out of his seat frequently. When the teacher gets him to sit in his seat and do his work, she notices his hands and feet are very "fidgety" and he makes careless mistakes. He seldom turns in assigned homework. His grandparents try to get him to read for them, but he says: "I don't want to." They find it nearly impossible to get him to sit and play quietly. The family and the teacher have all noticed that he is easily distracted by anything happening in his environment. He is an attractive child with a handsome smile. People tend to like him even though they don't like some of his behavior.

Case Study

Marty and his father have come to the community mental health center. Several people have suggested to the father that Marty might have ADHD. If he has this disorder, the father wants to see if the child psychiatrist will prescribe some medication and/or offer other help to increase Marty's attention span and slow him down a bit. Marty is into everything in the waiting room. He takes things out of the trash receptacle, throws some toys at the desk, climbs over and under chairs, turns the lights off and on, and then he runs behinds the desk and grabs one of the donuts the nursing staff have for coffee break. The father says to the nurse: "I'm sorry. Do you think he has ADHD?"

The nurse weighs Marty, measures his height, and gets vital signs and a preliminary history. The psychologist does some testing and asks a lot of questions and verifies the diagnosis of ADHD. The child psychiatrist also sees Marty and his father and prescribes methylphenidate hydrochloride (Concerta). The nurse does some teaching with the father and answers his questions. Next, the nurse asks the father about Marty's mother. The father reveals that the mother has custody of the child, but that the child lives with him. The nurse gets a release of information from the father so the treatment team can share information and obtain information from the mother. The nurse contracts the mother in regard to the medication. The mother says, "I don't want Marty to have Ritalin or any other drug that messes with his mind. I won't sign giving permission for him to be on drugs." She says: "I have read that Ritalin is prescribed for kids that don't need it. Marty just has more energy than most kids his age. He will grow out of it."

Questions

1. If you were the nurse in this case, what would you say to the father when he asks: "Do you think he (Marty) has ADHD?"

2. If you were the nurse in this case, what could you and other staff members do to make the time in the waiting room easier for the father and this very active child?

3. What behaviors does Marty have that match the criteria for Attention-Deficit/Hyperactivity Disorder (ADHD)? Looking at the criteria, what type of ADHD do you think he would most likely have?

4. What would you tell the father about Concerta, the medication prescribed for his son?

5. If you had the opportunity, what would you say to the mother who is refusing to allow Ritalin for Marty and stating he just has more energy than other boys and will grow out of his hyperactivity?

6. Discuss the debate as to whether ADHD is overdiagnosed and Ritalin and similar stimulants are overprescribed for ADHD. Is Ritalin or other psychostimulants sometimes necessary for children? Why or why not?

7. What other medications besides Ritalin could the health care provider prescribe for ADHD?

8. The father asks: What causes ADHD? How would you answer this question?

9. Marty's father shares an observation that all the children he knows that have ADHD seem to be boys. He asks: "Do girls also have ADHD? What is the ratio of girls to boys who have ADHD?" How would you answer this father?

10. If you were to help write a care plan for this client, what information would you like to gather?

11. What nursing diagnoses and goals would you likely write for this client? What interventions, other than medication, do you think would be helpful for this client?

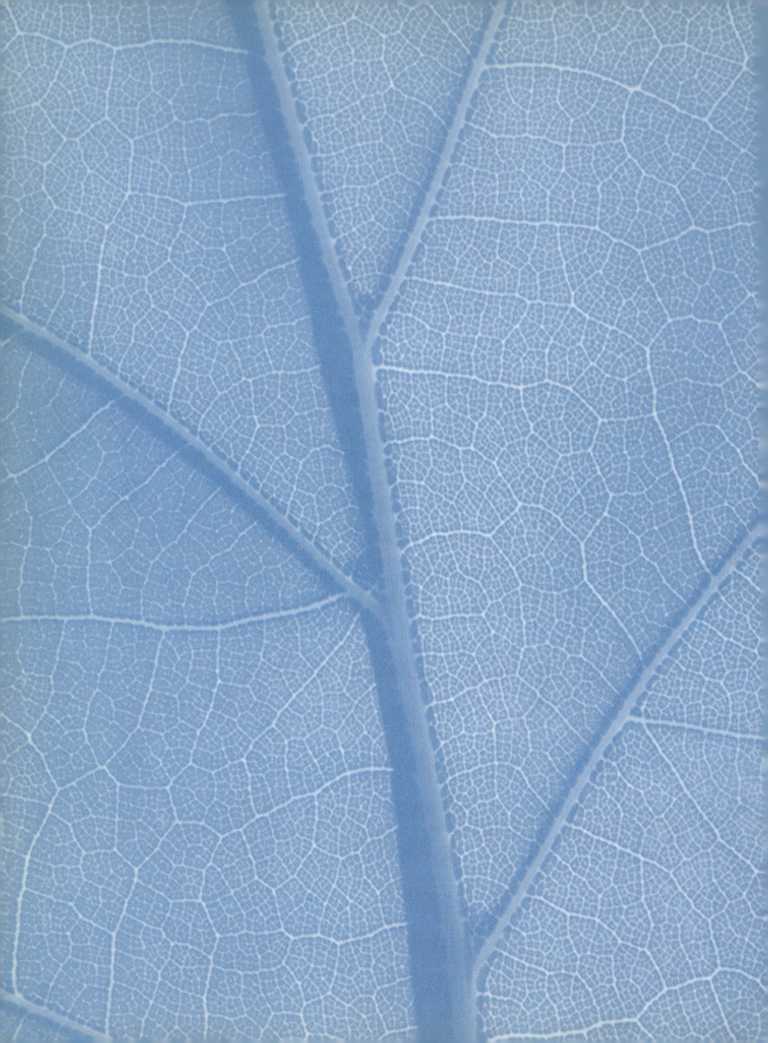

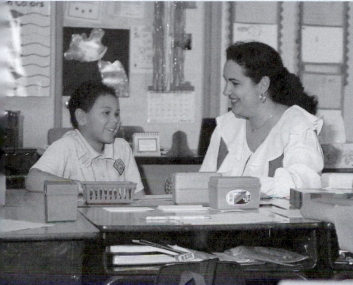

## PART NINE

Survivors of
Violence or
Abuse

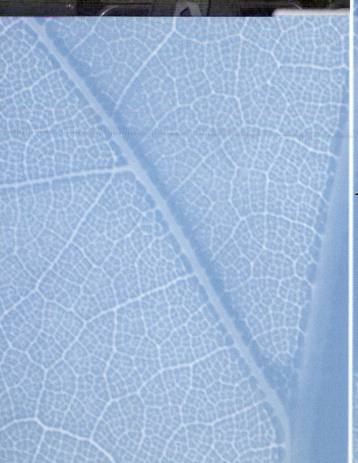

Reata

GENDER

Female

AGE

10

SETTING

- Home setting with visit by home health nurse

ETHNICITY

- White American

CULTURAL CONSIDERATIONS

- Southern
- Rural
- Military

PREEXISTING CONDITIONS

COEXISTING CONDITIONS

COMMUNICATION

DISABILITY

SOCIOECONOMIC

- Lower middle class

SPIRITUAL/RELIGIOUS

- Belongs to Seventh-Day Adventist church but not attending

PHARMACOLOGIC

PSYCHOSOCIAL

LEGAL

- Legal requirement to report "suspected" abuse
- Confidentiality

ETHICAL

- Child and mother's need to report suspected child abuse to ensure safety.

ALTERNATIVE THERAPY

PRIORITIZATION

DELEGATION

PHYSICAL ABUSE OF A CHILD

Level of difficulty: Moderate

Overview: Requires understanding of what constitutes child abuse and critical thinking to determine if there is sufficient evidence to warrant a suspicion of abuse. Requires knowledge of the legal requirements and process for reporting child abuse.

Client Profile

Reata is a 10-year-old girl living with her parents in their rural home. Her mother suffers from Manic Depression and Panic Disorder with Agoraphobia and smokes two packages of cigarettes a day. When agitated or angry, the mother hits Reata or burns her with cigarettes and tells her that she was/is an unwanted child. Reata's mother was raised in the Seventh-Day Adventist Church by the grandparents who live in a nearby city and still attend church. Reata's mother does not attend due to her Agoraphobia and her mental illness, which, combined with living in a rural area, greatly isolates the family.

Reata's father is a member of a military guard unit and is gone from home for long periods of time. When the father is home, he punishes Reata for such things as not doing chores perfectly, not having better grades, imperfect table manners, and for many small infractions of his strict rules. She is beaten with his belt and sent to her room hungry. One time she tried to run away, but her father killed her dog and put his head on the fence for her to see when he found her and brought her back home. She is afraid of her father and more so of his belt.

During the time that the father is gone, Reata tries to stay away from home as much as possible and to hide from her mother when she is at home. She feels safer when the visiting nurse is in the home and comes out of hiding due to curiosity and in hopes of getting some food or candy without being beaten or burned.

Case Study

The visiting nurse knocks on the door, which is opened by Reata, who is wearing a cast on her arm. The nurse is a visiting nurse from the county health department who has come to care for Reata's mother. The nurse asks Reata: "How are you today?" The child whispers in a low voice: "Hungry." The mother yells: "I heard that. It is not mealtime yet. Go get the nurse and me a glass of ice water, you stupid girl." The mother tells the nurse: "She just wants to eat all the time. I can't fill her up no matter how hard I try."

The nurse says: "Reata seems very thin." The mother does not respond, and the nurse asks how much Reata weighs. The mother responds: "Oh, I don't know how much she weighs, but the worthless child eats all the time and just runs it all off. She is always running. Don't worry about her. Take my blood pressure." The nurse starts getting out her stethoscope and sphygmomanometer. She quietly slips Reata a sandwich from her bag while the mother is walking toward her chair and not looking. The nurse can see Reata in the next room, sitting under the table and eating the sandwich in a few quick bites, without her mother being aware of it.

Midway through the visit, the nurse says: "I notice that Reata has a cast on." The mother does not reply, and the nurse says: "Tell me about the cast." The mother explains: "She is a clumsy girl. Always climbing trees and falling out. She also climbs out her window and jumps off the roof [one-story roof]." The nurse notices a burn on the dorsal side of Reata's left hand, but says nothing about it at this time, focusing instead on the client, Reata's mother. Just before leaving, the nurse says: "Reata has a burn on her hand." "Just a cooking accident because she is stupid," replies the mother.

Questions

1. If you were the nurse in this case, making a first visit and not knowing what was going on in the family, what would you think when you see Reata's cast and her thinness and hear her say she is hungry? What would you think as you hear the mother's explanations for these observations and for the burn on the child's hand?

2. If you were the nurse, would your visit focus only on the mother's care or would you be concerned with her child? Did the nurse do the right thing in giving the child a sandwich, and what did the nurse learn by doing this?

3. Briefly describe the therapeutic communication tools used by the nurse in this home visit and a rationale for using them. What strategy does the nurse use to get information about the daughter from the client? Do you agree with this strategy, and if so, why? If not, what strategy would you like to use?

4. If you were the nurse in this case, what would you do to build a trusting relationship with Reata and help her other than reporting your suspicion of abuse? Provide a rationale for your actions.

5. Discuss the federal act that names and defines four major classifications of maltreatment of children. As the nurse in this case, your observations and assessment in the home would best support a suspicion of which one or more of the four types of abuse described in the federal act?

6. What are some of the common characteristics of parents who abuse or neglect children? Do Reata's parents or family have any of these characteristics?

7. What are some behaviors frequently found in children who are abused? What conditions could a child have that might mislead a nurse into thinking the child was being abused when they are not experiencing abuse?

8. What short-term and long-term effects could occur if this child is being abused and neglected and this continues because you don't report your suspicions to the proper authorities?

9. Are all nurses legally obligated to report suspected child abuse? Does the nurse have to gather sufficient data to prove child abuse? Are you as a nurse protected from civil and criminal liability if, acting in the interest of a child, you report suspected child abuse or neglect? How can you find out the procedure to follow to report child abuse and neglect?

10. What do you think bothers nurses the most about reporting suspicion of abuse and neglect? If you report that you suspect Reata is being abused and neglected and she is taken from the family and placed in foster care, how would you feel? On the other hand, if you report suspected abuse and neglect and the authorities decide your suspicions are unwarranted or that the child is in no danger and better off staying with her parents, how would you feel and what would you do?

11. What other means of getting information can you think of to confirm your suspicion of physical abuse and neglect, or to rule it out?

12. Making the child as well as the mother, who is the official client of the nurse, the focus of nursing process, what additional assessments would you do? What nursing diagnoses and goals would you likely write for this child if you continue working with the family and child? What interventions would be helpful?

GENDER

Male

AGE

77

SETTING

- Gerontologist's office

ETHNICITY

- White American

CULTURAL CONSIDERATIONS

PREEXISTING CONDITION

COEXISTING CONDITION

COMMUNICATION

- Hard of hearing; has hearing aides

DISABILITY

SOCIOECONOMIC

- Middle income

SPIRITUAL/RELIGIOUS

PHARMACOLOGIC

- haloperidol (Haldol)

PSYCHOSOCIAL

- Daughter controls access of client to others

LEGAL

- Legal requirement in most, if not all, states for nurses to report abuse/neglect of elderly
- Confidentiality
- Right to make decisions unless declared incompetent

ETHICAL

- Professional manner with a person suspected of abusing the elderly
- Daughter giving client medication without his consent

PRIORITIZATION

DELEGATION

DIFFICULT

PHYSICAL ABUSE OF ELDERLY CLIENT

Level of difficulty: High

Overview: Requires knowledge of signs and symptoms of elder abuse. Requires keeping an open mind while using therapeutic communication skills to determine if there is enough evidence to warrant reporting suspected elder abuse.

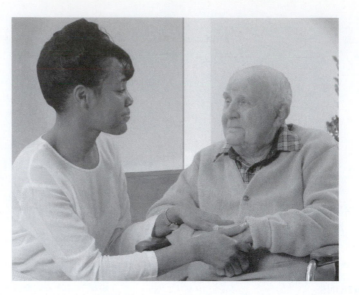

Client Profile

Francis, described as a cantankerous old man by family and neighbors, lived alone until recently, when he reluctantly moved to another city to live with his daughter Alline. He has five living children, none of whom particularly like him, remembering him as being humorless and even mean to them when they were growing up. Francis feared going to a nursing home and got his daughter Alline to promise to keep him out of nursing homes by saying he would leave her some money when he dies.

Alline thought it was a good idea to have her father move in with her, but it soon became evident that he required a lot of care, could not be left alone safely, and was never quite satisfied with anything she did for him. Alline also had to care for his dog that he brought with him, and she did not like the dog. Alline began to resent her siblings not helping her with their father's care. One day she became so angry with her father, the dog, her siblings, and the situation that she shoved her father. He fell, broke his glasses, broke a bone in his foot, and acquired a few bruises. There was some question about whether the foot was broken or not, but Alline decided it probably was not broken. She thought it would be a lot of trouble to get the foot x-rayed, so she did not. A few days later Alline lost control again and hit her father several times, giving him even more bruises. Francis has hearing aids, but his daughter has not put batteries in them. He is usually restrained in a wheelchair when his daughter goes to the store to get groceries. Francis often feels like he is drugged and wonders if his daughter is slipping something into his pudding to calm him down. He usually slips the dog at least half his pudding. Francis is correct in his suspicions. Alline's neighbor gave her a bottle of Haldol after her husband died and no longer needed it. Alline has been putting half a crushed Haldol pill into the pudding.

Case Study

Francis's daughter and a younger brother, who came from another state on an unannounced visit, bring Francis to a gerontologist's office. The brother tells the nurse that he is concerned about Francis's swollen foot, his complaint of pain, the bruising, and Francis thinking it had been at least three years since he had last seen a doctor. The brother mentions that Francis cannot see well because his glasses were broken and he does not hear well because his hearing aids don't work. After weighing Francis, the nurse tells the family she is taking him to an examination room for his physical examination. Alline jumps up to go with them. Francis yells, "No, don't come!" Alline insists on accompanying her father and says: "The nurse will have trouble understanding you and you will have trouble understanding and remembering, so I had better come too."

Questions

1. What are some possible reasons this elderly client might not want his daughter with him during his physical examination?

2. The client is hard of hearing. What actions will you take to enhance his ability to hear you?

3. What approach will you take with this client whom you suspect might be the victim of elder abuse? Are there questions that need to be asked of the caregiver and the client separately? If so, what are these questions and what is your rationale for interviewing the client and others separately?

4. Define elder abuse, elder physical abuse, and elder neglect. Give examples of caretaker behavior that constitutes elder physical abuse and elder neglect. What is the incidence of elder abuse? Are more men than women victims of elder abuse?

5. What are the risk factors for elder abuse? Which of these risk factors are present in this case? What are the signs and symptoms of elder physical abuse that you would look for? What are the signs and symptoms of neglect you would be observing for?

6. If this client says nothing to you (the nurse) or to the health care provider about abuse and he is being abused, why isn't he telling you about the abuse and getting it stopped? Are you as a nurse required to report suspected elder abuse, and how do you report it?

7. If you report suspected elder abuse and it is substantiated, can the abuser be punished by the legal system? What percentage of reported suspected elder abuse cases are substantiated, and what is the type of elder abuse most often substantiated?

8. If the client and his daughter hold firm in that nothing abusive is occurring in the household, what is your course of action?

9. The client says he thinks his daughter is putting pills in his pudding. Alline admits to getting the deceased neighbor's Haldol (haloperidol) and putting it into her father's food. What actions do you need to take? Given what you know and suspect about how Alline is treating her father, how would you now feel about working with Alline and her father?

10. Nurses in some health care providers' offices may not write care plans; however, some likely nursing diagnoses will come to your mind. What are those nursing diagnoses? What goals and interventions would be helpful to this client?

11. What do you especially need to document in this and other cases of suspected abuse?

Chuy

GENDER	**DISABILITY**
Male	■ Congenital deafness
AGE	**SOCIOECONOMIC**
11	■ Upper middle class
SETTING	**SPIRITUAL/RELIGIOUS**
■ Deaf school infirmary	■ Catholic
ETHNICITY	**PHARMACOLOGIC**
■ Mother is White American; father is Hispanic American	**PSYCHOSOCIAL**
CULTURAL CONSIDERATIONS	**LEGAL**
■ Hispanic	■ Legal requirements to report suspected child abuse
PREEXISTING CONDITION	**ETHICAL**
■ Waardenburg Syndrome (WS)	■ Unethical to ask questions out of curiosity rather than need to know
■ Possible Hirschsprung Disease associated with WS	**ALTERNATIVE THERAPY**
COEXISTING CONDITION	**PRIORITIZATION**
■ Urine infection with low grade fever	**DELEGATION**
COMMUNICATION	
■ Congenital deafness; uses American Sign Language	

SEXUAL ABUSE OF A CHILD

Level of difficulty: High

Overview: Requires critical thinking, as well as knowledge of the laws pertaining to reporting of suspected sexual abuse of a child, to determine a course of action to take when a deaf child describes experiences that suggest sexual abuse by his father. Requires knowledge of the communication needs of deaf children and critical thinking to determine how to meet those needs.

DIFFICULT

Client Profile

Chuy, an 11-year-old boy, was born deaf in both ears. At first both eyes looked the same color, but after awhile it was very noticeable that one eye was bright blue and the other brown. His father, a third-generation Hispanic American, blamed the mother for this problem, saying she had bad genes. The paternal grandfather blamed his estranged sister for putting the evil eye on the boy. The neonatologist and the otologist blamed it on Waardenburg Syndrome (WS); their assessments found the father carries the trait, and several members of his family, including the boy's grandfather, have a variety of signs associated with WS, but none are deaf like Chuy.

The father physically and emotionally abused the mother. He was angry with her for producing an imperfect child and angry at the child for not being perfect. The father began to sexually abuse Chuy at about age 4. When the boy went to a residential school for the deaf, the mother went to work, separated from the father, and eventually divorced him. The court decision was joint custody. The mother knew of the sexual abuse, but did not report it or use it in the divorce trial.

Case Study

Chuy is admitted to the school infirmary for observation because he complains of a stomachache and he has a low grade fever. He is found to have urine infection. The infirmary nurse has two other children under her care, and they are isolated with chicken pox. The nurse is able to assess Chuy in a private area of the infirmary. She first plays a game of "Go Fish" and gets him to take turns with her telling "silly jokes." She then takes his vital signs and listens to his heart and lungs and lets him listen to his own heartbeat. The nurse listens for bowel sounds and palpates the stomach, inquiring about pain and about when he had last "pooped." Chuy says maybe three days ago when he was home with his father, but since coming back to school, he is having a hard time pooping. "So it was easier to 'poop' at home," the nurse says. Chuy reveals that his father puts his finger up his "butt" and puts other objects up there to stretch the "butt" and help the "poop" come out. "So he helps you …" the nurse says, and Chuy responds: "He helps other people too by taking pictures of how he does this so they will learn to do it, and he sometimes lets them practice on me or do other things with my wee wee and takes pictures. Oh, I am not supposed to tell. My dad told me to keep it secret. He said other people won't understand and they will be jealous. I won't be punished for telling will I, nurse? Dad says I will be punished if I tell and my mom will get real sick and die if I tell. Please don't tell anyone."

Questions

1. Describe Waardenburg Syndrome (WS), including signs and symptoms.

2. What possible reason or reasons did the nurse in this case have for beginning an assessment by first playing "Go Fish" and taking turns telling silly jokes with this client?

3. What do you suppose could be the cause of this child's constipation? What assessments could you do if you were the nurse in this case?

4. What do you think the nurse in this case might think or feel as the child describes his father's behavior associated with his (the client's) genitals? What techniques did the nurse in the case study use in examining the client and why?

5. How would you define sexual abuse of a child? Are there some gray areas about what is sexual abuse and what is not sexual abuse?

Questions (continued)

6. Do you need to ask this client questions about the sexual abuse to make sure the child was sexually abused and to get more specific details of the abuse (i.e., take a sexual abuse history)? If yes, what is your rationale? If no, should someone else do this, and if so, who and why?

7. What do you need to do and say in response to the child's request that you tell no one about the things his father did to him? What thoughts do you have about documentation of the child's statements in regard to his treatment by his father? Should you take notes while the child is talking?

8. What reasons could the mother have for not reporting the sexual abuse of her son? Should you ask her? Do you need to know the reasons?

9. If this client is to have an anogenital examination, what preparation would be helpful to the child? What is usually done in an anogenital examination? What would it mean if the anogenital examination were negative for evidence of sexual abuse?

10. What behavioral symptoms do sexually abused children display? Will all children who have been sexually abused display behavioral symptoms? What are some thoughts and feelings children have identified in regard to their sexual abuse?

11. What is the incidence of sexual abuse of children? Do you think the incidence is similar or different in other countries? Do you think culture plays any role in this case?

12. Are sexual abuse rates the same for boys as for girls? Do you think that sexual abuse rates are higher for disabled children? If yes, why do you think this is so?

13. When children are sexually abused, who is often the perpetrator? Is this the same for other forms of abuse?

14. What nursing diagnoses and goals would you likely write for this client? What interventions do you think would be helpful for this client?

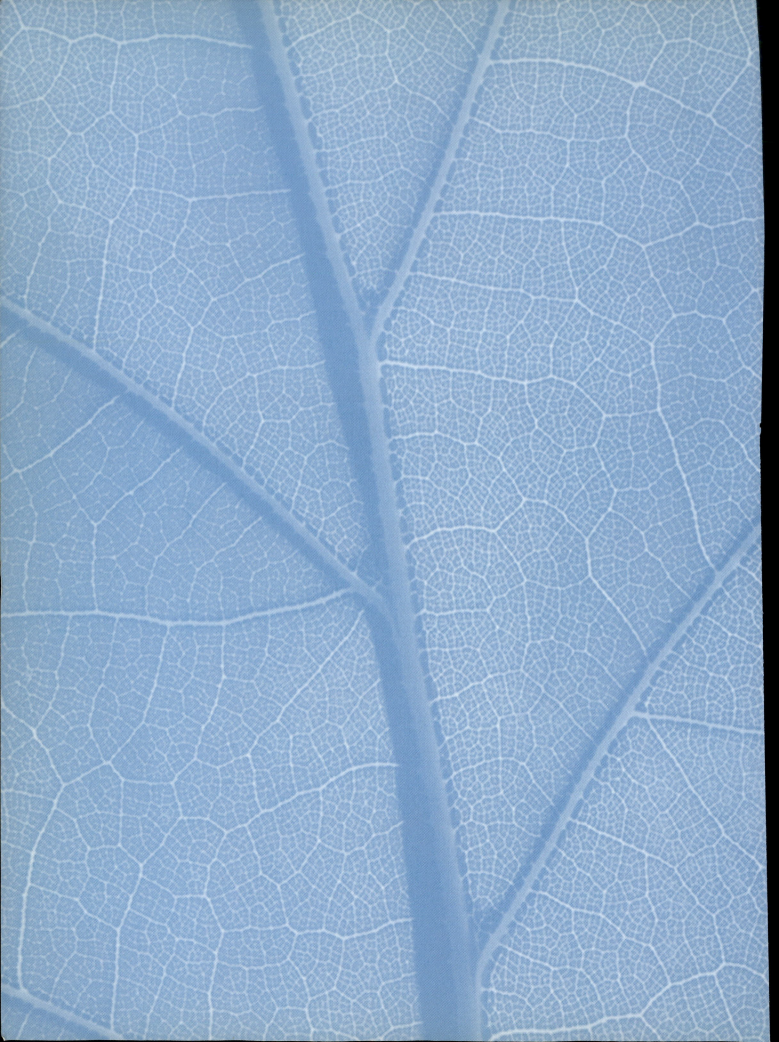

Index